Physical Fitness

The Pathway to Healthful Living

Physical Fitness

The Pathway to Healthful Living

EIGHTH EDITION

ROBERT V. HOCKEY, Ed.D.

Professor
Department of Physical Education and Athletics
Trinity University
San Antonio, Texas

with 242 illustrations

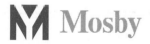 Mosby

St. Louis Baltimore Boston Carlsbad Chicago Naples New York Philadelphia Portland
London Madrid Mexico City Singapore Sydney Tokyo Toronto Wiesbaden

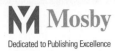

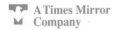

Editor-in-Chief: Jim Smith
Acquisition Editor: Vicki Malinee
Developmental Editor: Jennifer Hartman
Project Manager: Linda McKinley
Production Editor: Catherine Bricker
Manuscript Editor: Rick Dudley
Designer: Elizabeth Fett
Manufacturing Supervisor: Linda Ierardi
Cover Art: © Stephen Simpson/FPG

EIGHTH EDITION

Printed in the United States of America

Composition by Top Graphics
Printing/binding by Courier Companies, Inc.

Mosby–Year Book, Inc.
11830 Westline Industrial Drive
St. Louis, Missouri 63146

Library of Congress Cataloging in Publication Data

Hockey, Robert V.
    Physical fitness : the pathway to healthful living / Robert
V. Hockey. —8th ed.
       p.   cm.
    Includes bibliographical references and index.
    ISBN 0 8151 4479 2
    1. Aerobic exercises.   2. Physical fitness.   3. Health.
I. Title.
RA781.15.H63   1996
613.7—dc20   95-50586
                                                          CIP

96 97 98 99 00 / 9 8 7 6 5 4 3 2 1

Foreword

In this ever-changing world, many complex factors contribute to the state of one's health and fitness. Dr. Robert V. Hockey has so brilliantly captured the essence of teaming physiological training concepts with the field of nutrition. He has combined the best of two disciplines into a practical and concise work.

Society has been desperate for logical guidance and direction in health maintenance and achievement. Last year corporate America spent 50% of its current operating profits on medical and health-related problems. Nothing is as powerful as the idea whose time has come. "Medicine + Fitness = The Winning Edge to Health Care." Physical fitness programs together with sound scientifically based nutrition guidance provide the answer to solving the health care dilemma. Dr. Hockey has developed a splendid contribution to help solve this problem.

Physical Fitness: The Pathway to Healthful Living is a real pearl. The practical approach to making complicated medical and physiological data understandable is unique. The graphically displayed concepts reward the reader with the opportunity to structure his or her own personal lifetime wellness program.

Since the days of Hippocrates, who wrote that "sudden death is more common in those who are naturally fat than in lean," we have struggled with obesity. Today, more than ever before, each of us needs a personal guidebook for fitness and nutrition. Although we have had astounding recent medical breakthroughs in research, hypokinetic disease plagues our society. We do not engage in enough physical exercise to live a quality life. This book provides the knowledge and keen insight to alleviating a national health care crisis.

The two chapters on cardiovascular endurance and training include information on the benefits of aerobic conditioning and provide a succinct review of what is needed to achieve and maintain an optimal level of cardiovascular endurance. In Dr. Hockey's new chapter, Exercise and Wellness, the conceptual information is displayed so that you can easily make lifelong decisions for enhancement of your human performance.

Research has contributed tremendous knowledge to the field of nutrition in recent years. Leading scientists and nutritional experts agree that a change in certain Recommended Dietary Allowances would produce long-range health benefits, including emphasis on the antioxidant vitamins—vitamin C, vitamin D, and betacarotene.

The great philosopher, Socrates, believed that all individuals had an obligation to society to take care of their own health. The real challenge in helping people to change is to find ways by which mass media can be utilized to get people to live healthier lifestyles. It is time that all segments of society awaken to these responsibilities.

Dr. Hockey has beautifully designed very complex issues into a most readable book. It is a must for your personal and professional growth.

Larry Thirstrup, M.D., M.Ed.
Founder of Medical Fitness Centers of America

Preface

Most Americans are now aware that they can achieve optimal health if they assume responsibility for their lifestyle in an attempt to decrease their risk of disease, sickness, disability, and premature death. The everyday decisions that they make relative to exercise, nutrition, and other health-related issues are very important. However, it is apparent that many of them either do not know what to do or else they just lack the motivation to do it.

"I would like to exercise regularly and eat better, but I just can't get myself to do it." I hear this statement almost every day from students who have a hard time finding time to exercise regularly and who are often fighting to control their body weight. Many of them have been on one diet or another, yet they have experienced very little success because they lack the discipline necessary to establish consistent habits relative to exercise and nutrition.

One problem is that there is so much conflicting information available that the average person has a hard time knowing what to believe. *Physical Fitness: The Pathway to Healthful Living* contains accurate, scientific information about exercise, nutrition, health, and fitness.

By understanding the material presented in this book, the reader should:

- **Become more knowledgeable concerning exercise, nutrition, health, and fitness.** Your success will basically depend on the everyday choices you make. By becoming more knowledgeable, you will be able to make better choices.
- **Be able to assess his or her habits and status relative to each of these.** As you study the consistency of your habits, you should be able to identify specific habits that need to be changed.
- **Be able to plan strategies as to how to change these habits.** You will have to make appropriate changes in your lifestyle if you are to attain optimal health and wellness.
- **Be able to implement these changes.** The consistency with which you implement these changes will determine how successful you will be. Worksheets are included that can be used to monitor the consistency of your exercise and eating habits.

With the increased mechanization of modern society, the body does less and less physical work. Therefore everyday tasks must be supplemented with a systematic exercise program. The emphasis throughout this book is on aerobic fitness—activities that stimulate the heart and circulatory system and develop cardiovascular endurance. The added health benefits associated with an optimal level of cardiovascular fitness are clearly identified. Although the primary emphasis is on cardiovascular fitness, the other health-related physical fitness components of strength, muscular endurance, flexibility, and body composition are also discussed in detail. In addition, the importance of nutrition and stress management is emphasized.

Physical Fitness: The Pathway to Healthful Living is one of the few physical fitness textbooks currently on the market that has enjoyed the success of seven previous editions.

AUDIENCE

Many universities and colleges across the country offer introductory courses emphasizing the scientific approach to exercise and fitness. These classes have titles such as "Concepts of Lifetime Fitness" and often combine lectures and laboratory experiences. This book is designed primarily for use in these classes. In addition, it provides useful background information for students interested in exercise physiology and/or sports medicine.

The growing interest in recent years in health and wellness has prompted a tremendous increase in the number of health clubs and exercise facilities. Because of the lack of knowledge by participants, these clubs have been forced to offer classes in weight management and physical fitness. Very few books with accurate scientific information in this field have been written for the general public. Most have been written specifically for college students. The material presented in this book is designed to serve the needs not only of college students but also of all those interested in fitness and nutrition, regardless of their background and experience. What people like most about this book is the simple way that complex information is presented.

FEATURES OF THIS EDITION

The eighth edition of *Physical Fitness: The Pathway to Healthful Living* has been planned carefully, and comments and suggestions from the many instructors who have used this book have been implemented in this revision. Several features have been incorporated in an attempt to make the material more meaningful.

New Chapters: Chapter 1: Exercise and Wellness, and Chapter 2: Physical Fitness: Basic Concepts, allow for a greater discussion of wellness issues.

New Topics: Updated studies such as Healthy People 2000, NHANES III, and the 1994 nationwide survey results from the *Prevention Magazine* Index are included.

Laboratory Experiences: Self-assessment laboratory information is included at the end of each chapter to ensure greater continuity within each chapter. These include questionnaires, worksheets, and simple practical tests that readers can take to see how they rate. There are a total of 33 Laboratory Experiences included, with at least one for every chapter.

Photographs and Drawings: The inclusion of over 240 line drawings and photographs makes it easy for students to understand the instructions for the various exercises that are included in the text.

Objectives: Objectives are included at the beginning of each chapter. These help to identify important concepts. They are stated in terms of what each student should be able to do when he or she understands the material contained in each chapter.

Summary: A summary at the end of each chapter helps students review the important concepts.

Key Terms: Key terms are defined in each chapter. These assist each student in understanding new terminology and make it easier to understand the text.

Boxes: Boxes are used throughout the text to provide additional information or to summarize important concepts. Four different boxes are frequently included. These are:

Facts & Figures: These boxes highlight updated facts and figures that "stand out" so that each student can quickly grasp the information.

In Summary: These boxes present a summary of a key concept or concepts.

Fitness Flash: These boxes highlight new information on health and fitness research and present such topics as health risks and fitness trends.

Let's Get Started: These boxes provide motivational messages and ideas for starting and maintaining a fitness program.

Self-Assessment: These boxes provide exercises to reinforce the material in the text.

Year 2000 Objectives: These boxes present health goals for the nation and give updates on our current status.

Appendixes: Three appendixes are included in this text. These are as follows:

Appendix A. Food Exchange Lists: Updated information relative to each of the six exchange lists. This information can be used both to plan and to analyze meals.

Appendix B. Nutritional Information for Selected Foods: Basic nutritional information is provided for a variety of common foods so that students can evaluate their food intake in terms of calories, carbohydrates, fat, protein, cholesterol, and sodium.

Appendix C. Nutritional Information for Selected Fast-Food Restaurants: Nutritional information is presented for foods from 11 popular fast-food restaurants. Of particular interest to students should be the information pertaining to fat and sodium.

SUPPLEMENTS

Instructor's Manual and test bank

An Instructor's Manual is available for use with this textbook. It contains a course outline, a proposed schedule of classes, and suggestions for grading. The materials should help the instructor to organize the class. A section is included on each chapter, including a chapter summary, identification of important topics, proposed class activities, discussion topics, and a series of short answer, essay, and multiple choice questions that can be used to evaluate the students.

Computerized test bank

Available to qualified adopters, this software enables the instructor to select, edit, delete, or add questions, as well as construct and print tests and answer keys. Available in IBM DOS and Macintosh formats.

Laboratory activity software

The laboratory activities throughout this text are also available on computer diskette. This convenient software program allows students to assess their health and fitness levels and record their progress. Available free to qualified adopters and for a nominal fee to students. Available on IBM. See your Mosby sales representative for details about additional assessment programs.

Mosby's NutriTrac software

Your students can analyze diets with the click of a button. This easy-to-use program allows you to add foods for breakfast, lunch, dinner, and snacks for any number of days. The program then provides an intake analysis for an individual food, meal, or day or for an entire intake period. The database includes more than 2200 foods and 33 nutrient values. Available free to qualified

Chapter One **Exercise and Wellness**

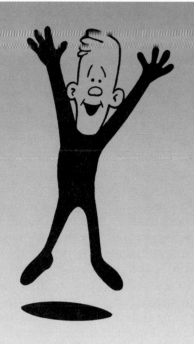

HEALTH AND WELLNESS

During the last decade, we have discovered that good health is no longer a matter of chance but a matter of choice. If *you* choose to take responsibility for your health by exercising regularly and by consistently practicing other positive lifestyle habits, you will not only promote better health, but you will also decrease your risk of disease, disability, and premature death. Perhaps this is the reason an enthusiasm for exercise and fitness and an interest in nutrition are presently at an all-time high in the United States.[8]

Most Americans recognize the importance of regular exercise and good nutrition and are aware that they can greatly influence their health by the decisions they make each day, particularly the ones relating to diet, nutrition, and exercise. However, there is a basic problem in that many people either do not know the way to achieve a healthier lifestyle or they lack the motivation to do so. "I know I should exercise regularly and eat better, but I just can't get myself to do it." I hear this statement almost every day from college students who seldom find time to exercise and often blame college life for their poor eating habits. I also hear the same statement from adults enrolled in weight management programs who have not found time to exercise consistently and have continuously been dieting with very little success.

Facts and Figures

Following are the results from a recent national survey[20]:

	Agree	Disagree
"I can do more for my health by what I do and what I eat than anything doctors or medicine can do."	95%	5%
"If I exercise and eat right, I am almost certain to stay healthy."	85%	15%

To many people the term **health** still means simply "the absence of disease," and a large percentage of people who have no obvious signs of disease or sickness consider themselves to be healthy. A recent survey conducted by Friedman[4] supports this conclusion. His study showed that 90% of the people surveyed considered themselves to be in good health. However, a risk-appraisal survey revealed that 62% of the same people needed to improve their health habits, and 25% of them were in such poor health that they needed to be referred to their physicians for treatment. It is unfortunate that many of these people rely on annual physical examinations to determine their levels of health. In most cases the examinations are not very thorough and people are given "clean bills of health." This reinforces their existing lifestyles regardless of whether they incorporate healthy or unhealthy practices.

The word *health* should be associated with the term **wellness** rather than being associated with an absence of disease. The relationship between these two terms will be clearer if we imagine health as existing on a continuum. In the center of this continuum is a neutral point reflecting a state of no discernible disease or illness. Many people find themselves at the neutral point of the continuum most of the time (Figure 1-1).

Moving to the left of the neutral point indicates a progressively deteriorating state of health where the signs and symptoms of illness appear. If medical treatment is sought, it can usually alleviate the symptoms and return the person to the neutral point. If medical treatment is not sought, the condition usually gets worse and in many cases results in premature death.

Simply being at the neutral point and free from disease and illness is not actually the goal. Move beyond the neutral point and constantly strive for optimal health. The opposite side of the continuum is often referred to as the *wellness side* and involves a personal approach to health with individuals accepting responsibility for their own lifestyles as they try to prevent illness and disease and strive for optimal wellness[22] (Figure 1-2).

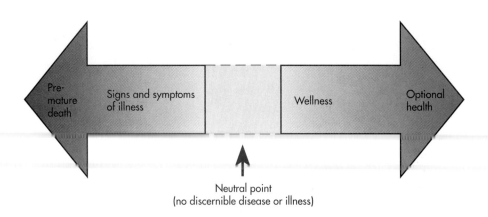

Premature death — Signs and symptoms of illness — Wellness — Optional health

Neutral point
(no discernible disease or illness)

Figure 1-1   Illness-wellness continuum.

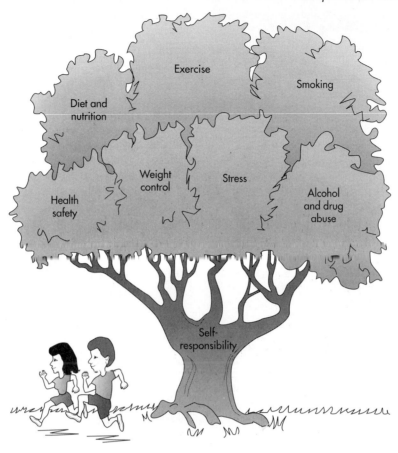

Figure 1-2   The wellness umbrella.

WHY WELLNESS?

Attaining a high level of health should be extremely important in today's world, where the most prominent health problems can be considered lifestyle induced. The 10 leading causes of death are identified in Table 1-1. The table's statistics indicate that almost 60% of all deaths in the United States are related to cardiovascular disease and cancer. A large percentage of these deaths were lifestyle induced and could have been prevented. The three major factors contributing to deaths in the United States have been identified in Table 1-2. Note that all three of these are related to lifestyle choices.

Consider the following additional facts:
1. Sedentary lifestyles have been linked to 23% of deaths resulting from leading chronic diseases.[5]

The balancing of the choices we make each day determines our position on the health continuum. Some of our choices will negatively affect our position, whereas others will move us closer to the wellness side. By becoming more knowledgeable about health-related topics and developing consistently positive lifestyle behaviors, we can approach an optimal state of health.

In today's world there is a lot we can do to influence our health. For example, consider the following quote from Dr. Richard Winter, chairman of the board for National Health Services, which appeared in *Newsweek:* "Prevention is still the best medicine. Quite simply, if you take care of yourself, most probably someone else won't have to. All that it requires is learning some very basic health and fitness principles, and then applying them—with common sense—to everyday living. It's hardly a high price to pay for our greatest asset . . . good health."[28]

Health: Balancing all aspects of a lifestyle to achieve a higher quality of existence.

Wellness: Engaging in behaviors that enhance the quality of life, reduce the incidence of disease, and maximize personal potential.

In Summary
Unfortunately, many of us spend more time worrying about our health than taking steps to improve it.

Table 1-1	**The 10 Leading Causes of Death in the United States, 1993**

Diseases	Percentage of Deaths
1. Diseases of the heart	33.1
2. Cancer	23.9
3. Stroke	6.5
4. Chronic obstructive pulmonary disease	4.2
5. Accidents/injuries	3.9
6. Pneumonia and influenza	3.5
7. Diabetes mellitus	2.3
8. Suicide	1.4
9. AIDS	1.4
10. Homicide	1.2

From U.S. National Center for Health Statistics: *Vital statistics of the United States—annual vital statistics report*, 1994, The Center.

Table 1-2	**Actual Causes of Death in the United States, 1990**

Cause	Estimated Number
Tobacco use	400,000
Diet/activity patterns	300,000
Alcohol	100,000

From U.S. Department of Health and Human Services, Washington, DC, and Carter Presidential Center, Atlanta, Ga, 1993.

2. Current studies estimate that 25 million men (28.1%) and 23 million women (23.5%) smoke. Cigarette smoking accounts for approximately 400,000 deaths each year, including approximately 30% of cancer deaths and 21% of cardiovascular-disease deaths.[14]
3. Cigarette smoking has also been associated with 87% of all deaths from lung cancer.[1]
4. The risk for developing cardiovascular disease for smokers is almost triple that of nonsmokers.[16]
5. High blood pressure *(hypertension)* is a well-established contributing factor to cardiovascular disease. As many as 50 million Americans over 6 years of age have high blood pressure, and approximately 35% are not aware of this fact. Hypertension is easily identifiable and in most cases can be controlled with the appropriate treatment.[10]
6. Highway accidents account for almost 50,000 deaths annually. The majority of these deaths are attributed to not using seat belts, excessive alcohol consumption, and/or excessive speed.[27]
7. Alcohol misuse accounts for approximately 100,000 deaths each year.[14]
8. The suicide rate is increasing rapidly in the United States. High stress levels are the major determining factors in the majority of these cases. Fifty-seven percent of U.S. adults report that they experience at least moderate amounts of stress every 2 weeks, and 41% felt that stress had at least some effect on their health.[27]
9. Approximately 60% of American adults currently exceed their recommended weights, which presents another risk factor for developing cardiovascular disease. In most cases, excessive weight is caused by a lack of exercise and/or poor eating habits.[21]
10. The overall risk of having a heart attack is 40% lower for people who exercise regularly than those who do not.[17]
11. Type II diabetes accounts for approximately 90% of all cases of diabetes and afflicts approximately 10 million Americans. Eighty-five percent of individuals with Type II diabetes are obese or overweight. Regular exercise can reduce the incidence of Type II diabetes by as much as 42%.[12,13]

HEALTH OBJECTIVES FOR THE YEAR 2000

In 1990 the Public Health Service published a document entitled *Healthy People 2000: National Health Promotion and Disease Prevention Objectives.* The basic premise was that adults could assume personal responsibility for their health by adopting habits that promote good health, which in turn would enable them to live full and active lives and prevent premature death and disabilities by reducing their incidences of disease.

Specific objectives were formulated for a variety of health-related factors, including physical activity and fitness, nutrition, tobacco, alcohol and drugs, and certain chronic lifestyle-related diseases. At appropriate places throughout this chapter and other chapters, references are made to these objectives.[9]

EXERCISE AND HEALTH

Frequently, people who exercise regularly become more health conscious. It appears that an increase in fitness leads to an increase in self-esteem, and people who feel better about themselves are much more likely to have a greater sense of control over the factors that influence their health.

Two different surveys showed that individuals who worked out regularly were much more likely to implement other health practices.[6,7] For example, a larger percentage of exercisers than nonexercisers were able to quit smoking, reduce their sugar intake, reduce their body weight, increase their fiber intake, and control their level of stress. The differences between the two groups were significant for each of these variables.

Another interesting finding from one of these surveys was that the amount of exercise was very important. It appears that "the more you sweat, the more leverage you have on your habits." The advantages were far greater for those who exercised for 5 hours or more per week compared with those who exercised for only 1 to 1½ hours per week. This might be due to the discipline learned from participating in a regular exercise program. The discipline of exercise results in positive feedback and possibly in a greater sense of control. "Lack of discipline" was one of the top three reasons given for nonparticipation by those who recognized that they do not get sufficient exercise.

It should be emphasized that regular exercise alone does not necessarily ensure better health or reduce the risk of certain diseases. Consider the following case study:

Case Study

DON

Don is a 30-year-old man who exercises regularly, running 4 or 5 miles at least 5 days each week. He takes great pride in his accomplishments and has no problems maintaining his weight at a desirable level. However, Don smokes two packs of cigarettes a day and has an extremely high level of stress and some very poor eating habits. He also figures that because he exercises just about every day, he can reward himself by drinking a six-pack of beer each day. Because of his eating and drinking habits, his cholesterol level is dangerously high. Despite the fact that Don exercises regularly and maintains a desirable weight, he still has other poor habits that negatively influence his health.

CURRENT TRENDS IN EXERCISE AND FITNESS

The present exercise-fitness revolution is now almost 25 years old. It was probably initiated in part by Dr. Kenneth Cooper's first book, *Aerobics,* which was published in 1968. This book helped the American public to understand the importance of aerobic fitness and challenged them to counter the epidemics of heart disease, obesity, and other health-related problems.

Early in the 1970s, a national survey indicated that almost 60% of all adults in the United States did not participate in any form of physical activity.[19] From that time on, it appears as if millions of Americans have taken up the exercise challenge in an attempt to get in shape and improve their health[8] (Figure 1-3).

The results from surveys such as the one in Figure 1-4, however, tend to be misleading. A closer look at the most recent statistics shows that the average num-

ber of days of participation was fewer than 6 per month for each participant. This is insufficient for the development of aerobic fitness and would tend to support the conclusion made by Brooks that "most Americans are not knowledgeable about the frequency, duration and intensity recommended for exercise to strengthen the heart and lungs."[2] The results from her survey show that approximately 60% of adults do not exercise regularly, yet more than 80% of them consider themselves to be active and are "somewhat" or "very" satisfied with their fitness level.

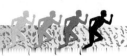
Fitness Flash

Figures released in 1993 by the U.S. Department of Health and Human Services showed that less than 5% of persons over 18 years of age knew that exercise needed to be performed at least three times per week and maintained for 20 minutes or more per session to increase the efficiency of the heart and circulatory system.[27]

Several other surveys have been completed, but many of them lack consistency relative to the procedures involved. Probably the most consistent survey has been the nationwide survey conducted by *Prevention* magazine, which has used the same procedures for the last 11 years. The results for 1994 are summarized in Figure 1-4 and compared with the results for 1983, the first year this survey was done.[21]

Note that although the number of people who do not exercise at all has hardly changed during this time, the percentage of those who exercise three or more times per week has increased from 34% to 40%.

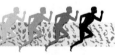
Fitness Flash

Based on information from all the surveys reviewed, the following summary best depicts the situation that presently exists for adults in this country:

- Approximately 40% exercise on a regular basis at the required intensity and duration to result in maximal aerobic development.
- Approximately 30% exercise less frequently and at a lower level of intensity, probably not frequently enough and not strenuously enough to develop or maintain desirable levels of aerobic fitness.
- Approximately 30% participate less than 1 day per week or do not participate at all in any organized physical activity and could be classified as sedentary.

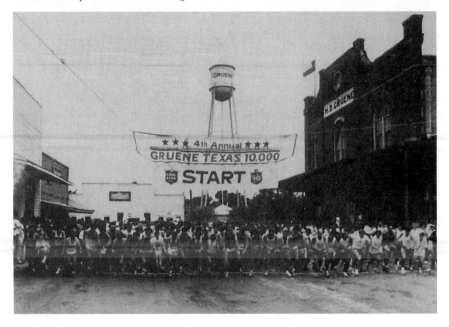

Figure 1-3   More people than ever before are participating in some form of exercise.

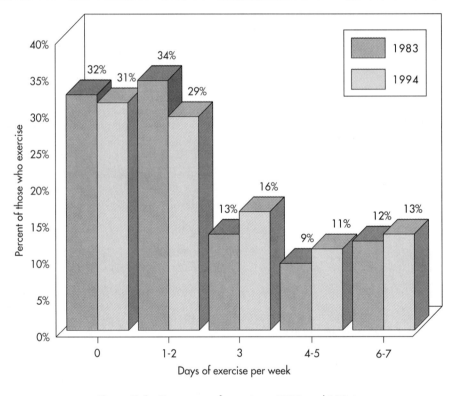

Figure 1-4   Frequency of exercise—1983 and 1994.

In Summary

Despite the widespread fitness boom, far too few Americans get sufficient strenuous exercise and the average American is far from fit.

Why so many Americans are unfit

Most Americans are aware of the benefits that can be derived from regular exercise, and many of them intend to exercise more, but for various reasons they just do not. One problem with changing habits is that the present lifestyle has little effect on current health. The ab-

Year 2000 Objectives Exercise

To increase physical activity and fitness by the year 2000 . . .

	Current Status
To increase to at least 30% the proportion of adults who participate regularly, preferably every day, in moderate physical activity, for at least 30 minutes per day	13%—6 or 7 days/wk 24%—4 or more days/wk
To reduce to no more than 15% the proportion of adults who engage in no leisure-time physical activity	31% presently are "inactive"

sence of any immediate effect is a serious barrier to change. However, individuals must remember that they are laying the foundation for what their health will be 20, 30, or 40 years from now.

Excuses for nonexercise More than half of the people who recognize the importance of exercise never actually take the time to exercise on a regular basis. There are many excuses used in an attempt to justify this:

Excuses for Not Exercising
"I don't have the time."
"I work hard all day, and I am too tired."
"It is inconvenient."
"My lifestyle is busy enough; I don't need exercise."
"I am too old."
"I am out of shape."
"I just don't enjoy exercise."
"I don't like to sweat."
"Exercise will mess up my hair."
"When I exercise I get sore muscles."
"It is too late to change the way I live."

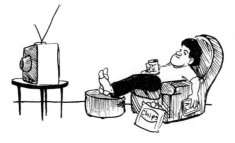

The number-one reason for inactivity given by those who recognize that they do not get enough exercise is "insufficient time."

Lack of sufficient time is by far the most common excuse. All it takes is a minimum of 20 minutes of aerobic exercise every other day to stay in reasonable shape. If a person believes strongly enough in exercise, he or she will make time available to participate in an activity on a regular basis. Unfortunately, too few Americans believe strongly enough to do this. Lack of time is obviously not as big a problem as lack of desire or lack of self-discipline.

The President's Council on Physical Fitness suggests several ways to persuade people to exercise regularly:

- Show them how to fit exercise into their busy schedules.
- Convince older people that age is not a barrier to exercise.
- Appeal to their concern for health and an attractive appearance.
- Convince them that exercise can be enjoyable.
- Present more information to them on the types of exercises that are best and the amount of exercise necessary to develop and maintain adequate fitness.

For most people the major problem is finding time to exercise. When the schedule gets tight and there are specific things to do at school, work, or home, exercise is usually the first activity to skip. We rationalize by saying that we will get back to it tomorrow or the day after when things settle down. Unfortunately, for many of us this never happens. There is no reason why you cannot schedule exercise each day just like you schedule other activities.

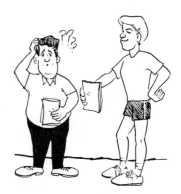

Each of us can program our daily activities to positively influence our health and well-being.

It is now well documented that people who are well informed about exercise and nutrition tend to be more active than those who are not, and they also make more intelligent decisions each day. It should be emphasized, however, that having knowledge is not enough. More than 95% of entering college freshmen indicate that exercise is important to them. These students also claim that the attainment of an "adequate" level of physical fitness is a worthwhile objective. However, when these issues are investigated further, the results are rather confusing. Less than 30% of these same students exercise regularly, and even a lower percentage believe that they presently have an adequate level of physical fitness.

Let's Get Started

Consistency is important in any exercise program. Don't wait until you "find" time to exercise. Schedule exercise into your daily lifestyle. Get started today.

Finding time to exercise is a problem for many college students. Classes, study, assignments, dating, and other commitments place heavy demands on their time, and part-time jobs make it even more difficult to find time to exercise regularly. In many cases, students who do not exercise regularly find that they have a higher level of stress, tend to gain weight more readily, and are frequently sick. These problems can detract from their success, and college life often becomes a struggle. On the other hand, exercise can contribute to their success by making them more alert and productive, reducing their level of stress, and making college life in general more enjoyable.[18]

In Summary

Whether or not you exercise regularly will be determined by whether or not you believe strongly enough that exercise is important to you. If you do, you will find the time necessary to participate on a regular basis.

THE IMPORTANCE OF EXERCISE

In recent years, because of increased mechanization, the need for regular exercise has increased; however, because of our busy lifestyle, many of us do not make time available for exercise. Because of this, we never achieve an adequate level of physical fitness, and we frequently suffer from diseases associated with inactivity. One of the basic problems is that there is so much conflicting information available, we have a hard time knowing what to believe, and in many cases we just do not know what to do. Because of this, we wind up doing nothing. Almost 80% of the American adult population admit that they need assistance if they are to make a commitment to change their exercise and eating habits.

The following are three good reasons why exercise should be important to you:

1. The body functions more efficiently if it is active.
2. Many of our leisure activities are sedentary in nature.
3. Inactivity contributes to many of the prominent health problems that exist today.

Efficiency of an active body

Modern technology has resulted in a substantial decrease in the number of tasks that require a significant expenditure of energy:

- Driving has replaced walking in certain situations. Note the number of people who have become so lazy that they will circle the parking lot several times to obtain a parking place near where they are going.
- The majority of the working population is now involved in positions requiring mental rather than physical work.
- People use escalators or elevators at airports, stores, and office buildings rather than walking up or down stairs.
- Many daily household tasks have become mechanized. For example, mowing the yard and washing dishes or clothes are now done using appliances.

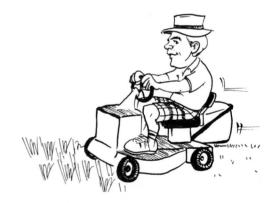

Lack of activity is prevalent in today's society.

The tasks of daily life no longer provide sufficient vigorous activity to develop and maintain adequate levels of physical fitness, and we must now go out of our way to "program" exercise back into our lifestyle. This is important because the body was designed and constructed for movement and vigorous activity, not for rest. It functions more efficiently when it is active. Notice what happens when an arm or leg is placed in a cast and not used for an extended period: the muscle mass decreases in size, resulting in loss of strength, endurance, and flexibility. It is obvious that as far as the body is concerned, that which is used becomes stronger and that which is not becomes weaker.

Many factors are involved in helping the body to become stronger and more efficient. However, the underlying principle is that the functioning of the body requires energy, which in turn depends on the ability of the heart, lungs, and blood vessels to process oxygen and deliver it to the muscles, where it becomes the fuel for energy.

If you exercise regularly, your body is able to process and use greater amounts of oxygen because the intake and supply channels have become more efficient. Some of the changes in the body that result in an increase in efficiency are summarized in Figure 1-5.

Stated simply, a person who does not exercise regularly may lack sufficient energy to perform simple everyday tasks such as sitting, standing, and walking. This is because the body functions inefficiently and is therefore forced to "overwork" to provide the energy necessary for the performance of these tasks. A person who exercises regularly will have an extra energy reserve because of the increase in efficiency of the functioning of the body. This person will have more drive and increased energy, will feel good, and will possibly be more productive.

Most people take better care of their automobiles than they do their own bodies. They depend on their cars, and they want them to look good, go fast, and last a long time. Yet, unlike the automobile, the human body comes with no guarantees or trade-ins in case it wears out prematurely.

There are many people who frequently neglect the preventive maintenance necessary for their bodies to function efficiently. The old saying "If you don't use it, you lose it" certainly applies to your body in relation to physical fitness.

The sedentary nature of leisure activities

With increased mechanization, many tasks that once required physical work and a considerable amount of time can now be accomplished very quickly by pushing a button or setting a dial. Additional time is therefore available for leisure activities. The problem, however, is that many of our leisure activities are sedentary.

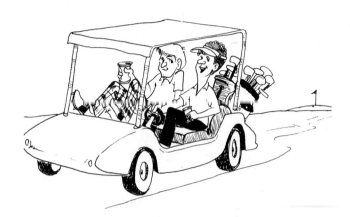

Many of our leisure activities have suddenly become inactive

Adults and children spend a considerable amount of leisure time using the home computer or playing video games. Previously, much of this time was spent more actively. Because of increased mechanization and changes in the use of our leisure time, it is now important to program vigorous, sustained physical activity into our daily schedules if we are to achieve and maintain an optimal level of physical fitness.

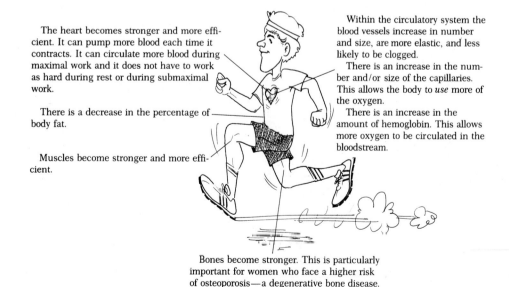

The heart becomes stronger and more efficient. It can pump more blood each time it contracts. It can circulate more blood during maximal work and it does not have to work as hard during rest or during submaximal work.

There is a decrease in the percentage of body fat.

Muscles become stronger and more efficient.

Within the circulatory system the blood vessels increase in number and size, are more elastic, and less likely to be clogged.

There is an increase in the number and/or size of the capillaries. This allows the body to *use* more of the oxygen.

There is an increase in the amount of hemoglobin. This allows more oxygen to be circulated in the bloodstream.

Bones become stronger. This is particularly important for women who face a higher risk of osteoporosis—a degenerative bone disease.

Figure 1-5 With regular exercise, our bodies function more efficiently.

Prominent health problems associated with inactivity

The sedentary way of life has had a negative effect on the human body and has been associated with many serious health problems. These are often referred to as **hypokinetic diseases.** The following are of specific interest:

- Cardiovascular disease
- Hypertension
- Obesity
- Diabetes
- Low back pain
- Osteoporosis

Cardiovascular disease   During the 1980s and the early 1990s there were major declines in death rates attributable to heart disease and stroke. Much of this is associated with a reduction in risk factors and early detection and treatment. However, the most recent figures released by the American Heart Association indicate that approximately 34% of all deaths in this country can be attributed to **cardiovascular** diseases.[10] This is true despite the fact that there are almost 300,000 coronary bypass operations per year.

Research has clearly shown that regular vigorous physical activity is associated with a reduced overall risk of coronary heart disease and that the rate of sudden cardiac death is lessened in those who exercise regularly compared with those who are inactive. The positive effects of exercise have been shown to be independent of such other risk factors as smoking, obesity, and hypertension.[25] An analysis of over 40 studies shows that cardiovascular disease is 1.9 times more likely to develop in physically inactive people than in active people. This is comparable with 2.1 for hypertension, 2.4 for elevated cholesterol, and 2.5 for smoking.[26] However, physical inactivity possibly has a greater impact than any of the other risk factors simply because there are more people at risk for developing coronary heart disease resulting from lack of regular exercise.

Hypertension   An estimated 60 million Americans have consistently elevated blood pressure, thereby placing them at an increased risk of death and illness. They are at 2.1 times the risk of developing coronary heart disease[26] and at approximately 7 times the risk of having a stroke when compared with people with normal blood pressure.[3] Several research studies have shown that regular physical activity can reduce the risk of developing **hypertension** and that exercise can also be used to control hypertension.

Obesity/overweight   Sixty-eight percent of the American adult population currently exceed their recommended weight range. The percentage of those who are 20% or more above this recommended range has increased from 25.4% to 33.3% during the last 10 years.[11] Substantial research shows that physical activity is positively associated with weight control, and it is well established that those who are more active weigh less than those who are sedentary.

Diabetes   Diabetes is one of the most common afflictions of modern society. Approximately 12 million Americans suffer from some form of this disease. The majority of the diabetes cases are classified as Type II diabetes. Two separate studies—one involving men[12] and the other women[13]—have shown conclusively that

Fitness Flash

Cardiovascular disease

	Incidence	Death Rate	Treatment/Cost
Heart Disease	7 million with coronary artery disease	500,000 deaths/yr	Coronary bypass surgery: 284,000/yr at an average cost of $30,000 each
Stroke	600,000 strokes/yr	150,000 deaths/yr	Rehabilitation—average cost: $22,000

Data from *Healthy People 2000, national health promotion and disease prevention objectives,* US Department of Health and Human Services, Public Health Service, Pub No (PHS) 91-50213, Washington, DC, 1991, US Government Printing Office.

Year 2000 Objectives Cardiovascular Disease

To reduce heart disease and stroke by the year 2000 . . .	Current Status
To reduce coronary heart disease deaths to no more than 100 per 100,000 population	135/100,000 population
To reduce stroke deaths to no more than 20 per 100,000 population	33/100,000 population

Year 2000 Objectives Hypertension

	Current Status
To increase to at least 50% the percentage of people with high blood pressure who can control it	25%

Year 2000 Objectives Obesity/Overweight

	Current Status
To decrease to no more than 20% the percentage of adults who are 20% or more overweight	33%

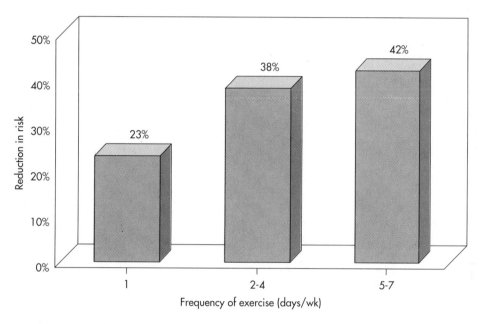

Figure 1-6   Reduction in incidence of Type II diabetes with various amounts of exercise.

exercise can significantly reduce the risk of Type II diabetes. Figure 1-6 presents data pertaining to men.

Despite the fact that over 80% of adult-onset diabetes occurs in individuals who are obese and/or overweight, regular exercise may be the only practical way of preventing diabetes, since obesity is much more difficult to control. The reason why physical activity is important is that it results in certain metabolic and hormonal changes within the body that might prevent or postpone the development of certain forms of diabetes.

Low back pain   The incidence of low back pain in the United States continues to increase. It has been estimated that 75 million Americans suffer from low back pain, with a resulting cost of over $1 billion in lost productivity and $250 million in workers' compensation each year. It has also been estimated that

over 80% of all low back pain problems are caused by improper muscle development. People suffering from low back pain frequently avoid exercise, thinking that it may cause further damage. However, research shows that physical activity can reduce the incidence of low back pain by increasing strength, muscular endurance, and flexibility of the muscles responsible for the pain.[24]

Cardiovascular: Pertaining to the heart and circulatory system.

Hypertension: Consistently high blood pressure.

Hypokinetic disease: A disease related to or resulting from lack of sufficient activity or exercise.

Osteoporosis Osteoporosis is a chronic disease that frequently occurs in late–middle-aged women and involves a decrease in bone mass and density. It is responsible for over 1 million bone fractures each year. Exercise plays an important role in both the prevention and treatment of osteoporosis.[15]

In Summary

It can clearly be seen that several of today's most serious health problems are the result of our sedentary way of life and that indeed exercise may be the cheapest preventive medicine in the world.

PERSONAL BENEFITS OF EXERCISE

Many advantages result from the development of an optimal level of physical fitness. Several of these are difficult to measure objectively; however, people who exercise regularly report the following:

They feel better and have more energy. Physical fitness promotes a feeling of increased vitality because more energy is available to perform daily tasks. Those who are fit are usually eager to get up in the morning and experience more drive throughout the day. They exhibit a "zest for life."

They look better. People who are physically fit usually have an improved personal appearance. They are usually stronger and have better muscle tone, decreased weight, and reduced body fat. These factors contribute to better posture and an increased efficiency in the functioning of the body, and they may result in a delay of the aging process.

They have a reduced level of stress and tension. Those who are fit can usually cope better with daily problems such as worry, anxiety, pressure, frustration, anger, and fear. They are more able to relax; many work off their tension with some form of exercise.

They are more productive in their everyday tasks. Physically fit people can do more work with less effort and are thus more efficient. Fitness also promotes alertness and self-confidence. Thus they are more successful and less susceptible to mistakes and accidents that often result from fatigue.

They exhibit a better sleeping pattern. Not only do physically fit people require less sleep, but they usually fall asleep sooner, sleep more soundly, and wake up more refreshed.

They experience fewer physical complaints. People who are physically fit usually have a better resistance to disease. For example, low back pain and the common cold occur less frequently among those who are fit. The benefits are obvious—reduced medical expenses and less time off from work.

They enjoy life more. Those who are physically fit have sufficient energy left at the end of the day to participate in active recreational activities rather than falling asleep in front of the television.

They experience improved psychological benefits. Fitness usually promotes self-confidence and results in enhanced self-esteem and improved body image. The result is an increased feeling of well-being.

Many other specific benefits that result from participation in regular exercise are related to cardiovascular disease and to each of the components of physical fitness. Information on these benefits is presented in later chapters.

MAKING CHOICES

Despite the fact that more people than ever before are concerned about their health and are now aware of the importance of regular exercise and good nutrition, this knowledge does not always translate into action. How successful you will be depends on the balance that exists between the choices that you make each day. These choices basically relate to the following:

- Diet and nutrition
- Exercise
- Weight control
- Stress
- Smoking
- Alcohol and drugs
- Health and safety

Prevention magazine has identified 21 key health-promoting behaviors that can be controlled by each individual and that have been shown to affect disease or disability. Each of these behaviors was then rated for its health impact on a scale ranging from 1 to 10 by a group of experts.[21] These behaviors and ratings are listed in Figure 1-7. Note that a score of 9.78 for smoking indicates that this behavior has the greatest affect on a person's health, whereas getting 7 to 8 hours of sleep per night with a score of 6.71 is viewed as having much less of an impact. However, it should be noted that all behaviors do significantly influence your health.

A composite score based on all the behaviors on a scale of 1 to 100 is calculated. This is referred to as *The Prevention Index.* A score of zero would therefore mean that nobody has adopted any of these positive behaviors, and a score of 100 would indicate that everyone was carrying out all 21 of them.

Standardized national surveys were conducted each year from 1984 to 1994. A summary of the obtained scores for each year is presented in Table 1-3. Notice that there has been a consistent increase in the score over the past 11 years. This indicates that more people than ever before are trying to positively influence their health. However, investigators concluded that if our index scores were a grade, we would still barely be pass-

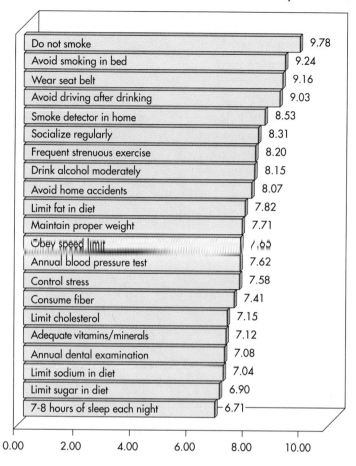

Behavior	Rating
Do not smoke	9.78
Avoid smoking in bed	9.24
Wear seat belt	9.16
Avoid driving after drinking	9.03
Smoke detector in home	8.53
Socialize regularly	8.31
Frequent strenuous exercise	8.20
Drink alcohol moderately	8.15
Avoid home accidents	8.07
Limit fat in diet	7.82
Maintain proper weight	7.71
Obey speed limit	7.65
Annual blood pressure test	7.62
Control stress	7.58
Consume fiber	7.41
Limit cholesterol	7.15
Adequate vitamins/minerals	7.12
Annual dental examination	7.08
Limit sodium in diet	7.04
Limit sugar in diet	6.90
7-8 hours of sleep each night	6.71

Figure 1-7 Health promoting behaviors and ratings—Prevention Index.

Table 1-3	**Prevention Index Scores 1984-1994**
Year	**Average Score**
1984	61.5
1985	63.2
1986	64.1
1987	65.2
1988	64.8
1989	65.4
1990	66.2
1991	66.5
1992	66.5
1993	67.3
1994	66.8

ing. However, since 1984, we have been moving in the right direction.

The frequency of the adults who claim to be practicing each of these behaviors in 1994 is presented in Figure 1-8.

You can determine your Personal Prevention Index by completing Laboratory Experience 1-2. This questionnaire includes the 21 questions used by *Prevention* magazine to assess health in the United States.

CHANGING YOUR LIFESTYLE

Lifestyle changes are a matter of choice. You must learn to control those habits that are detrimental to your health. Most of these lifestyle changes, however, do not come easy because although good health is seen as a desirable goal, the steps that one must take are often viewed as "unpleasant." We must learn to focus on what we will gain rather than on what we need to give up.

Making changes and being successful will take motivation and dedication; however, the results should more than compensate for the effort involved. You will almost certainly look and feel better, you will have more energy, and you will reduce your risk for certain diseases. If you have weight or body fat to lose, maintaining consistent good eating habits and exercising regularly should allow you to gradually and steadily lose the weight or body fat.

In Summary

Although people today know more about healthful living, many of them do not put into practice what they know.

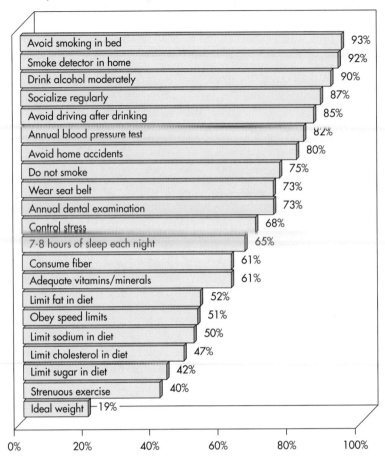

Figure 1-8   Percentage practicing each behavior

By understanding the material in this book, you will become more knowledgeable regarding health, physical fitness, and exercise and nutrition, and you will learn how you can positively influence your health. However, in addition to learning what to do, you must be willing to implement these changes in your lifestyle. This will take motivation and dedication, but the end result will be worthwhile. You will be a winner.

Let's Get Started

To be successful, you need to adopt a healthy lifestyle—one you can live with for the rest of your life. There are six steps involved in this process:

1. **Become more knowledgeable about health and wellness.** The choices you make determine your everyday habits. By understanding the material in this book, you will become more knowledgeable and learn how you can positively influence your health. You will also be able to make better decisions each day concerning these issues.
2. **Assess your existing habits.** By determining your Personal Prevention Index (Laboratory Experience 1-1) and completing the Health and Wellness Questionnaire (Laboratory Experience 1-2), you will get a good assessment of your current habits.
3. **Identify those habits that need to be changed.** You should now be able to identify specific habits that negatively affect your health. For example, you may find that you skip meals frequently, drink too much alcohol, and exercise far too infrequently. In the Self Assessment at the end of this chapter (Laboratory Experience 1-3), you can make a list of the specific habits that negatively affect your health.
4. **Set realistic objectives.** Much time and effort can be wasted unless specific objectives are established. For example, you may determine that you want to:

- Reduce your body weight by 10 lb.
- Exercise at least three times each week for 30 minutes in some kind of aerobic exercise.
- Eat a nutritious breakfast each morning.
- Limit your alcohol consumption to a maximum of two drinks a day.

Make your own list of specific objectives and include these in Laboratory Experience 1-3.

5. **Implement planned changes.** Not only do you need to know where you are going, but you must also have a plan as to how to get there. It is important to establish a systematic and carefully designed step-by-step approach. It is helpful if this plan is in writing so that it can constantly be revised and updated if necessary and modified if it does not work. It is important to remember to be patient rather than wanting everything at once. The plan should include specific weekly objectives that will contribute to your overall success. As these specific objectives become part of your daily lifestyle, new ones can be added.

6. **Monitor the consistency of these changes.** How consistent you are will determine how successful you will be. You need to work *constantly* rather than sporadically at achieving each of these objectives.

Chapter Summary

The following summary will help you to identify some of the important concepts covered in this chapter:

- Enthusiasm for exercise and fitness and interest in nutrition are at an all-time high in the United States.
- A large percentage of Americans are unfit because they lack motivation and self-discipline.
- Most college students "believe" that exercise is important, but the majority of them just do not "find" time to exercise regularly.
- The body functions more efficiently if we exercise regularly.
- Because of today's "inactive" lifestyle, we must now take time to "program" exercise into our busy schedules.
- Many of the serious health problems that exist in this country are "lifestyle induced" and could be prevented.
- In today's world, our everyday decisions greatly influence our health.
- Regular exercise does not necessarily ensure good health. We must also be concerned with other health-related practices.
- There are many advantages associated with working hard to build a healthy lifestyle around exercise, physical fitness, and good nutrition.

References

1. American Cancer Society: *Cancer facts and figures: 1994*, New York, 1994, The Society.
2. Brooks CL: Are Americans fit? Survey data conflict, *The Physician and Sportsmedicine* 14(11):24, 1986.
3. Dawber TR: *The Framingham Study: the epidemiology of artherosclerotic disease*, Cambridge, Mass, 1980, Harvard University Press.
4. Friedman G: *Group health analysis for standard population*, Tempe, Ariz, 1985, Health Advancement Services.
5. Hahn RA et al: Excess deaths from nine chronic diseases in the United States, *JAMA* 264:2654-2659, 1990.
6. Harris TG, Gurin J: Look who's getting it all together, *American Heart*, pp 42-47, March 1985.
7. Harris TG, Gurin J: Taking charge: the happy health confidants, *American Heart*, pp 53-57, March 1987.
8. *Health: choice or chance?* Chicago, Ill, 1991, American Dietetic Association.
9. *Healthy People 2000, national health promotion and disease prevention objectives*, US Department of Health and Human Services, Public Health Service, Pub No (PHS)91-50213, Washington, DC, 1991, US Government Printing Office.
10. *Heart facts-1994*, Dallas, Tex, 1994, American Heart Association.
11. Kucjmarski RJ et al: Increasing prevalence of overweight among US adults, *JAMA* 272(3):205-211, 1994.
12. Manson JE et al: A prospective study of exercise and incidence of diabetes among US male physicians, *JAMA* 268(1):63-67, 1992.
13. Manson JE et al: Physical activity and incidence of non–insulin-dependent diabetes mellitus in women, *Lancet* 338:774-778, 1991.
14. McGinnis JM, Foege WH: Actual causes of death in the United States, *JAMA* 270(18):2207-2212, 1993.
15. Munnings F: Osteoporosis: what is the role of

exercise? *The Physician and Sportsmedicine* 20(6):127-138, 1992.

16. Neaton JD, Wentworth D: Serum cholesterol, blood pressure, cigarette smoking and death from coronary heart disease, *Arch Intern Med* 152:56-64, 1992.

17. Powell KE et al: Physical activity and the incidence of coronary heart disease, *Annu Rev Public Health* 8:253-287, 1987.

18. Prentice W: *Fitness for college and life,* ed 4, St Louis, 1994, Mosby.

19. President's Council on Physical Fitness and Sport: *National adult physical fitness survey,* Newsletter, pp 1-27, May 1973.

20. *Prevention Index '91,* Emmaus, Penn, 1991, Rodale Press.

21. *Prevention Index '94,* Emmaus, Penn, 1994, Rodale Press.

22. Robins G, Powers D, Burgess S: *A wellness way of life,* ed 2, Dubuque, Iowa, 1994, Brown & Benchmark.

23. Rosato FD: *Fitness and wellness: the physical connection,* St Paul, Minn, West Publishing.

24. Schwade S: Get your back on track: how to enjoy fitness and sport again, even with a bad back, *Prevention* 46(4):67-70, 1994.

25. Siscovick DA et al: Habitual vigorous exercise and primary cardiac arrest: effect of other risk factors on the relationships, *Journal of Chronic Disease* 37:625-632, 1984.

26. Sopko G, Obarzanek E, Stone E: Overview of National Heart, Lung and Blood Institute Workshop on physical activity and cardiovascular health, *Med Sci Sports Exerc* 24(6):5192-5195, 1992.

27. *Vital and health statistics: health promotion and disease prevention 1990,* US Department of Health and Human Services, April 1993.

28. Winter RE: A message from the executive health group, *Newsweek,* 1987.

Laboratory Experience 1-1

Your Personal Prevention Index

Name _____ Section _____ Date _____

The Prevention Index takes stock of the nation's health, but you can also score your own prevention profile by taking the test below. Carefully check "yes" or "no" in each of the following questions:

	YES	NO
1. Do you have your blood pressure taken at least once a year?	___	___
2. Do you go to the dentist at least once a year for treatment or a checkup?	___	___
3. Is your body weight within the recommended range for your gender, height, and bone structure?	___	___
4. Do you exercise strenuously (so that you breathe heavily and your heart rate is accelerated for a period lasting at least 20 minutes) 3 days or more a week?	___	___
5. Do you smoke cigarettes now?	___	___
6. Do you consciously take steps to control or reduce stress in your life?	___	___
7. Do you usually sleep a total of 7 or 8 hours during each 24-hour day? (If you usually sleep either more or less than this, please mark "no.")	___	___
8. Do you socialize with close friends, relatives, or neighbors at least once a week?	___	___
9. In general, when you drink alcoholic beverages, do you consume less than 14 drinks a week and less than 5 drinks on any single day? (Mark "yes" if the answer to both parts is "yes." If you never drink at all, also mark "yes.")	___	___
10. Do you wear a seat belt all the time when you are in the front seat of a car?	___	___
11. Do you drive at or below the speed limit all the time? (If you don't drive please mark "yes.")	___	___
12. Do you ever drive after drinking? (If you don't drink, please mark "no.")	___	___
13. Do you have a smoke detector in your home?	___	___
14. Does anyone in your household ever smoke in bed?	___	___
15. Do you take any special steps or precautions to avoid accidents in and around your home?	___	___
16. Do you try to avoid eating too much salt or sodium?	___	___
17. Do you try to avoid eating too much fat?	___	___
18. Do you try to eat enough fiber from whole grains, cereals, fruits, and vegetables?	___	___
19. Do you try to avoid eating too many high-cholesterol foods such as eggs, dairy products, and fatty meats?	___	___
20. Do you try to get enough vitamins and minerals in foods or supplements?	___	___
21. Do you try to avoid eating too much sugar and sweet food?	___	___

NOTES: A drink is defined as a shot of hard liquor, a can or bottle of beer, or a glass of wine.
The healthy answer for questions 5, 12, and 14 is "no."
The healthy answer for all the other questions is "yes."
Scoring: Add up your total number of healthy responses and then divide that number by 21, which tells you the percentage of the 21 Prevention Index Behaviors that you practice.

Number of Healthy Responses = ____
Personal Prevention Index
= Number of Healthy Responses/21
= ____ /21
= ____

Compare your score with the national average (See Table 1-3).

Health and Wellness Questionnaire

Name _____ Section _____ Date _____

Please answer each question as honestly as possible. When completed, add together the total points for each of your responses.

Diet and Nutrition

1. How often do you consciously limit both your salt and sodium intake by not adding salt to prepared foods and by selecting foods that are low in sodium?
   - _____ (2) Frequently (almost every day)
   - _____ (1) Sometimes (every few days)
   - _____ (0) Rarely (once a week or less)

2. How often do you eat a well-balanced nutritious breakfast?
   - _____ (4) 7 days each week
   - _____ (3) 5 or 6 days each week
   - _____ (2) 3 or 4 days each week
   - _____ (1) 1 or 2 days each week
   - _____ (0) Never

3. During your waking hours, how often do you go longer than 5 hours without eating something nutritious?
   - _____ (0) Frequently (almost every day)
   - _____ (1) Sometimes (every few days)
   - _____ (2) Rarely (once a week or less)

4. How often do you drink at least six 8-oz glasses of water?
   - _____ (3) Frequently (almost every day)
   - _____ (1) Sometimes (every few days)
   - _____ (0) Rarely (once a week or less)

5. How often do you eat at fast-food restaurants?
   - _____ (0) Often (three or more times a week)
   - _____ (1) Occasionally (one or two times a week)
   - _____ (3) Seldom (maybe once a month)

6. Foods that are usually high in fat include cheese, chips, mayonnaise, salad dressings, red meat, Mexican food, fried foods, butter, margarine, and nuts. How would you describe your fat intake?
   - _____ (0) High (I usually eat at least two of these foods just about every day.)
   - _____ (1) Moderate (I usually eat one of these foods just about every day.)
   - _____ (3) Low (Most days I do not eat any of these foods.)

7. Food that are usually high in simple sugar include candy, cookies, cakes, pastries, ice cream, and sodas. How would you classify your intake of simple sugars?
   - _____ (0) High (I usually eat at least one of these types of foods each day.)
   - _____ (1) Moderate (I usually eat these types of foods two or three times each week.)
   - _____ (3) Low (I hardly ever eat foods that are high in sugar.)

8. Caffeine is contained in coffee, tea, and many soft drinks. How many 8-oz cups of caffeinated beverages do you drink in an average day?
   - _____ (4) None
   - _____ (3) 1 or 2
   - _____ (2) 3 or 4
   - _____ (1) 6 to 10
   - _____ (0) More than 10

9. How many days do you eat a well-balanced diet that includes at least two servings from each of the following food groups: milk or dairy products, fruits, vegetables, bread or grains, and meat or meat substitutes?
   - _____ (3) Every day
   - _____ (2) 5 or 6 days
   - _____ (1) 3 or 4 days
   - _____ (0) Less than 3 days

Healthy Lifestyle Changes

Name _____ Section _____ Date _____

Compile a list of specific habits that negatively affect your health:

Compile a list of objectives that includes changes you would like to incorporate in your lifestyle that would positively influence your health:

Chapter Two **Physical Fitness: Basic Concepts**

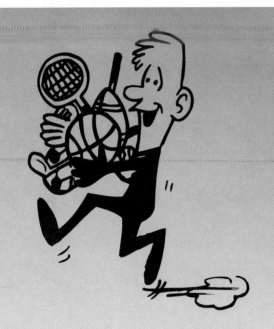

CHAPTER OBJECTIVES

Check off each objective you achieve.

☐ Define physical fitness, and identify and define each of the health-related components.

☐ Understand fully the benefits of striving to achieve an optimal level of physical fitness.

☐ Explain why it is important to exercise regularly to achieve even an adequate level of physical fitness.

☐ Define the terms *overload* and *progression*, and understand how to apply each of these in planning a simple exercise program.

☐ Devise a strategy to make regular exercise a part of your lifestyle.

☐ Subjectively determine whether you have an adequate level of physical fitness.

PHYSICAL FITNESS: DEFINITION

Despite the widespread interest in physical fitness, it is still difficult to define. The average person does not know exactly what physical fitness is, what level of fitness he or she needs to achieve, how to develop that level of fitness, or how to evaluate his or her present level of physical fitness.

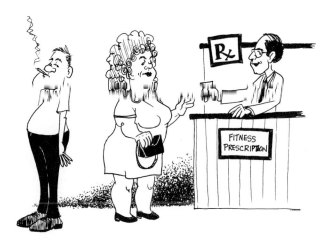

If fitness came in a pill, it would be the most widely prescribed medicine by far.

Physical fitness has been defined as "the ability to carry out everyday tasks with vigor and alertness, without undue fatigue, and with ample energy to enjoy leisure-time pursuits and to meet unforeseen emergencies."[1] The problem with this definition is that our modern way of life has changed. We have seen that many of our everyday tasks now require very little energy expenditure, and several of our leisure-time pursuits that once involved a reasonable amount of energy expenditure now require considerably less.

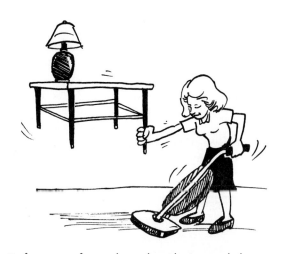

Performance of everyday tasks with vigor and alertness.

It would appear that a high level of fitness may no longer be needed to work in today's world dominated by technological innovations.[5] Therefore if physical fitness is defined as the level of fitness needed to function in modern society, a large percentage of the American adult population would be considered physically fit. As you can see in this chapter, this definition can be used to define what would be considered an *adequate* level of physical fitness.

Physical fitness means different things to different people. It must be viewed as an individual matter and as such has little meaning unless considered in relation to the specific needs and interests of each individual. Consider what physical fitness means to the following five people:

1. Shirley, a 21-year-old secretary, participates four times each week in an aerobic dance class. She is single, and her major reason for exercise is to maintain a neat, trim figure.
2. Jim is a 30-year-old construction worker. He is very strong, has well-developed muscles, and appears to have very little body fat. He does not participate in any organized exercise program because he feels that he gets all the physical activity he needs each day at work.
3. Jean is a 40-year-old avid runner. Her objective is to someday complete a marathon in less than 3 hours. She runs between 40 and 50 miles each week.
4. George is a 45-year-old man who is presently recovering from heart bypass surgery. His exercise program consists of 20 minutes of slow walking 4 days per week to improve the functioning of his cardiorespiratory system.
5. Ann is a 20-year-old varsity tennis player who feels that if she is going to reach her potential and compete at the national level, she must practice her skills on the tennis court 2 to 3 hours per day, at least 5 days per week.

To each of these people, physical fitness appears to be important, but it is apparent that each of them views it somewhat differently. They would probably all agree with the statements that "regular exercise is good for you" and that "it is good to be physically fit." It should also be clear that physical fitness is not the same for everyone.

In Summary

Physical fitness is a desirable quality that can be developed in numerous ways for a variety of reasons.

PHYSICAL FITNESS CONTINUUM

It may be beneficial to find a way to quantify physical fitness. A logical approach might be to consider physical fitness as existing on a scale or continuum. A person who is seriously ill and needs help to function would possess a very minimal level, whereas a highly conditioned person would be close to the maximal level. This concept is suggested by Clarke and Clarke,[1] who state that "physical fitness is a positive and dynamic quality extending on a continuum from 'death' to 'abundant life.'" This concept is illustrated in Table 2-1, where physical fitness is represented on a 10-point scale. The table is arbitrarily divided into the following five categories: maximal, high, adequate, minimal, and very low.

Notice that specific criteria are presented relative to each of these categories, and an attempt is made to relate each category to the amount of exercise that is possible and to performance on the physical fitness tests.

We have seen that there is an optimal level of efficiency for the functioning of the body and that it is only through regular, sustained physical activity that this can be achieved. To achieve this, your level of physical fitness would have to be classified as "high" or "maximal" according to the criteria presented in Table 2-1. These are the levels of fitness for which everyone should strive.

COMPONENTS OF PHYSICAL FITNESS

There has been much confusion in past years as to what the components of physical fitness actually are. To clarify the situation, existing components have been grouped into two categories—health-related and skill-related.

Health-related physical fitness components

It is now generally agreed that only those components that contribute to the development of health and increase the functional capacity of the body will be classified as health-related physical fitness components. These are identified in Figure 2-1.

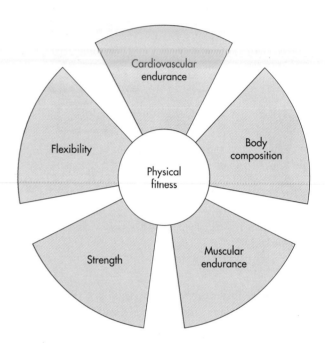

Figure 2-1   Health-related physical fitness components.

Table 2-1	**Physical Fitness Continuum**		
Criteria	Category	Rating*	Activity Criteria
Highly conditioned person with maximum functional capacity	Maximal	10 9	Excels in all physical fitness components and able to complete an hour or more of moderate to high intensity aerobic activity and still have energy left
Increased energy and vitality for a well-rounded life	High	8 7	High ratings on physical fitness components and able to complete at least an hour of moderate aerobic activity and not feel tired at the end or after the exercise
Ability to function normally without undue fatigue and be able to make the most out of what life has to offer and have energy left at the end of the day	Adequate	6 5	Average ability on physical fitness components and able to complete at least 30 minutes of aerobic activity; may be tired or fatigued at the end or after the activity
Barely able to perform everyday tasks with little or no energy left at the end of the day; tires easily in completing daily tasks	Minimal	4 3	Unable to complete 30 minutes or more of continuous aerobic activity and performs less than average on several of the physical fitness components
Unfit for work and frequently needs help to function; often seriously ill	Very low	2 1	Cannot complete most of the physical fitness tests and unable to participate in any form of exercise on a regular basis

*Circle the score that you feel best represents your level of physical fitness.

Skill-related physical fitness components

There are several essential components for the successful execution of various sport skills, often referred to as *skill-related* or *performance-related:*

1. Agility
2. Balance
3. Coordination
4. Speed
5. Power
6. Reaction time

Highly skilled athletes possess an extremely high level of these components. It should be emphasized, however, that a high degree of athletic ability is not essential for the development and maintenance of physical fitness because there are many activities that can be included in your physical fitness program that require minimal amounts of skill. However, for those who thrive on competition and who have a reasonable level of skill, several activities are excellent for the development of physical fitness. Racquetball is an excellent activity for the development of aerobic fitness, provided that you have an "adequate" level of skill (Figure 2-2).

Health-related physical fitness components defined

To clarify the meaning of physical fitness, each of the health-related physical fitness components is defined and identified briefly in this chapter and discussed in detail in the following chapters.

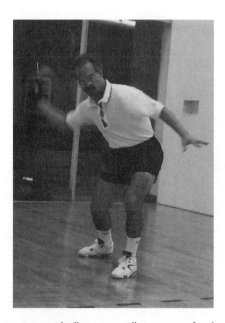

Figure 2-2 Racquetball is an excellent activity for the development of aerobic fitness, provided that you have an "adequate" skill level.

Cardiovascular endurance

Cardiovascular endurance may be defined as the ability to perform heavy physical work involving large muscle groups continuously for an extended period of time. The performance of such tasks largely depends on the ability of the body to deliver oxygen to the working muscles and the ability of these muscles to extract and use this oxygen. The level at which you can participate in such activities as cycling, running, swimming, and a variety of other **aerobic activities** depends on the efficiency of your circulatory and respiratory systems. When insufficient oxygen is delivered to the muscles, their ability to perform work diminishes greatly.

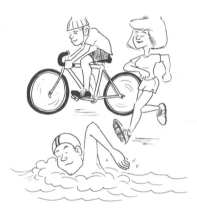

The level at which you can participate in such activities as cycling, running, swimming, and a variety of other aerobic activities depends on the efficiency of your circulatory and respiratory systems.

Because aerobic processes account for the majority of the energy produced in the body, the ability to take in and deliver oxygen to the working muscles is an important factor in determining how much work can be performed. The more oxygen the body is able to take in and use, the more work a person should be able to perform before fatigue and exhaustion occur. Cardiovascular endurance may therefore be defined more simply as the maximum amount of work an individual is capable of performing continuously where the work in-

Cardiovascular endurance: The maximal amount of work that can be performed continuously involving large muscle groups that is dependent on the efficiency of the heart and circulatory system. Also referred to as *aerobic fitness.*

Aerobic activity: Any organized activity that is continuous and involves large muscle groups. Examples include walking, jogging, swimming, and stair-stepping.

volves large muscle groups. It is often referred to as *physical work capacity.* The 12-minute run test is a simple practical test used to measure cardiovascular endurance. The maximum amount of work a person can perform is determined by how far he or she can run in 12 minutes.

The circulatory and respiratory systems must function efficiently if a high level of cardiovascular fitness is to be achieved. It is therefore often referred to as **cardiovascular endurance** or **aerobic fitness.** Because of the various health benefits associated with the development of a high level of cardiovascular endurance, it is by far the most important physical fitness component.

Flexibility

Flexibility is recognized as one of the important health-related components of physical fitness. It can be defined as the capacity of a joint to move freely through a full range of motion without undue strain.

The amount of movement possible at a joint is usually determined by the length of the muscles, ligaments, and tendons, and by the structure of the joint. The most important of these appears to be the length of the muscles. When muscles are not used, they tend to become shorter and tighter and the range of motion at the specific joint is reduced significantly.

Having a full range of motion at each of the major joints of the body is advantageous. Without flexibility, movement is impossible. With limited flexibility, there is a decrease in the efficiency with which you can perform everyday activities such as walking up a flight of stairs, bending to pick up a newspaper, tying shoes, or getting in or out of the back seat of a two-door car. It is interesting to note that people with poor flexibility tend to be accident-prone and to tire very quickly when performing simple tasks such as walking.

Certain activities tend to shorten muscles and thus reduce flexibility. This may often result in muscle tear or strain. As the body grows older, this may become a very serious problem. It is therefore very important not to neglect the development of flexibility.

Strength

Strength can be defined as the ability of a muscle or muscle group to exert force against a resistance. It is measured by determining the maximum one-time force that can be exerted. This is referred to as *one repetition maximum* (1 RM).

Each person needs a certain level of strength. Without this, it would be impossible to carry out many of the simple everyday tasks such as lifting a heavy suitcase, picking up a bag of garbage, or even maintaining an upright posture. In some cases the development of strength of specific muscles reduces the incidence of joint injury. For example, well-developed abdominal muscles and strong lower back muscles can contribute significantly to the reduction of many low back pain problems.

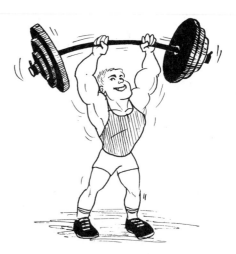

Strength is the maximum force that can be exerted at one time by a muscle or muscle group.

Muscular endurance

Muscular endurance can be defined as the ability of a muscle or muscle group to apply force repeatedly, or the ability of a muscle or muscle group to sustain a contraction for a period of time.

There is of course a close relationship between strength and muscular endurance. For example, you need a certain level of strength to lift an object such as a suitcase. Your level of muscular endurance determines how long you can carry the suitcase. If you are constantly experiencing sore or aching muscles, this is probably an indication that you need to improve your level of muscular endurance.

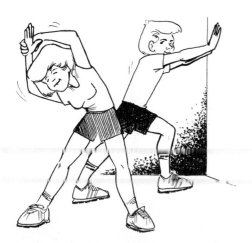

Flexibility is frequently overlooked and often misunderstood.

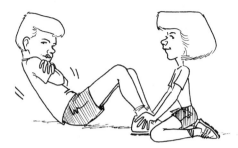

Muscular endurance is the performance of a maximum number or repetitions.

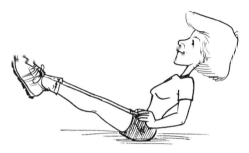

Muscular endurance is sustaining a given contraction.

Body composition

Body composition is also included as one of the health-related physical fitness components. It refers to the relative amounts of fat and **lean body weight** (or fat-free mass) that comprise your body. Your fat-free weight consists of all the tissues of the body other than fat. When you have an excessive amount of fat, you can be classified as obese. An obese person has an increased risk for several serious medical problems such as various cardiovascular diseases and diabetes. In addition, excess fat limits the amount of work that you can perform and may contribute to a decrease in the performance of various sports skills. The percentage of total body weight attributable to body fat is referred to as your **percentage of body fat.**

In Summary

Aerobic fitness is the most important health-related physical fitness component. Achieving a maximal level has many benefits.

EXERCISE AND PHYSICAL FITNESS

The human body was designed to be active and functions more efficiently when it is active. The basic problem is that today's lifestyle requires very little activity to accomplish the everyday tasks that we perform. This is discussed in Chapter 1. It is very important to remember that you must exercise regularly for your body to function efficiently. This principle applies to each of the physical fitness components.

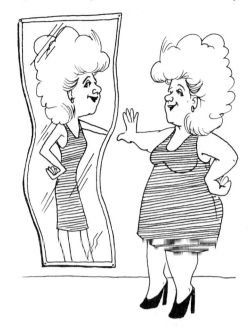

When you exercise, you force your body to work at a level slightly higher than what it is accustomed to working at because you are placing additional stress on the body. Over time, if the exercise is performed regularly, your body will adapt to the increased workload and will therefore function more efficiently. The case study on the following page demonstrates this point.

Important exercise principles

There are three principles that you must apply when designing any exercise program. These are as follows:

Overload. Overload involves subjecting the body to a task slightly beyond its normal level so that sufficient stress is placed on the body to stimulate the desired response.

Flexibility: The range of motion that is possible at a joint.

Strength: The amount of force a muscle or muscle group can exert with a single contraction.

Muscular endurance: The ability of a muscle or muscle group to sustain a contraction or to repeat contractions continuously.

Body composition: The relative proportion of fat weight to lean body weight in the body.

Lean body weight: The total amount of body weight that is not attributable to fat; this includes muscle, ligaments, tendons, bones, and fluids.

Percentage of body fat: The percentage of your total body weight that is attributable to fat.

Case Study

JON

Jon was a student in my aerobic fitness class in the fall of 1993. He was 20 lb overweight and had not exercised regularly for the previous 5 years. He started walking on the treadmill at a speed of 3.5 mph, and he could walk for only 20 minutes before becoming fatigued and having to stop. After exercising regularly for 4 weeks, not only could he complete 30 minutes without stopping, but the task that at first was very difficult suddenly became quite easy. He could not only increase the length of time that he exercised but also the speed at which he was walking.

Progression. The body will adapt to the increased level of resistance as improvement takes place. For this reason, it is necessary to increase the workload frequently. This can be incorporated easily in an aerobic exercise program by carefully checking the heart rate at frequent intervals and adjusting the intensity of the exercise to ensure that you are exercising at the right intensity. This is discussed in detail in Chapter 4.

Specificity. To improve a particular physical fitness component, an exercise must be performed for that particular component. This is referred to as the principle of specificity. For example, jogging is a good activity for the development of cardiovascular endurance but has little effect on the development of flexibility, strength, and muscular endurance.

Specific programs are presented throughout this book for each of the physical fitness components.

Specific Exercise Programs

Cardiovascular fitness	Chapter 4
Strength	Chapter 5
Muscular endurance	Chapter 5
Flexibility	Chapter 6
Body composition	Chapters 8 and 9

WHY PEOPLE EXERCISE

The reasons as to why people exercise can be grouped into three major categories:

Fitness. The overall objective for many people who exercise regularly is to increase their level of fitness so that their body functions more efficiently.

Weight management. Many people exercise primarily to reduce their body weight or percentage of body fat to a desirable level or to maintain their present level.

Health. Many regular exercisers are aware of the health benefits associated with regular exercise, and their major objective is to add years to their life expectancy by reducing the risk of certain diseases.

In designing any exercise program you must be able to answer the following questions:

- How often do I need to exercise?
- How long must each exercise session last?
- How hard must I exercise?
- Which activities are best for me?

The answer to each of these questions will vary according to your overall objective. Those wishing to obtain the maximal health benefits will need to do more exercise than those who exercise to increase the efficiency with which their body functions. Specific information is presented throughout this book pertaining to the **frequency, duration,** and **intensity** for each type of exercise program.

In Summary

The amount of exercise that is necessary and the intensity of the exercise will vary for each of the physical fitness components.

GETTING MOTIVATED TO EXERCISE

We have seen that regular exercise is important if you are to achieve even an adequate level of physical fitness, and the achievement of an optimal level will take dedication and motivation. If you do not presently exercise regularly, you need to get started.

It is very easy for obstacles to get in your way when it comes to exercise. If you have tried exercise and lack the consistency that is necessary to be successful, it may be because:

- An injury or illness caused you to stop exercising.
- A change in schedule resulted in less time being available.
- You became bored with your exercise program.
- You failed to lose weight.
- You were disappointed with your progress.

The following suggestions may help you to make exercise a permanent part of your lifestyle:

1. If a busy schedule limits the amount of time you have for exercise, try to build more physical activity into your daily routine. Try to walk or ride a bicycle as frequently as you can instead of driving a car, and climb the stairs rather than using the elevator. You will then need to schedule fewer exercise sessions because you will be more active throughout the day.

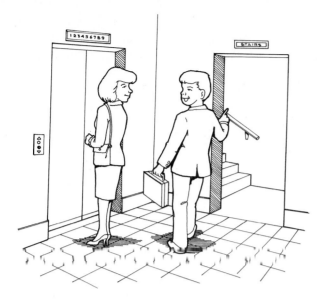

3. Try to make exercise more enjoyable. It may be necessary to vary your routine so that you do not become bored. For jogging, walking, or cycling, try a different route or listen to music. If you are exercising on a treadmill, stationary bicycle, or stepping machine, watch television as a diversion.

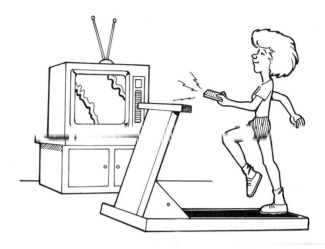

2. Schedule exercise into your lifestyle just like you schedule appointments, classes, etc. If your lifestyle is such that you frequently just do not have time to exercise, you may need to get up an hour earlier than normal so that you will have time to exercise.

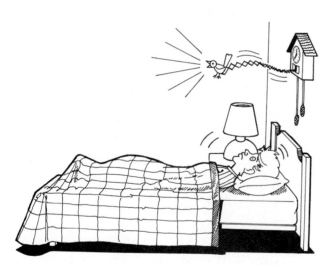

4. Try exercising with another person or with a group of people, or if you enjoy exercising by yourself, you can simply enjoy the solitude.

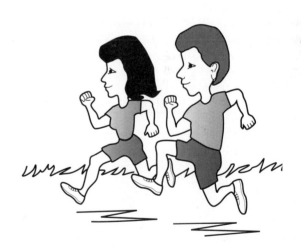

Frequency: The number of exercise sessions per week.

Duration: The length of each exercise session.

Intensity: How strenuous each exercise is.

Let's Get Started

If you have not exercised regularly for some time, the following beginning walking program designed to get you to walk 3 miles in 45 minutes may help you to get started. By making small manageable goals, monitoring your progress, and making a commitment to follow this program for 3 or 4 weeks, you should experience some of the benefits of regular exercise and you may find that exercise will become a healthy addiction.

Step 1. Get in your car and measure a half-mile distance from where you live or from where you might start walking.

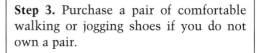

Step 2. Schedule a time for 4 or 5 days for the first week that you are going to set aside to exercise. Mark this on a calendar on your bathroom mirror or refrigerator.

Step 8. You are now ready to start on your final goal of walking 3 miles in 45 minutes. By now you know what to do and you should have seen the benefits of setting specific goals, achieving these goals, and recording your progress on a calendar. When you achieve your final goal, you should know how to build further progression into your exercise program.

Step 3. Purchase a pair of comfortable walking or jogging shoes if you do not own a pair.

Step 7. Concentrate on keeping a steady pace, and gradually increase your speed until you reach your second goal of 2 miles in 30 minutes.

Step 4. Walk the half-mile at a comfortable pace without stopping, and turn around and walk back to the start. Note how long it takes you to walk the mile. Record this time and place a big check mark on the calendar for having completed the exercise for that day.

Step 6. When you can walk 1 mile comfortably in 15 minutes, you are ready to increase the distance to 2 miles. Either measure a new course or walk the 1-mile course twice.

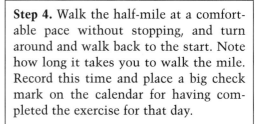

Step 5. Walk the same course each exercise day. Note the time it takes and mark your calendar each time you complete the distance.

Chapter Summary

The following summary will help you to identify some of the important concepts covered in this chapter:

- Health-related physical fitness relates to the efficiency with which the body functions, and it is only through regular, sustained exercise that a desirable level can be achieved.
- The components of health-related physical fitness include cardiovascular endurance, flexibility, strength, muscular endurance, and body composition.
- Because of the health-related advantages, attainment of an optimal level of cardiovascular endurance is advantageous.
- Physical fitness is important to everyone and can be developed in a variety of ways for many different reasons.
- A high level of skill is not necessary for the development and maintenance of physical fitness.
- A high level of cardiovascular endurance depends on the efficient functioning of the circulatory and respiratory systems.
- A person who has excess fat will be less active and at an increased risk for certain chronic diseases.
- Achieving a maximal level of aerobic fitness has many advantages; however, with strength, muscular endurance, and flexibility, most people need only an adequate level to function in today's world.
- It is important to build progression into any exercise program because your body will adapt to the increased level of exercise.

References

1. Clarke HH, Clarke DH: *Application of measurement to physical education,* Englewood Cliffs, NJ, 1987, Prentice Hall.
2. Fahey TD, Insel PM, Roth WT: *Fit and well,* Mountain View, Calif, 1994, Mayfield Publishing.
3. *Healthy people—AFLC focus on wellness,* Scarsdale, NY, Oct 1989, Health Management Communications.
4. *Hope health appraisal,* Seattle, Wash, 1987, The Bob Hope International Heart Research Institute.
5. Nieman DC: *Fitness and sports medicine fitness: an introduction,* ed 3, Palo Alto, Calif, 1995, Bull Publishing.

Laboratory Experience 2-1

Subjective Evaluation of Present Level of Physical Fitness

Name _____ Section _____ Date _____

How do you know if you have an adequate level of physical fitness? You may be able to subjectively determine this by answering the questions below:

	YES	NO
1. Do you feel tired when you wake up in the morning and often do not really want to get out of bed?	____	____
2. Do you yawn regularly throughout the day?	____	____
3. Do you become fatigued from tasks requiring minimal energy such as climbing several flights of stairs or walking around in a shopping mall?	____	____
4. Do you run out of energy by the middle of the day or early afternoon and often wish that you had time to lie down and take a nap?	____	____
5. When you look at yourself, do you wish you weighed less or had less fat in specific areas of your body?	____	____
6. Do you frequently fall asleep in the evenings while reading or watching television?	____	____
7. Are you often too tired to participate in active leisure activities?	____	____
8. Are you vulnerable to frequent aches and pains?	____	____
9. Do you often drive around a parking lot looking for a parking space close to the entrance?	____	____
10. Do you buy a new pair of shoes every year or so because the old ones are dirty rather than worn out?	____	____

Overall Evaluation: Do you generally lack energy and vitality?

If several of your responses are "yes," then you may have less than an adequate level of physical fitness.

Chapter Three Cardiovascular Endurance

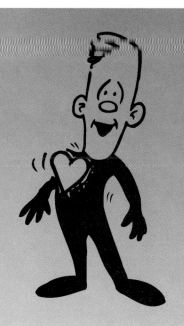

CHAPTER OBJECTIVES

Check off each objective you achieve.

- ❏ Explain why cardiovascular endurance is the most important component of physical fitness.
- ❏ Differentiate clearly between aerobic and anaerobic work.
- ❏ Determine your resting heart rate (Laboratory Experience 3-1).
- ❏ Define each of the terms associated with the cardiovascular system, and be able to discuss their importance in relation to cardiovascular endurance.
- ❏ Describe the relationship between oxygen consumption and energy expenditure.
- ❏ Define maximal oxygen consumption, and discuss the changes that take place in the body as a result of regular aerobic exercise, which positively influences this variable.
- ❏ Design and evaluate an exercise program specifically planned to develop your level of aerobic fitness.
- ❏ Calculate your target-zone heart rate.
- ❏ Calculate your critical heart rate.
- ❏ Understand the importance of the target-zone heart rate and the critical, or threshold, heart rate in the development of cardiovascular endurance.
- ❏ Complete Laboratory Experience 3-2: Measurement of blood pressure.
- ❏ Complete Laboratory Experience 3-3: Determination of exercise heart rate for various activities without the use of a heart rate monitor.
- ❏ Complete Laboratory Experience 3-4 or 3-5: Measurement of cardiovascular endurance—the 12-minute run test or the 1.5-mile run test.
- ❏ Complete Laboratory Experience 3-6: Measurement of cardiovascular endurance—the 5-minute step test.
- ❏ Define each of the key terms.

Cardiovascular endurance, which is also referred to as physical work capacity or aerobic fitness, is the most important component of physical fitness. Attaining a high level of cardiovascular endurance has many health benefits and will result in an increase in the efficiency with which your body functions. You will be able to exercise at a higher level of intensity, and you will be able to sustain this level for a longer period of time.

Cardiovascular endurance depends on how efficiently the lungs, heart, and blood vessels can provide the necessary oxygen to the working muscles and how efficiently these muscles can use this oxygen. Cardiovascular endurance can therefore be defined as the efficiency with which you can perform heavy, continuous physical work involving large muscle groups and lasting for an extended period. The more oxygen that can be supplied and used, the higher the level of work that an be sustained (Figure 3-1).

In Summary

The amount of continuous work you can perform before you become fatigued and the level at which you can work both reflect your level of cardiovascular endurance.

EFFICIENCY OF PERFORMANCE

The intensity of effort required for an activity can be measured by your heart rate response. This reflects the efficiency with which you perform the task. A person with a low level of cardiovascular endurance will have a higher heart rate response to a submaximal standardized task compared with that of a fit person and will fatigue much faster (Figure 3-2).

Efficiency of performance is reflected by a fit person's ability to:

- Work at a higher intensity level than an unfit person without fatigue. For example, a fit person may be able to run at 7 mph on the treadmill for 30 minutes to get an aerobic workout, whereas an unfit person may only be able to walk at 3.5 mph.

- Perform more work than an unfit person before reaching exhaustion. For example, a fit person may be able to run 2 miles in 12 minutes, whereas an unfit person may only be able to cover 1 mile in the designated time.

- Recover faster than an unfit person after exercise. A fit person's heart will return to its resting rate much faster than that of an unfit person.

ANAEROBIC AND AEROBIC WORK

Within the body there are two systems that can supply energy—the anaerobic system and the aerobic system.

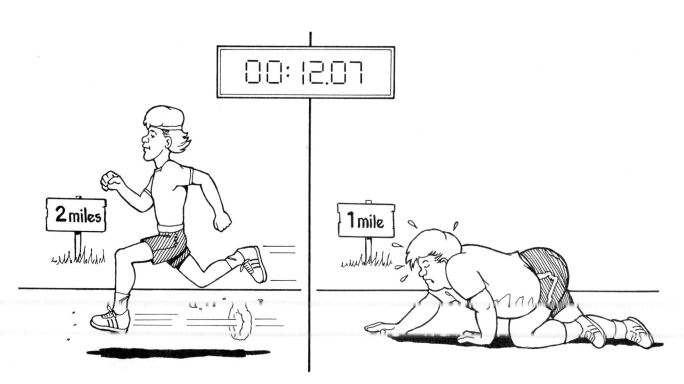

Figure 3-1   A fit person's body functions more efficiently, and a fit person can run farther than an unfit person in the same amount of time.

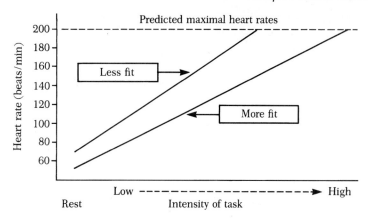

Figure 3-2 Comparison of heart rate patterns for individuals with different fitness levels.

The type of task you perform determines which system makes the major contribution.

Anaerobic system

The anaerobic system provides energy for tasks requiring a high rate of energy expenditure for a short period of time. The 100-yard dash is an example. With this system a large amount of energy is released to supply the immediate needs of the body. The amount of **anaerobic work** you can perform is limited, and you will usually be able to perform this type of exercise for only up to 2 minutes. Lactic acid is produced with this process, and an accumulation of lactic acid in the body contributes to muscle fatigue.

Aerobic system

The aerobic system provides energy for **submaximal tasks** requiring a lower rate of energy expenditure over a longer period of time. Walking and jogging are examples of **aerobic work.** Tasks such as these depend on a constant amount of oxygen being available for use by the muscles performing the work. The amount of oxygen taken in and used by the body must be sufficient to provide the energy required for the task.

The length of time and intensity of the exercise determines the relative contribution of each of these energy systems. This relationship is summarized in Figure 3-3. This graph shows that during a 1-minute run,

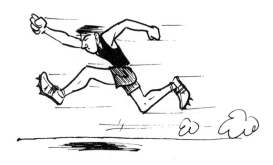

Anaerobic task.

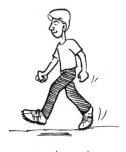

Aerobic task.

Figure 3-3 Relative roles of anaerobic and aerobic processes for supplying oxygen.

Anaerobic work: A high-intensity activity that can be sustained for only a short period in which energy demands are greater than the capacity of the heart and circulatory system to supply the energy.

Aerobic work: Activities using large muscle groups at an intensity that can be sustained for a long period of time in which the body is able to provide sufficient energy aerobically.

Submaximal task: A task performed aerobically at an intensity where the body can supply the necessary energy aerobically.

more than 60% of the work is performed anaerobically. When the time of the task exceeds 10 minutes, the anaerobic system becomes less important and accounts for no more than 5% of the oxygen required.

In Summary

Aerobic tasks include jogging, swimming, walking, and stair-stepping, where you participate at a rate that can be sustained for at least 10 minutes. Anaerobic tasks including sprinting and running at a fast pace, can be sustained for 2 minutes or less.

BASIC PHYSIOLOGICAL INFORMATION

Knowledge of the heart and circulatory system is necessary to understand cardiovascular endurance and the changes that occur in your body that will allow you to function more efficiently.

The Heart as a muscular pump

The heart is simply a muscular pump that provides the force to keep blood circulating throughout the network of arteries. This hollow, muscular organ is located between the lungs and the diaphragm in what is known as the *medial sternal space.* It is mostly to the left of the midline of the body with its apex pointing down.

The heart actually consists of two pumps. A thick muscular wall known as the *septum* divides the heart cavity down the middle into the right side and the left side. On each side is an upper chamber known as the **atrium** and a lower chamber called the **ventricle.** Each

atrium is separated from the ventricle by a valve that regulates the flow of blood. These are atrioventricular valves.

The right side of the heart receives blood that has completed its cycle through the body. This blood collects in the right atrium of the heart. This used blood reaches the heart by way of two large veins—the superior and inferior venae cavae. The superior vena cava returns blood from the head and arms, whereas the inferior vena cava drains blood from the trunk and legs. A third opening into the right atrium is the coronary sinus. This returns blood that is used by the heart muscle itself. From the right atrium, blood enters the right ventricle through the tricuspid valve. Blood is pumped from the right ventricle through the pulmonary arteries to the lungs, where it picks up fresh oxygen and gives up carbon dioxide. The function of the right side of the heart, then, is to pump blood to the lungs, where oxygen is picked up and carbon dioxide is eliminated. The blood flow associated with the right side of the heart is illustrated in Fig. 3-4, *A.*

The left side of the heart receives reoxygenated blood, which is returned through the pulmonary veins. This blood collects in the left atrium and passes from this upper chamber to the lower through the mitral, or bicuspid, valve. It is this left ventricle that pumps blood out of the heart. Blood passes through the aorta—the largest artery in the body—to all parts of the body. Fig. 3-4, *B,* illustrates blood flow associated with the left side of the heart.

Valves of the heart

The valves play an important role in regulating the flow of blood. Besides the two atrioventricular valves that have been explained previously, two other valves are lo-

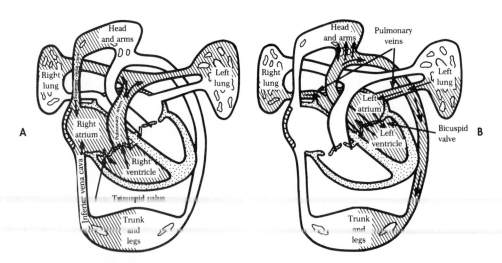

Figure 3-4 A, Blood flow associated with the right side of the heart. Note that the major purpose of the right side of the heart is to pump blood to the lungs where oxygen is picked up and carbon dioxide is eliminated. **B,** Blood, associated with the left side of the heart. Blood is pumped to all parts of the body by way of the aorta.

cated where the pulmonary artery and aorta join the ventricles. These valves, as well as the two atrioventricular valves, allow blood to flow in only one direction, thus preventing the backward flow of blood during diastole, when the heart is relaxed. The heart sounds that may be heard with a stethoscope are caused by the closing of the valves of the heart. The sounds could be described as *lubb-dupp*. The first of these sounds, *lubb*, is caused by the atrioventricular valves as they close, when the contraction of the ventricles takes place. At this time the other two valves, the aortic and pulmonary valves, are open as blood is being ejected from the heart. The *dupp* sound is made by the closing of the valves in the aorta and pulmonary arteries as the heart again is filling with blood. If heart valves do not function properly, blood is used to flow in the valves and abnormal sounds may be heard. These are referred to as *heart murmurs*.

Blood vessels

A clear distinction is necessary between arteries and veins. Any vessel taking blood away from the heart is an **artery,** whereas any vessel returning blood to the heart is a **vein.** The muscular wall of the normal artery is much thicker than that of the vein. This allows the arteries to be elastic so that when blood is ejected from the heart, they can expand to receive the blood. During the relaxation phase of the cardiac cycle, the muscular walls of the arteries contract to keep blood moving through the arterial system. As fatty deposits accumulate on the inner arterial walls, they tend to lose their elasticity and become smaller. This decreases the circulatory system's ability to function efficiently and increases the possibility of cardiovascular problems. This is discussed in detail in Chapter 11.

Arterial branches become smaller and smaller as they are distributed throughout the body. The smallest branches are known as **capillaries.** It is here that oxygen and nutrients leave the blood to enter body cells and carbon dioxide and metabolic wastes leave the cells to be picked up by the bloodstream.

Blood is returned to the heart through the network of veins. As indicated previously, veins do not have the thick, muscular walls that most arteries have. For this reason there is less pressure in veins. This does not create a problem for blood returning from the upper parts of the body, since gravity will assist in the return of blood to the heart. However, blood in the arms and legs must rely on the squeezing action of the muscles to be returned to the heart. There is a system of valves in veins that allows blood to flow only toward the heart. These veins are located between skeletal muscles, and when these muscles contract, veins are "squeezed" and blood flows toward the heart. If too much time is spent standing in one place, it is not uncommon for a person to experience fatigue and pass out. Blood is not returned

from the lower parts of the body to the heart, and it "pools" in these lower areas. Varicose veins may result from failure of used blood to be returned to the heart fast enough. The accumulated blood causes the veins to swell. Varicose veins often occur in individuals whose jobs require them to stand still or to remain seated for extended periods of time.

TERMS ASSOCIATED WITH THE CARDIOVASCULAR SYSTEM

There are four basic terms associated with the cardiovascular system that you will need to know to understand the changes that occur in your body as a result of a good aerobic exercise program. These are: (1) heart rate, (2) stroke volume, (3) cardiac output, and (4) blood pressure.

Heart rate

For an average person at rest who does not exercise regularly, the heart will beat about 70 to 75 times per minute. This is the **heart rate,** or pulse. It is caused by the impact of blood on the arteries as the heart contracts. The heart rate is determined by counting the number of times your heart contracts in a certain period and then converting this number to the standard measure in beats per minute.

Measuring your heart rate   Your heart rate can be determined by placing your finger or fingers on your lower arm at the base of the thumb or on one of the arteries in the front of the neck. Make sure that you press just firmly enough to feel the pulse. Pressing too

---

Atrium: An upper chamber of the heart. Blood returning to the heart first enters the right or left atrium.

Ventricle: The lower chamber of the heart. It is responsible for pumping blood away from the heart.

Artery: A blood vessel that transports blood away from the heart.

Vein: A blood vessel that returns blood to the heart.

Capillary: The smallest blood vessel in which the exchange of gases takes place between blood and tissues.

Heart rate: The number of times the heart contracts per minute.

hard may interfere with the rhythm. The procedures for this are given in the following self-assessment.

Self-Assessment

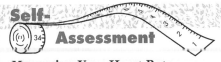

Measuring Your Heart Rate

Your heart rate can be determined by counting the number of times your heart contracts in a given period and converting this to beats per minute. Make sure that you press just firmly enough to feel the pulse. Pressing too hard may interfere with the rhythm.

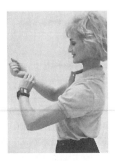 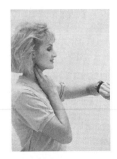

Your pulse can be detected by placing a finger or fingers on your lower arm near the base of the thumb.

Your pulse can also be easily detected over the carotid artery in the front of the neck.

The procedures for determining your resting heart rate and for interpreting your scores are presented in Laboratory Experience 3-1.

Changes with regular exercise   With regular aerobic exercise, your heart becomes stronger and more efficient, which should result in a reduction in your resting heart rate.

Stroke volume

Each time the heart contracts, blood is ejected. This is referred to as the **stroke volume.** For an average person at rest, the stroke volume is about 70 ml. A physically trained person, with a stronger heart, can pump as much as 100 ml with each contraction.

Cardiac output is the amount of blood the heart circulates each minute. It is determined by how many times the heart contracts each minute (heart rate) and the amount of blood ejected with each contraction (stroke volume). The resting cardiac output for most people will range from 5 to 6 liters and is not dependent on fitness level. The following example clearly shows the relationship between cardiac output, stroke volume, and heart rate.

> For an untrained person who has a resting heart rate of 72 beats/min and a stroke volume of 70 ml, the resting cardiac output is calculated as follows:
>
> Cardiac output = Heart rate × stroke volume
> = 72 × 70
> = 5040 ml/min
> = 5.04 L/min
>
> (NOTE: 1000 ml = 1 L)

As the heart becomes stronger with regular exercise, it can pump more blood each time it contracts, and it therefore does not have to beat as frequently to circulate the same amount of blood. The following example will clarify this relationship.

> If the person in the previous example, through regular exercise, is able to change the resting stroke volume from 70 ml to 90 ml, the anticipated change in resting heart rate would be calculated as follows:
>
> Cardiac output = Heart rate × stroke volume
> 5.04 liters = Heart rate × 90
> Heart rate = 5.04/90
> = 5040 ml/90
> = 56 beats/min
>
> CONCLUSION: The resting heart rate should drop from 72 to 56 beats/min, with the cardiac output remaining steady at 5.04 L/min.

Blood pressure

Blood pressure is the amount of force that blood exerts against the artery walls. It is generated by the heart as it contracts and is maintained by the elasticity of the arterial walls.

Blood pressure changes constantly during each cardiac cycle. Each time the heart contracts, blood pressure goes up as more blood is forced from the heart into the arterial system. The contraction phase of the cardiac cycle is called **systole,** which creates the systolic blood pressure. The relaxation phase of the cardiac cycle is called **diastole** and creates the diastolic blood pressure.

Blood pressure is measured in millimeters of mercury (mm Hg) and is written as systolic/diastolic. For example, 120/80 indicates that the systolic blood pressure is 120 mm Hg and the diastolic blood pressure is 80 mm Hg. It is difficult to define "normal" blood pressure. However, a score of 140/90 is usually considered to be the highest pressure that could be classified as normal. Blood pressure that is consistently higher should be is called **hypertension.** This condition is discussed in Chapter 11 as one of the risk factors associated with cardiovascular disease. Suggestions are given in that chapter for the control of blood pressure.

The procedures for measuring your blood pressure and for interpreting your scores are presented in Laboratory Experience 3-2.

In Summary

The heart is obviously the key to the entire cardiovascular system. Its major function is to circulate blood constantly throughout the body.

ENERGY AND PERFORMANCE

The major function of the cardiovascular system during exercise is to deliver oxygen to the working muscles. Because aerobic processes account for most of the energy produced in the body, the amount of oxygen that can be supplied directly determines the amount of work that can be performed. Cardiovascular endurance depends on how efficiently the lungs, heart, and blood vessels take oxygen from the air you breathe in, process it, and deliver it to the muscles where it is used. Efficient performance depends on:

- Availability of sufficient oxygen in the inspired air
- Ability of oxygen and carbon dioxide to diffuse across the pulmonary membrane into and out of the blood
- Chemical binding of oxygen with **hemoglobin** in the blood
- A blood flow through the lungs geared to pick up and carry the amount of oxygen required by the body
- Ability of the cells to pick up oxygen from the capillaries in exchange for carbon dioxide and other waste products

The relationship between oxygen consumption and energy expenditure can be summarized as follows:
- Each activity requires energy. Even simple activities such as sitting and sleeping require energy.
- To produce energy, oxygen is necessary. Energy is provided by food, but oxygen is the necessary fueling agent.
- The body can store food, but it cannot store oxygen. A person must breathe to live. If the oxygen supply is discontinued, the body will die quickly, since the oxygen supply in the body will last for only a short time.

When demands for oxygen increase within the body, such as during strenuous exercise, the ability to take in and deliver oxygen to the working musculature will be important in determining how much work can be performed and how efficiently it can be performed. The more oxygen the circulatory and respiratory systems are able to deliver, the longer the person will be able to exercise before becoming fatigued or exhausted. The reason a person becomes fatigued is that he or she reaches the point at which the body cannot process enough oxygen to supply the energy needed.

MAXIMAL OXYGEN CONSUMPTION

The rate at which oxygen is delivered and used by the body is referred to as *oxygen consumption.* It is expressed as a volume of gas per unit of time and is abbreviated as $\dot{V}O_2$.

V = Volume (usually expressed in liters or milliliters)
O_2 = Oxygen gas
• = Per unit of time (usually expressed in minutes)

The more oxygen your body is able to process and use, the more work you should be able to perform before becoming fatigued. The maximal rate at which oxygen can be used by your body is therefore important and is considered by most experts to be the best indicator of cardiovascular (or aerobic) fitness. It is called **maximal oxygen consumption** and is abbreviated $\dot{V}O_2$ max.

Stroke volume: The amount of blood pumped from the left ventricle each time the heart contracts.

Cardiac output: The amount of blood circulated by the heart each minute.

Blood pressure: The force exerted by the blood against the walls of the blood vessels.

Systole: The contraction phase of the cardiac cycle, occurring when the ventricles contract.

Diastole: The relaxation phase of the cardiac cycle when the heart is not contracting.

Hypertension: Blood pressure that is consistently higher than it should be.

Hemoglobin: The iron-containing protein found in blood that is responsible for the transportation of oxygen.

Maximal oxygen consumption: The maximal amount of oxygen the body is capable of processing and using. It is considered to be the best measure of cardiovascular endurance. It is also referred to as maximal oxygen uptake, aerobic capacity, and physical work capacity.

Your rate of oxygen consumption is measured in liters per minute, but because those who weigh more will have a higher total score resulting from their larger size, this score must be adjusted to account for individual differences in size. Comparisons can then be made between individuals of different body weights. Table 3-1 should help you to understand this concept. Note that by dividing the total oxygen consumption (ml) by the body weight (kg), the amount of oxygen available for each unit of body weight can be determined. This is expressed as milliliters of oxygen per kilogram of body weight per minute (ml/kgbw/min); the higher this value, the more oxygen there is available for each unit of body weight and thus the more work that you can perform before exhaustion.

The sample data in Table 3-1 clearly shows that Subject 2 can provide more oxygen for each kilogram of body weight (53.65) than Subject 1 (49.94) even though the total oxygen consumption is less.

With regular participation in a good aerobic exercise program, a person can increase his or her maximal oxygen consumption by as much as 30% over a 12-week period, depending on his or her initial level of fitness. The following changes in the body may contribute to this:

■ An increase in the amount of hemoglobin in the blood, which results in an increase in the amount of oxygen that can be transported in the blood

■ An increase in the maximal cardiac output as the heart becomes stronger and more efficient; this means that you can circulate more blood to the working muscles

■ An increase in the amount and/or size of the capillaries, allowing for a more efficient exchange of gases, which in turn allows the muscles to *use* more of the oxygen circulated

In Summary

An efficient body can process and use more oxygen and will be able to work at a higher intensity level and perform more work before reaching exhaustion.

DEVELOPMENT OF CARDIOVASCULAR ENDURANCE

A high level of aerobic fitness is an important objective of most exercise programs. Your body was designed to be active, and if you achieve a high level of aerobic fitness and maintain this level, your body will function more efficiently and you can reduce your risk of cardiovascular disease. To achieve this, it is important to determine if your program is too hard, too easy, or just right.

In designing an aerobic fitness program, you must be able to answer the following questions:

■ How hard must I exercise? (intensity)

■ How long must each exercise session last? (duration)

■ How often do I need to exercise? (frequency)

■ Which activities are best for me? (mode of exercise)

In Summary

To obtain maximal benefits from aerobic exercise, you must incorporate the principles of frequency, intensity, and duration into your program.[1]

Intensity of exercise

Intensity of exercise refers to how vigorous an exercise must be to contribute to the development of aerobic fitness. Many people do not understand this concept and exercise at a level that is too high or too low. When you exercise, your heart rate increases in proportion to the energy required for the performance of the task. As the task increases in intensity, there is a corresponding increase in your heart rate. Your exercise heart rate can therefore be used to determine the amount of physiological stress placed on the body. It is easy to measure and has become universally accepted as the standard way to determine exercise intensity. Your heart rate response to exercise is obviously an individual matter and will depend on the efficiency of your heart and circulatory system. Figure 3-5 compares the heart rate responses for two people of about the same age and body weight running at the same speed.

Table 3-1	**Comparison of Maximal Oxygen Consumption for Individuals of Different Body Weights**	
Variable	Subject 1	Subject 2
$\dot{V}O_2$ max (L/min)	4.2 L/min = 4200 ml/min	3.9 L/min = 3900 ml/min
Body weight	185 lb = 84.1 kg	160 lb = 72.7 kg
$\dot{V}O_2$ max (ml/kgbw/min)	4200/84.1	3900/72.7
	49.94	53.65

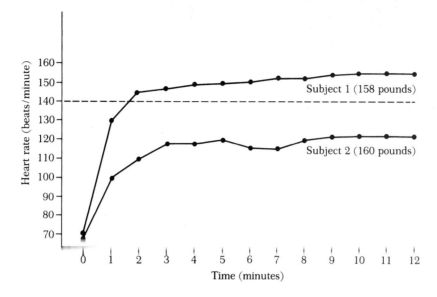

Figure 3-5 Comparison of heart rate responses for 20-year-old subjects running on a treadmill at 6 mph for 12 minutes.

With regular aerobic exercise, your cardiovascular system will function more efficiently and you will have a lower heart rate response for the same task. It is apparent from Figure 3-5 that Subject 2 has a higher aerobic fitness level than Subject 1.

For a 20-year-old person, the minimum intensity of exercise needed for an increase in aerobic fitness is a level of work that will produce a heart rate of about 140 beats/min. For Subject 1, running at a speed of 6 mph would be sufficient, but Subject 2 would have to run faster to obtain the desired results.

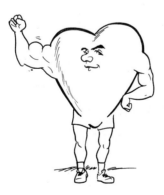

Since the heart is a muscle, like any other muscle, stress is necessary for it to function more efficiently. Unless sufficient stress is used, the changes will be minimal. If a person exercises too intensely, it may be dangerous and he or she will probably not be able to continue long enough to produce desirable results. High levels of exertion often result in muscular injuries.

Target-zone heart rate For a safe and effective workout, the intensity of the activity must be regulated so that your heart rate is elevated to a predetermined level.[27] This is called your *training heart rate,* or more commonly the **target-zone heart rate.** Your target-zone heart rate is 70% to 85% of your maximal heart rate. Maintaining your heart rate within this range for an extended time will result in optimal development of aerobic fitness. Procedures for calculating target-zone heart rate are included in the self-assessment on p. 42.

People who are extremely unfit or overweight may have difficulty in working at an intensity where their heart rate exceeds the lower level of their target zone. They may be able to work at a lower intensity and still achieve beneficial results. The appropriate level for these people might be 60% to 70% of their maximal heart rate.

Predicted maximal and target-zone heart rates for different age groups are summarized in Figure 3-6. The heart rates corresponding to 60% of the maximal heart rate are also included for people who need to work at this intensity.

When you are exercising and not using a heart rate monitor and you want to determine your heart rate, you can stop and count your pulse for 10 seconds.[8] Procedures for this are given in Laboratory Experience 3-3. Table 3-2 allows you to quickly equate your 10-second pulse count to that necessary for reaching the required target zone.

> **Target-zone heart rate:** The heart rate necessary for maximum development of cardiovascular endurance. It ranges from 70% to 85% of the maximal heart rate.

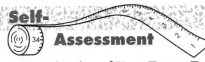

Self-Assessment

Determination of Your Target-Zone Heart Rate

To determine your target-zone heart rate, you must first estimate your maximal heart rate. This is not influenced by gender or level of fitness. It is almost entirely related to age.

For practical purposes your maximal heart rate can be estimated by subtracting your age (in years) from 220. This will usually be accurate within 10 beats/min.

Maximal heart rate = 220 − age (years)

(Estimated) = 220 − ____

= ____ beats/min

Calculate your target-zone heart rate:

Lower level = 0.70 × Maximal heart rate
(70% maximal heart rate) = 0.70 × ____

= ____ beats/min

Upper level
= 0.85 × Maximal heart rate
(85% maximal heart rate) = 0.85 × ____

= ____ beats/min

Critical or threshold heart rate

An alternate method to evaluate the intensity of an exercise is to determine **the critical, or threshold, heart rate** that must be exceeded if maximum development of cardiovascular fitness is to result.[16] With this method, you obtain a value that you must exceed rather than the range of values you get with the target-zone heart rate method.

Your critical, or threshold, heart rate represents the minimal heart rate needed for the development of cardiovascular endurance. It is determined by calculating 60% of the difference between your maximal and resting heart rates and then adding this value to your resting heart rate (Figure 3-7).

In Summary

The target-zone heart rate or critical heart rate can be used to determine if the intensity of the exercise is sufficient to result in the development of cardiovascular endurance.

Use of a heart rate monitor

Various heart rate monitors can be used to determine your heart rate while you are exercising. An advantage of these is that you do not have to stop exercising to determine your heart rate. By knowing your heart rate while exercising, you can adjust the intensity of your workout to sustain

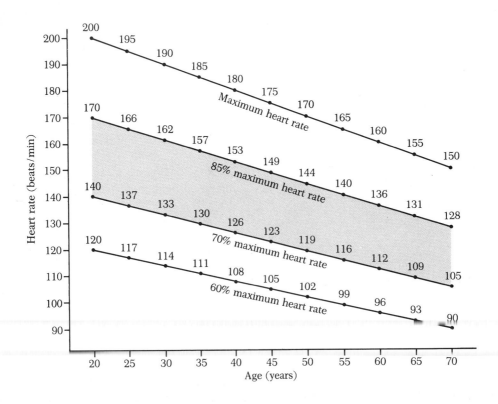

Figure 3-6 Maximal heart rate and target-zone heart rate in relation to age. Also included is the corresponding 60% level of maximal heart rate.

Table 3-2	**Determination of the Target-Zone Heart Rate for Specified Age-Groups**		

| | Target-Zone Heart Rate | | |
Age Range	Lower Limit (Beats/Min)	Upper Limit (Beats/Min)	Number of Beats/ 10 Seconds
20-29	140	162	23-27
30-39	133	154	22-26
40-49	126	145	21-24
50-59	119	137	20-23
60-69	112	128	19-21

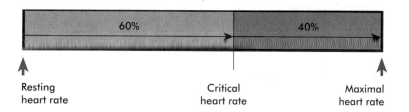

Figure 3-7 Critical heart rate in relation to resting heart rate and maximal heart rate.

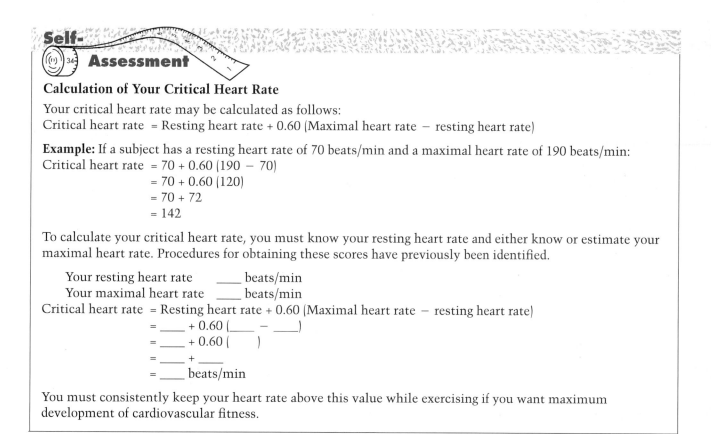

Self-Assessment

Calculation of Your Critical Heart Rate

Your critical heart rate may be calculated as follows:

Critical heart rate = Resting heart rate + 0.60 (Maximal heart rate − resting heart rate)

Example: If a subject has a resting heart rate of 70 beats/min and a maximal heart rate of 190 beats/min:

Critical heart rate = 70 + 0.60 (190 − 70)
= 70 + 0.60 (120)
= 70 + 72
= 142

To calculate your critical heart rate, you must know your resting heart rate and either know or estimate your maximal heart rate. Procedures for obtaining these scores have previously been identified.

Your resting heart rate ____ beats/min
Your maximal heart rate ____ beats/min

Critical heart rate = Resting heart rate + 0.60 (Maximal heart rate − resting heart rate)
= ____ + 0.60 (____ − ____)
= ____ + 0.60 (   )
= ____ + ____
= ____ beats/min

You must consistently keep your heart rate above this value while exercising if you want maximum development of cardiovascular fitness.

your heart rate at the desired level. Most monitors provide a continuous digital readout of the heart rate.

The Polar Vantage Heart Watch (Figure 3-8) allows you to store heart rates into memory so that you can play them back and record them later. With this moni-

Critical or threshold heart rate: The minimal heart rate necessary for the development of cardiovascular endurance.

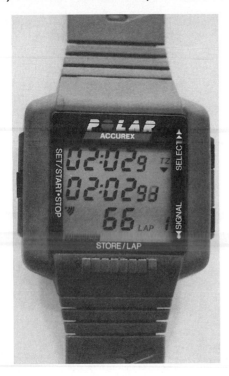

Figure 3-8   A Polar heart rate monitor. Using a monitor such as this takes the guesswork out of exercise.

Table 3-3	**Rate of Perceived Exertion Scale**	
Number	**Perceived Exertion**
6	
7	Very, very light
8	
9	Very light
10	
11	Fairly light
12	
13	Somewhat hard
14	
15	Hard
16	
17	Very hard
18	
19	Very, very hard
20	

tor, after you have finished your workout, you can see exactly what your heart rate was at any time during your exercise session. In addition, the monitor will alert you if you are exercising at a level that is too low or too high. This takes the guesswork out of exercise.

Computer programs are available to analyze scores from heart rate monitors. These can be used to compare heart rate responses for different activities and to measure aerobic fitness improvement. Figure 3-9 contains a sample printout from one of these computer programs.

Rate of perceived exertion   Despite the fact that the heart rate is used most often for evaluating intensity of exercise, it does have the following limitations:

- Some people have difficulty finding their pulse or counting it accurately.
- Errors in estimation of maximal heart rate result in calculation errors of the desired heart rate.
- Several factors can change your heart rate, including room temperature, level of stress, medication, altitude, and smoking.

Because of these limitations, an alternate method has become popular: the rate of perceived exertion (RPE), developed in the 1960s by Borg.[3] It uses a scale of numbers from 6 to 20, and each odd number is related to a subjective evaluation of exercise intensity (Table 3-3). This technique is based on the premise that you have the ability to determine how hard your body is working during exercise. To use this method, you need

to see the scale while exercising. Rate your exercise intensity based on how it feels. For college-aged students, adding a zero to the selected number should give an indication of the anticipated heart rate response for that level of work.[14]

Change in exercise heart rate   Your exercise heart rate must be checked regularly because regular participation in a good aerobic exercise program will cause a gradual reduction in the exercise heart rate for a standardized task as your heart becomes more efficient. It is necessary to increase the intensity of the task from time to time to maintain your heart rate at the desired level. This is why progression must be built into an exercise program.

Frequency

Research indicates that maximal development of cardiovascular endurance can be attained if you exercise regularly, between 3 and 5 days per week, with the days of rest interspersed with exercise days.[26] People who are starting an exercise program are advised against exercising more frequently than this. Rest periods are essential and need to be built into any exercise program. They result in both physical and mental relaxation. Exercising 6 or 7 days each week actually produces very minimal additional benefits and may result in poor adaptation by the muscles in the body. The incidence of injury is much higher in those who exercise this frequently compared with those who exercise three to five times each week. It is better to start gradually and take more time in reaching objectives than to start out at a high level and drop out because of injuries.

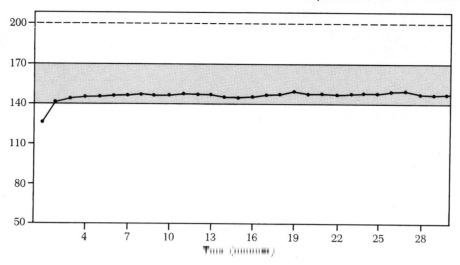

Name: Freddie Fitness   *Date:* 6/2/94
Mode: **Regular running time: 30 min**   *Total miles:* **3.00**

Exercise Heart Rate Summary

Name	Freddie Fitness
Date	6/2/94
Age (years)	21
Body Weight (lb)	165
Predicted maximal heart rate	199
70% maximal heart rate	139
85% maximal heart rate	169
Mode of exercise	Regular running
Time of exercise (minutes)	30
Total miles	3.00
Aerobic minutes of exercise	29
Average heart rate (beats/min)	144.27
Starting minute	1
Finishing minute	30
Standard deviation	3.71

Figure 3-9   Sample printout from Fitness Profile Software for the Heart Rate Monitoring Program.

Duration of exercise sessions

The length of each exercise session may vary according to the objectives. The plan proposed by the American Heart Association for development of cardiovascular endurance is adequate for most people. This association suggests that each exercise session be divided into three segments[27]:

1. A 5- to 10-minute warm-up and stretching session so that the heart and circulatory system are not suddenly taxed.
2. A sustained 20- to 30-minute exercise session in which the heart rate remains in the target zone.
3. A 5- to 10-minute cooldown session in which the intensity of the task is lessened before the exercise is completely stopped.

This plan is summarized in Figure 3-10. If you are training to compete in a marathon, or if your objective is to lose weight quickly, this plan would be inadequate. This is simply an exercise plan for optimal development of cardiovascular fitness.

The warm-up and cooldown phases of the program are important. A good warm-up gradually stretches the muscles and therefore reduces the chance of injury. In addition, it allows the heart to adjust to the increase in work. It can significantly reduce muscle soreness, which often results from a poorly planned exercise program.

The cooldown period is of equal importance. Blood relies on contraction of skeletal muscles to be returned to the heart from the lower extremities. If activity ceases abruptly and there is no contraction of these muscles, blood tends to pool in the legs and there may be insufficient blood returned to the heart for circulation. Any body movement involving your legs will assist in the return of blood and will be beneficial.

Many people who initiate a running program for fitness development feel that they must run a certain distance each week. However, the distance covered is not as important as making sure they continue long enough

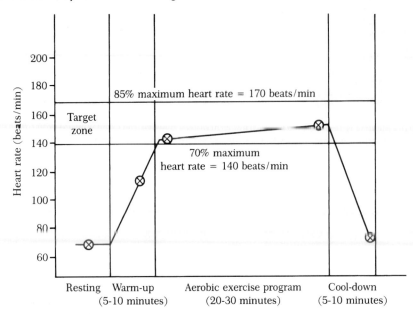

Figure 3-10   Suggested exercise training pattern for a 20-year-old.

at an intensity that is high enough to produce the desired results. Most beginning joggers who are 20 to 30 years old should be able to cover between 2 and 3 miles in 30 minutes of continuous work. If they exercise 5 days per week, which is the maximum that is recommended, they will cover 10 to 15 miles per week. Cooper[5] suggests that anyone who runs more than 15 miles per week is running for something other than fitness. The program previously described is consistent with his conclusion.

A question often asked is, "If 30 minutes of sustained exercise will result in a significant improvement in cardiovascular fitness, will exercising longer result in even greater improvement?" Exercising longer will result only in minimal additional changes. Stone, for example, presents information showing that 15 minutes of exercise resulted in an 8.5% increase in aerobic fitness, and with 30 minutes the increase was 16.1%. When the duration was increased to 45 minutes, the corresponding change was 16.8%. In this study the intensity of the work remained constant with subjects working within their target zones.[25]

You will not attain a high level of cardiovascular fitness without consistent effort. However, excessive effort can be wasted. The old saying "no pain, no gain" simply is not true. You must learn how to exercise for maximum development of aerobic fitness without pain or discomfort. The amount of exercise you need will depend on your present level of fitness and what your objectives are for exercise. Your exercise program should be fun.

Mode of activity

If the criteria for intensity, duration, and frequency are met, it makes no difference what aerobic exercise you use. Any activity that can be maintained continuously and that uses large muscle groups will be beneficial. Bicycling, swimming, walking, jogging, aerobics (aerobic dance), cross-country skiing, jumping rope, racquetball, basketball, and stair climbing (Figure 3-11) are examples of good cardiovascular activities.

With activities such as walking, jogging, and bicycling, the intensity is determined by how fast you move; skill level is of little significance. If your heart rate response is too low, increase your speed until you reach the desired heart rate level (Figure 3-6). With activities such as cross-country skiing and swimming, skill level is very important. To a large extent, this will determine how continuous the activity will be and how fast you will need to move to maintain your desired heart rate.

With racquetball and squash, not only is your skill level important but so is the skill level of your opponent. If you have a minimal amount of skill and you play an opponent who is at least at your skill level, you can get a good aerobic workout playing racquetball or squash. The case study on the following page will show how good an activity racquetball can be.

Most racquetball and squash players who have at least a minimal amount of skill are able to achieve and maintain their desired target-zone heart rate. For them, these activities provide a good aerobic workout. Tennis, however, is not nearly as good as racquetball or squash. In tennis the heart rate goes up and down, not remaining in the target zone long enough to bring about significant training effects. Even those who have an extremely high level of skill in tennis are rarely able to maintain their heart rate in the target zone. However, in racquetball, even beginners can usually achieve and maintain the desired heart rate.

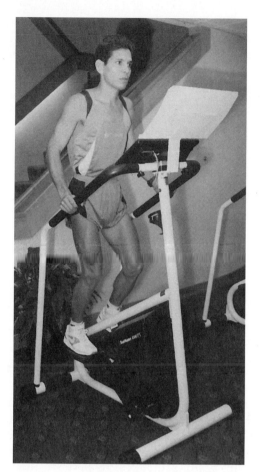

Figure 3-11 Stair climbing is an excellent form of exercise.

It is clear that not all activities are beneficial for the development of aerobic fitness. Remember that the activity must be continuous, involve a large amount of musculature, and result in a heart rate consistently high enough to produce a cardiovascular training effect. Activities that usually meet these criteria are considered to be good aerobic activities.

Good Aerobic Activities	
Aerobics (aerobic dance)	Rope jumping
	Rowing
Basketball	Running
Bicycling	Skating (ice and roller)
Cross-country skiing	Soccer
Handball	Squash
Jogging	Stair climbing
Racquetball	Stationary bicycling
Rebound running (mini trampoline)	Swimming
	Walking
Rollerblading	

Activities that do not meet these criteria are considered to be poor aerobic activities.

Poor Aerobic Activities	
Archery	Gymnastics
Baseball	Softball
Bowling	Tennis
Football	Volleyball
Golf	Weight training

We have seen that heart rate response to an activity will vary according to aerobic fitness level (see Figure 3-2). What might be a good aerobic activity for one person may not be good for another. The best way to be sure that the activities you select are beneficial is to determine their intensity by measuring your heart rate response. Procedures for this are identified previously in this chapter. Remember that this must be done regularly because a good aerobic program will change your heart response to a given activity. Laboratory Experience 3-3 outlines the procedures you can use to evaluate several of the activities in which you participate.

MAINTENANCE OF CARDIOVASCULAR ENDURANCE

When you have reached a desirable level of cardiovascular endurance, you must make a lifetime commitment to exercise to sustain it. If you stop exercising, your fitness level deteriorates quickly, with all gains lost within 5 to 10 weeks.[12] However, you may not have to exercise as often to sustain your fitness level as

Case Study

ROBERT

Robert is a 54-year-old who enjoys running and playing racquetball. He has participated regularly in these two activities for the last 10 years, not competitively, but simply to develop his level of aerobic fitness.

When running, because of his fitness level, Robert must run at about an 8½-min/mile pace, or 7 mph, to sustain his heart rate at the desired level (Figure 3-12). When playing racquetball, he does not feel that he gets as good an aerobic workout, but despite the start and stop nature of the activity, his heart rate usually averages 10 to 20 beats/min higher for each minute of racquetball than it does when he is running. These scores are compared in Figure 3-12.

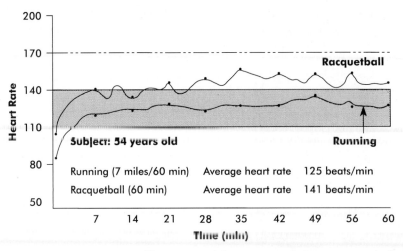

Figure 3-12 Comparison of heart rates while running and playing racquetball.

CHANGES IN THE BODY RESULTING FROM REGULAR AEROBIC EXERCISE

The human body was designed to be active, and when you exercise regularly, it will function more efficiently. There are a number of physiological adaptations occurring in the body that contribute to this increase in efficiency, including the following:

Change	Result
An increase in the strength of the heart muscle	An increase in resting stroke volume occurs, which means that the heart beats less frequently in circulating the same amount of blood. This also results in an increased maximal stroke volume, which means that your body is capable of circulating more blood when oxygen is needed by the muscles at a higher rate.
An increase in the number and/or size of the capillaries	A greater exchange of oxygen at the cellular level occurs between the blood and cells. Your body is able to use more of the oxygen that is circulated.
An increase in the amount of hemoglobin	Your body can carry more oxygen in the blood to the working muscles.
An increase in the amount of oxygen that your body is capable of using [$\dot{V}O_2$ max]	You can exercise longer and at a higher level before you become fatigued.

CARDIOVASCULAR FITNESS AND HEALTH

We have seen that the attainment of a high level of cardiovascular endurance will result in an increase in the efficiency with which your body functions, and you will be able to perform more work before becoming fatigued and exhausted. This will occur only if you participate regularly in an exercise program that incorporates the basic principles relative to frequency, intensity, and duration of aerobic exercise.

Regular aerobic exercise can also positively affect your health. Dr. J. Michael McGinnis, director of the Office of Disease Prevention and Health Promotion, stated, "Physical activity is related to the health of all Americans. It has the ability to reduce directly the risk of several major chronic diseases as well as to catalyze positive changes with respect to other risk factors for these diseases."[20]

Because of the importance of regular aerobic exercise and its relationship to health, national objectives have been established in an attempt to make people more aware of the benefits of regular exercise and to get more people to exercise. Unfortunately, despite the recent research pertaining to the many health benefits resulting from exercise, we have seen very little change in the last 10 years in the physical activity patterns among Americans.

Fortunately, it appears as if the intensity of the exercise or activity that is necessary to achieve health benefits may be less than that required to produce cardiovascular fitness. Many of the low-intensity everyday activities such as washing the car, gardening, and walking up or down stairs may have positive effects on these health benefits. Duncan, for example, studied whether the quantity and quality of walking necessary to decrease the risk of cardiovascular disease differed from that required to improve cardiovascular fitness. He concluded, "Walking at intensities that do not have a major impact on cardiorespiratory fitness may nonetheless produce equally favorable changes in cardiovascular risk profiles."[6]

MEASUREMENT OF CARDIOVASCULAR ENDURANCE

The best method to determine cardiovascular endurance is to measure $\dot{V}O_2$ max. This involves the use of a treadmill or bicycle ergometer; the heart rate, oxygen consumption, and other metabolic variables are monitored continuously during the test. The task is made progressively more difficult until a rate is reached where there is no further increase in oxygen consumption, even though the intensity of the task is increased. When this occurs, a person is said to have reached his or her maximal intake for that task. This relationship is illustrated in Figure 3-13.

The measurement of $\dot{V}O_2$ max is a difficult procedure that can only be conducted in a well-equipped laboratory. It is not practical with large groups or for class use. An alternate approach is to estimate aerobic capacity by measuring the maximal amount of work that can be performed over a period of time. The most commonly used tests involving this concept are the 12-minute run test and the timed 1.5-mile run.

Valid results can be obtained from these tests if you learn how to pace yourself and you give a maximal performance. If you do not run regularly, you will have a better chance of meeting these criteria if you take several days before the test and practice pacing yourself. Procedures to follow for the 12-minute run test are presented in Laboratory Experience 3-4 and for the 1.5-mile run test in Laboratory Experience 3-5.

You can also estimate your aerobic capacity by evaluating the efficiency of your heart and circulatory system. You can measure your heart rate response by a standardized task such as the step test. Laboratory Experience 3-6 presents the information you need to use this evaluation.

Fitness Flash

Aerobic exercise and health

Following is a summary of recent research that pertains to the health benefits associated with regular exercise:

- Those who are most active and have a high level of cardiovascular fitness have a lower incidence of coronary heart disease as compared with those who are inactive. If they do develop cardiovascular disease, it usually occurs at a later age and tends to be less severe.[10]

- The incidence of cardiovascular disease is almost twice as prevalent in those who do not exercise compared with those who do exercise.[2]

- Regular aerobic exercise results in decreased insulin production because of increased cell sensitivity to insulin.[17]

- Those who exercise regularly have higher levels of high-density lipoprotein, or HDL (good cholesterol), compared with those who are sedentary.[11]

- Regular aerobic exercise results in an increase in life expectancy of up to 2 years compared with the average life of the U.S. population.[24]

- Blood pressure and level of activity are inversely related, with less active and less fit individuals having a 30% to 50% greater incidence of hypertension.[23]

- Regular aerobic exercise results in a decrease of 10 mg/dl in both systolic and diastolic blood pressure for those who are borderline hypertensive.[n]

- The risk of developing Type II diabetes in men is twice as great in those who are less active as compared with those who are more active.[18]

- Women who exercise at least once each week are significantly less likely to develop Type II diabetes.[19]

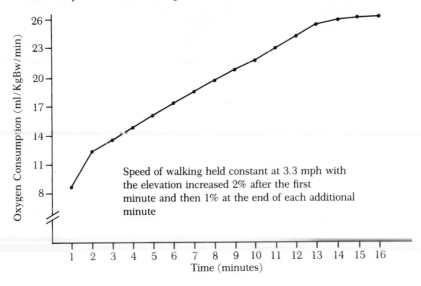

Speed of walking held constant at 3.3 mph with the elevation increased 2% after the first minute and then 1% at the end of each additional minute

Figure 3-13   Comparison of minute-by-minute oxygen consumption scores for a woman on the Modified Balke Treadmill Test. Note the linear relationship in oxygen consumption until the thirteenth minute and then the leveling off, which occurs at this time.

Chapter Summary

The following summary will help you to identify some of the important concepts covered in this chapter:

- Cardiovascular endurance is the most important physical fitness component.
- Your level of aerobic fitness will be reflected by how much work you can perform and at what level you can work.
- Anaerobic work is high-intensity work, which lasts for only a few minutes.
- Aerobic work is performed at a lower intensity than anaerobic work and can be sustained for a longer period.
- The heart and circulatory system must function efficiently if you are to attain a high level of aerobic fitness.
- The ability of your body to process and use oxygen will determine your level of cardiovascular endurance.
- To increase your aerobic capacity, you must exercise at the right intensity continuously for 20 to 30 minutes at least 3 days each week.

References

1. American College of Sports Medicine: *Guidelines for exercise testing and prescription*, ed 4, Philadelphia, 1991, Lea & Febiger.
2. Berlin JA, Colditz GA: A meta-analysis of physical activity in the prevention of coronary heart disease, *Am J Epidemiol* 132:612-628, 1990.
3. Borg GAV: Psychophysical cases of perceived exertion, *Med Sci Sports Exerc* 14:377-381, 1982.
4. Consolazio F, Johnson R, Pecora L: *Physiological measurement of metabolic function in man*, New York, 1963, McGraw-Hill.
5. Cooper KH: *The aerobics program for total well-being*, New York, 1982, M Evans & Co.
6. Duncan JJ: Women walking for health and fitness: how much is enough? *JAMA* 266:3295-3299, 1991.
7. Fletcher GES et al: Statement on exercise benefits and recommendations for physical activity programs for all Americans, *Circulation* 86:340-344, 1992.

8. Greer N, Katch F: Validity of palpation recovery pulse to estimate heart rate following four intensities of bench step exercise, *Res Q Exerc Sport* 53:340, 1982.
9. Hagberg JM: Exercise, fitness, and hypertension. In Bouchard C et al, editors: *Exercise, fitness, and health*, Champaign, Ill, 1988, Human Kinetics.
10. Haskell WL et al: Cardiovascular benefits and assessment of physical activity and physical fitness in adults, *Med Sci Sports Exerc* 24:S201-S220, 1992.
11. Haskell WL: The influence of exercise on the concentrations of triglyceride and cholesterol in human plasma, *Exerc Sports Sci Rev* 12:205-244, 1984.
12. Hickson RC, Rosenkoetter MA: Reduced training frequencies and maintenance of increased aerobic power, *Med Sci Sports Exerc* 13(1):13-16, 1981.

13. Hoeger WWK: *Principles and labs for physical fitness and wellness*, ed 3, Englewood, Colo, 1994, Morton Publishing.
14. Monahan T: Perceived exertion: an old exercise tool finds new applications, *The Physician and Sportsmedicine* 16(10):174-179, 1988.
15. Johannessen S et al: High frequency, moderate intensity training in sedentary middle-aged women, *The Physician and Sportsmedicine* 14(5):99-102, 1986.
16. Karvonen MJ: Effects of vigorous activity on the heart. In Rosenbaum MJ FF, Belknap EL, editors: *Work and the heart*, New York, 1959, Paul B Hoeber.
17. King DS et al: Insulin secretory capacity in endurance-trained and untrained young men, *Am J Physiol* 227 E1547E1541, 1990.
18. Manson JE et al: A prospective study of exercise and incidence of diabetes among US male physicians, *JAMA* 268:63-67, 1992.
19. Manson JE et al: Physical activity and incidence of non-insulin dependent diabetes mellitus in women, *Lancet* 338:774-778, 1991.
20. McGinnis JM: The public health burden of a sedentary lifestyle, *Med Sci Sports Exerc* 24:S196-S200, 1992.
21. Monohan T: Is activity as good as exercise? *The Physician and Sportsmedicine* 15(10):181-186, 1987.
22. Ong TC, Sothy SP: Exercise and cardiorespiratory fitness, *Ergonomics* 29(2):273-280, 1986.
23. Pfaffenbarger RS et al: Physical activity and hypertension: an epidemiological view, *Ann Med* 23:319-327, 1991.
24. Pekkanen JB et al: Reduction of premature mortality by high physical activity: a 20-year follow-up of middle-aged Finnish men, *Lancet* 1:1473-1477, 1987.
25. Stone WJ: *Adult fitness programs: planning, designing, managing and improving fitness programs*, Glenview, Ill, 1987, Scott, Foresman & Co.
26. Wenger HA, Bell GJ: The interactions of intensity, frequency and duration of exercise training in altering cardiorespiratory fitness, *Sports Med* 3:346-356, 1986.
27. Zohman LR: *Exercise your way to fitness and heart health*, Dallas, Tex, 1974, American Heart Association.

Laboratory Experience 3-1

Measuring Your Resting Heart Rate

Name	Section	Date

Your heart rate can be determined by counting how frequently your heart contracts during a given period and converting this number to the standard measure in beats/min. Make sure that you press just firmly enough to feel the pulse. If you press too hard, it may interfere with the rhythm.

Determination of Your Resting Heart Rate

There are many factors that influence your resting heart rate, including stress, food, excitement, room temperature, and previous physical exertion. Therefore your resting heart rate should be taken while sitting quietly and not after participating in vigorous activity. If possible, you should sit quietly for at least 30 minutes before measuring it. Take it several times to make sure it is stable.

Your resting heart rate should not be changing as rapidly as it does after exercise, so you can count for either 10 seconds and multiply by 6, 30 seconds and multiply by 2, or count for the full minute.

Most highly-trained endurance athletes have low resting heart rates. Most untrained subjects who participate regularly in a good aerobic fitness program will experience a decrease in their resting heart rates. Your score can be evaluated as follows:

Resting Heart Rate

Trial 1	_____	beats/min
Trial 2	_____	beats/min
Trial 3	_____	beats/min
Trial 4	_____	beats/min
Trial 5	_____	beats/min
Typical Score	_____	beats/min

Rating	Resting Heart Rate (beats/min)
Excellent	<60
Good	60-69
Average	70-79
Fair	80-89
Poor	>89

Laboratory Experience 3-2
Measuring Your Blood Pressure

Name _____ Section _____ Date _____

A sphygmomanometer is used to measure blood pressure (Figure 3-14). An airtight cuff is wrapped around the arm just above the elbow. The cuff is connected to a glass tube filled with mercury. Air is pumped into the cuff by squeezing a bulb. As the cuff becomes tighter, it compresses a large artery in the arm—the brachial artery. This temporarily cuts off the flow of blood to the forearm, and no heart sounds can be heard when a stethoscope is placed on the compressed artery just below the cuff. As the air pressure in the cuff is released, the mercury level drops. Eventually, a point will be reached at which the blood pressure in the artery is just greater than the air pressure in the cuff. Blood will now begin to flow through the artery, and the heart sound may be heard through the stethoscope. This is the systolic, or upper, pressure; it is the maximum pressure that can be produced by the heart. As air continues to be let out of the cuff, the sounds heard through the stethoscope will become louder as more blood flows through the artery. Finally, a point will be reached at which the distinct heart sound disappears as the blood is flowing steadily through the artery. At this point the height of the mercury shows the diastolic, or lower pressure, representing the least amount of pressure in the artery.

Results

Record your blood pressure figures in the space provided below.

Blood pressure ____/____

Classification _____

Interpretation

Your blood pressure scores can be evaluated by consulting Table 3-4.

Table 3-4	Classification of Blood Pressure Scores	
Score	**Classification**	**Values (mm Hg)**
Systolic	Good	<116
	Average	116-140
	Poor	>140
Diastolic	Good	<80
	Average	80-90
	Poor	>90

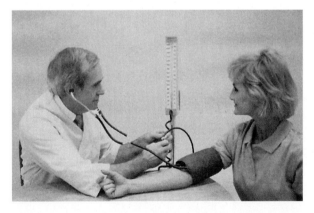

Figure 3-14 Measurement of blood pressure with a sphygmomanometer.

Laboratory Experience 3-3

Determination of Exercise Heart Rate without a Monitor

Name _____   Section _____   Date _____

If you do not use a heart rate monitor, it is usually not possible to count your heart rate accurately while participating in most activities. However, an accurate estimate of your exercise heart rate can be obtained if your heart rate is counted immediately after exercising. If you do not start counting within 10 seconds after stopping, the score is likely to be inaccurate.

Count the number of beats in 10 seconds and multiply this value by 6 to convert it to beats/min. Do not count for a longer time because your heart rate begins to slow down as soon as you stop exercising. The fitter you are, the quicker your heart rate will decrease after exercise.

Select several activities that you enjoy. Perform each for 5 minutes, working at a constant level or speed. Record heart rates for each of these activities.

Activity	Beats/10 Seconds	× 6 = Beats/Min
_____	_____ × 6 =	_____
_____	_____ × 6 =	_____
_____	_____ × 6 =	_____
_____	_____ × 6 =	_____
_____	_____ × 6 =	_____
_____	_____ × 6 =	_____
_____	_____ × 6 =	_____

Laboratory Experience 3-4

Measurement of Cardiovascular Endurance: 12-Minute Run Test

Name ______________________ Section ____________ Date ____________

Description

For 12 minutes, run as far as possible and try to maintain a steady pace until the last few minutes, when you should try to speed up slightly depending on how much energy you have left. The number of laps completed during this time is counted and recorded, and the distance covered is calculated.

Results

Record the results in the spaces provided.

Number of laps completed: _________
Distance of 1 lap: ____ feet
Distance covered = laps × distance
= ____ × ____ feet
= ____ feet
To convert to miles, divide by 5280.
Distance covered = distance covered (feet) / 5280
= ____/5280
= ____ miles (calculate to two decimal places)

Interpretation

The results of the 12-minute run test can be evaluated by consulting Table 3-5 (men) or Table 3-6 (women).

Table 3-5 Classification of Scores for 12-Minute Run Test (Men) Distance (Miles)

Category	Percentile Rank	Age (years) <20	20-29	30-39	40-49	50-59	>59
Excellent	95	2.04	1.91	1.79	1.70	1.58	1.49
	90	1.95	1.82	1.70	1.61	1.49	1.40
Good	80	1.85	1.72	1.60	1.51	1.39	1.30
	70	1.78	1.65	1.53	1.44	1.32	1.23
Average	60	1.72	1.59	1.47	1.38	1.26	1.17
	50	1.66	1.53	1.41	1.32	1.20	1.11
	40	1.60	1.47	1.35	1.26	1.14	1.05
Fair	30	1.54	1.41	1.29	1.20	1.08	0.99
	20	1.47	1.34	1.22	1.13	1.01	0.92
Poor	10	1.37	1.24	1.12	1.03	0.91	0.82
	5	1.28	1.15	1.03	0.94	0.82	0.73
Mean		1.66	1.53	1.41	1.32	1.20	1.11

			Age (years)				
Category	Percentile Rank	<20	20-29	30-39	40-49	50-59	>59
Excellent	95	1.70	1.62	1.54	1.44	1.37	1.28
	90	1.61	1.53	1.45	1.35	1.28	1.19
Good	80	1.51	1.43	1.35	1.25	1.18	1.09
	70	1.44	1.36	1.28	1.18	1.11	1.02
Average	60	1.38	1.30	1.22	1.12	1.05	0.96
	50	1.32	1.24	1.16	1.06	0.99	0.90
	40	1.26	1.18	1.10	1.00	0.93	0.84
Fair	30	1.20	1.12	1.04	0.94	0.87	0.78
	20	1.13	1.05	0.97	0.87	0.80	0.71
Poor	10	1.03	0.95	0.87	0.77	0.70	0.61
	5	0.94	0.86	0.78	0.68	0.61	0.52
Mean		1.32	1.24	1.16	1.06	0.99	0.90

Table 3-6 Classification of Scores for 12-Minute Run Test (Women) Distance (Miles)

Laboratory Experience 3-5

Measurement of Cardiovascular Endurance: 1.5-Mile Run Test

Name _____   Section _____   Date _____

Description

The 1.5-mile run test may be preferred to the 12-minute run test because it is easier to administer. You should try to cover 1.5 miles in the shortest time possible. Elapsed time is recorded in minutes and seconds.

Results

Record the results of the 1.5-mile run test in the spaces provided.

Time for 1.5-mile run ____ minutes ____ seconds.

Interpretation

The results for the 1.5-mile run test can be evaluated by consulting Table 3-7 (men) or Table 3-8 (women).

Table 3-7	Classification of Scores for 1.5-Mile Run Test (Men) Time (Min:Sec)						
	Percentile		Age (years)				
Category	Rank	<20	20-29	30-39	40-49	50-59	>59
Excellent	95	8:50	9:21	10:02	10:30	11:20	11:56
	90	9:17	9:53	10:39	11:11	12:10	12:52
Good	80	9:50	10:32	11:25	12:02	13:11	14:01
	70	10:15	11:00	11:58	12:38	13:56	14:51
Average	60	10:35	11:24	12:26	13:09	14:33	15:34
	50	10:54	11:46	12:52	13:38	15:08	16:13
	40	11:13	12:08	13:18	14:07	15:43	16:52
Fair	30	11:33	12:32	13:46	14:38	16:20	17:35
	20	11:58	13:00	14:19	15:14	17:05	18:25
Poor	10	12:31	13:39	15:05	16:05	18:06	19:34
	5	12:58	14:11	15:42	16:46	18:56	20:30
Mean		10:54	11:46	12:52	13:38	15:08	16:13

Table 3-8	Classification of Scores for 1.5 Mile Run Test (Women) Time (Min:Sec)						
	Percentile		Age (years)				
Category	Rank	<20	20-29	30-39	40-49	50-59	>59
Excellent	95	10:39	11:00	11:36	12:16	12:46	13:45
	90	11:16	11:46	12:30	13:14	14:00	15:07
Good	80	12:01	12:43	13:35	14:28	15:30	16:48
	70	12:34	13:24	14:22	15:22	16:36	18:01
Average	60	13:02	13:59	15:01	16:07	17:31	19:03
	50	13:28	14:37	15:39	16:49	18:22	20:00
	40	13:54	15:03	16:16	17:31	19:13	20:57
Fair	30	14:22	15:38	16:56	18:16	20:08	21:59
	20	14:55	16:19	17:43	19:10	21:14	23:12
Poor	10	15:40	17:16	18:48	20:24	22:44	24:53
	5	16:17	18:02	19:41	21:25	23:58	26:15
Mean		13:28	14:37	15:39	16:49	18:22	20:00

Laboratory Experience 3-6

Measurement of Cardiovascular Endurance: The Step Test

Name _____   Section _____   Date _____

Many versions of the step test are available. Probably the most common is the original 5-minute step test. This test and its variations are not as good as the 12-minute run test or the 1.5-mile run test, but because of practical considerations, it is often used, particularly with large groups of students.

An accurate measurement of the heart rate is necessary if the results from this test are to be meaningful. If you have trouble counting your heart rate, the results will not be accurate. For this evaluation the pulse will be counted for 30-second counts while remaining seated. Refrain from talking and unnecessary movement during periods when heart rates are being counted; these activities can influence your results.

Results should be recorded in the space below.

TRIAL	BEATS/30 SEC		BEATS/MIN
1	_____	× 2	_____
2	_____	× 2	_____
3	_____	× 2	_____
4	_____	× 2	_____

The step test is based on the premise that for all submaximal work the person with a higher level of cardiovascular fitness not only will have a smaller increase in heart rate but also will have a heart rate that returns to normal much faster after the task than it would in a person with a normal level.

Purpose

The purpose of this test is to obtain immediate knowledge of the level of cardiovascular efficiency.

Method

Do not perform any activity before this test; no warm-up is allowed. A 20-inch bench should be used for men, and a 16-inch bench for women. Step up to and down from this bench at the rate of 30 steps/min. The same foot must start the "step-up" each time, and an erect posture must be assumed. Continue the activity for a maximum of 5 minutes or until you are unable to maintain the set rate. The heart rate is counted for a 30-second period, starting exactly 1 minute after completion of the last step (that is, from 1 to 1.5 minutes after completion of the task).

Results

Record the results in the spaces provided.

Time of stepping ____ seconds

Heart rate ____ beats/30 sec (1 to 1.5 minutes of recovery)

The physical efficiency index (PEI) may be estimated by consulting Table 3-9, or it may be calculated using the following procedure.

Calculation of PEI

PEI = (Time of stepping [sec] × 100)/(5.5 × heart rate for 30 seconds)

= (____ × 100)/(5.5 × ____)

= (____) / (____)

= ____

Interpretation

The results are interpreted in Table 3-10.

Table 3-9 Scoring for the Harvard Step Test*

Duration of Test (Minutes)	Total Heart Beats 1-1½ Minutes Into Recovery (Score-Arbitrary Units)											
	40-44	45-49	50-54	55-59	60-64	65-69	70-74	75-79	80-84	85-89	90-94	95+
0-½	6	6	5	5	4	4	4	4	3	3	3	3
½-1	19	17	16	14	13	12	11	11	10	9	9	8
1-1½	32	29	26	24	22	20	19	18	17	16	15	14
1½-2	45	41	38	34	31	29	27	25	23	22	21	20
2-2½	58	52	47	43	40	36	34	32	30	28	27	25
2½-3	71	64	58	53	48	45	42	39	37	34	33	31
3-3½	84	75	68	62	57	53	49	46	43	41	39	37
3½-4	97	87	79	72	66	61	57	53	50	47	45	42
4-4½	110	98	89	82	75	70	65	61	57	54	51	48
4½-5	123	110	100	81	84	77	72	68	63	60	57	54
5	129	116	105	96	88	82	76	71	67	63	30	56

From Consolazio F, Johnson R, Pecora L: *Physiological measurement of metabolic functions in man*, New York, 1963, McGraw-Hill.
*INSTRUCTIONS:
1. Find the appropriate line for the time stepping was continued.
2. Find the appropriate column for the pulse count for the 30-second period; do *not* multiply this by 2—it is a 30-second count that is used.
3. Read the score where this line and the column intersect.

Table 3-10 Classification of Harvard Step Test Scores

Score	Cardiovascular Classification
55 or below	Very poor
56-64	Poor
65-79	Average
80-89	Good
90 or above	Excellent

Chapter Four
Development of Cardiovascular Endurance

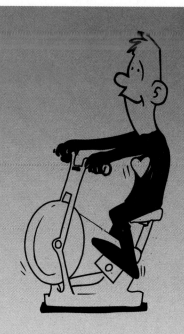

CHAPTER OBJECTIVES
Check off each objective you achieve.

❑ Identify the activities that can be used for the development of aerobic fitness, and know how to incorporate these activities into a good aerobic fitness program.

❑ Determine the level at which you need to exercise for each of the aerobic activities.

❑ Evaluate and compare the advantages and disadvantages of the various activities and programs.

❑ Discuss the advantages of circuit training as compared with a regular exercise program involving calisthenics.

❑ Design a program using weight-training activities that can contribute to the development of cardiovascular endurance.

HOW MUCH EXERCISE DO YOU NEED?

One of the most frequently asked questions pertaining to aerobic exercise is, "How much exercise do I really need?" The answer to this question depends on who is exercising, what their fitness level is, and what their objectives are. Consider, for example, the following two regular exercisers:

Case Study

JERRY

Jerry is a marathon runner, running anywhere from 60 to 100 miles each week. He is very thin with very little body fat. He has low blood pressure with a healthy heart, but he is running himself into the ground and is constantly fighting injuries and pain.

Case Study

BILL

Bill is also a regular exerciser who rides a stationary bike for 10 minutes, 3 days each week. The rest of his "exercise" time he spends relaxing in the steam room or the jacuzzi. Although his 10-minute workout may feel good, it is not enough to do much good for his body.

If Jerry is doing too much and Bill too little, what about all those regular exercisers somewhere between these two extremes? How much exercise should they be doing?

In Summary

The secret is to exercise enough so that you will be successful at achieving your goals yet not so much that it becomes an obsession or that you are constantly tired or frequently in pain or injured.

WHY PEOPLE EXERCISE

The reasons why most people participate in some form of aerobic exercise are identified in Chapter 2. These are:

Fitness The overall objective for many people who exercise regularly is to increase their level of cardiovascular fitness so that their bodies function more efficiently.

Weight management Many people use aerobic exercise to reduce their body weight or their percentage of body fat to a desirable level or to maintain their current level.

Health Many health benefits are associated with regular aerobic exercise. You can add years to your life by reducing your risk for developing cardiovascular disease, diabetes, hypertension, and osteoporosis. Information pertaining to the health benefits of exercise is presented in Chapters 1 and 11.

The amount of exercise necessary for attaining each of these objectives varies. This chapter provides information concerning several different aerobic activities or programs. By applying the scientific principles presented in Chapter 3, you will be able to achieve an optimal level of aerobic fitness together with the associated health benefits and you will know how to achieve and maintain a desirable body weight or percentage of body fat.

AEROBIC ACTIVITIES

Any activity that is continuous and involves large muscle groups can be classified as an aerobic activity. Aerobic activities that meet these criteria are listed below:

Continuous Aerobic Activities:	
Aerobic dance (aerobics)	Roller skating
Bicycling	Rollerblading
Cross-country skiing	Stair-stepping
Jogging/running	Stationary bicycling
Ice skating	Swimming
Rebound running	Walking
Rope jumping	

Because of the continuous nature of these activities, all you need to do is to determine at what **intensity** you need to participate to maintain your heart rate at the desired level.

The case study on p. 62 may help you to understand this concept and will help you to get started.

When participating in any of the aerobic activities previously listed, it is important to follow the same procedures as identified in the case study so that you can determine the correct level at which you should exercise. This will depend on your level of aerobic fitness, which basically reflects how efficiently your heart and circulatory system function. You must also keep in mind that over time your heart rate response to a specific task will change if you develop good, consistent

Intensity: The stress placed on the body by exercise. It can be determined by the heart rate response to the activity.

Case Study

JIM

Jim is a 20-year-old college student who wants to start an exercise program for the specific purpose of developing his level of aerobic fitness. He knows how to measure his heart rate, and after reading the previous chapter, he knows that if he is to be successful, he must exercise at such an intensity that his heart rate gets to and stays between 140 and 170 beats/min. However, he does not know how hard to exercise to achieve this. He decides to start out by walking. All he needs for this is a good pair of walking or jogging shoes and a watch.

He measures a distance that is exactly 1 mile and decides to walk this distance at a brisk pace. He finds that it takes him 15 minutes. On stopping, he immediately counts his pulse for 10 seconds and finds that his heart rate is 120 beats/min (20 beats in 10 seconds). He now knows that by walking a mile in 15 minutes, he is not exercising at a fast enough pace to maintain his heart rate in his target zone.

Jim decides to cover the same 1-mile distance again, but this time he decides to jog at a very slow pace. He finds that this time it takes him 12 minutes, and his heart rate at the end of the mile is 150 beats/min. Jim has now discovered the pace that he needs to maintain to achieve the right intensity for this type of workout.

---

exercise habits. For this reason, you need to periodically check your heart rate response to make sure that you are exercising at the right intensity.

There are also other aerobic activities that are not as continuous as those previously listed. Although these activities involve stop-and-start motion, because of the nature of the movements involved, many participants in these activities are able to sustain their heart rates in their target zones. These activities can therefore be classified as aerobic activities and include basketball, handball, racquetball, soccer, and squash. Information on several of these activities is presented in this chapter.

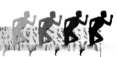

Fitness Flash

According to the results of a recent national survey, over 32 million Americans participate in jogging and running while an additional 13 million either walk or jog on a treadmill. The number of participants for these and for some of the fastest growing aerobic activities are presented in Table 4-1.

Table 4-1	Participants in Selected Aerobic Activities	
Activity	**Participants**	**Change (%)**
Running/jogging	32,875,000	0
Stair-climbing machines	17,140,000	+790
Treadmill—walking/jogging	13,580,000	+209
Cross-country ski machine	7,477,000	+119
Rollerblading	6,212,000	+103
Mountain biking	5,047,000	+232

From *Fifth annual study of U.S. sports participants*, 1992, American Sports Data.

STARTING YOUR PROGRAM

When initiating a program, it is important to start out at a low level and progress slowly. Many problems are caused by doing too much too soon. If you intend to become involved in a running program, most likely you will have to start out by walking and gradually build up your endurance and efficiency until you can run slowly.

Time must be taken in each session to **warm up** and **cool down.** If the correct procedures are followed, muscle soreness can be reduced and many injuries associated with exercise programs can be avoided. People who have had exercise-related injuries quickly learn to warm up and stretch the muscle groups they intend to use. Information pertaining to warming up and cooling down is presented in Chapter 6.

WALKING

Walking is fast becoming one of the most popular aerobic fitness activities. The results from two recent national surveys are summarized on p. 63.[17,18]

For a walking program, all you need is a good pair of shoes. You need little or no instruction, and you can walk almost anywhere either alone or with someone. Walking can be an enjoyable exercise, and although it is not as intense as jogging or running, it can be used by many people to develop cardiovascular fitness. Sustaining a steady brisk pace will maximize aerobic benefits.

If you use walking to develop your aerobic fitness level, it is important to learn how fast you must walk to sustain the desired heart rate. The normal pace for most people is 3 to 4 mph. You must walk fast enough to keep your heart rate in your target zone, but not so fast that you cannot carry on a conversation or that you are constantly fatigued. You should never walk so hard that you are unable to perform the same workout the next day. The procedures for initiating a walking program are included in Laboratory Experience 4-1.

If you use walking in your training program, it may be necessary to spend more than the 20 to 30 minutes per exercise session as suggested previously. This is particularly true if you wish to lose weight and develop cardiovascular endurance.

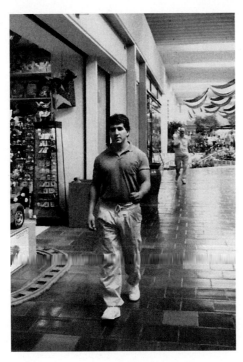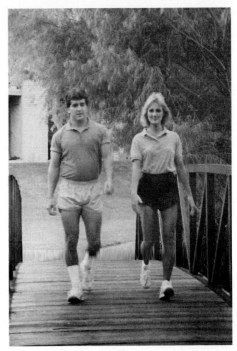

When the weather is inclement, walkers often use shopping malls for their aerobic workout. Many malls promote walking programs *(left)*. Walking is a form of movement in which at least one foot is in contact with the ground at all times *(right)*.

Your heart rate response to walking will depend on your aerobic fitness level. Heart rate responses for two 20-year-old women walking at 4 mph are compared in Figure 4-1. This speed is equivalent to walking a mile in 15 minutes. Even though each subject's weight is about the same, there is a significant difference in their heart rate responses to the same task. Subject 1 obviously has a higher level of cardiovascular fitness. Her heart is more efficient and therefore does not have to beat as frequently. This task is not of sufficient intensity for her heart rate to reach the target zone. However, for Subject 2, walking at the rate of 15 minutes per mile is sufficient to produce the training effect.

To initiate a good walking program you will need to:
- Know your current level of fitness.
- Have a good pair of walking or jogging shoes.
- Be able to calculate your target-zone heart rate.
- Be able to determine your pulse accurately.

Fitness Flash

- In 1991, over 73% of the adults surveys indicated that "during the past month" they had done some "walking for exercise." This is significantly higher than a previous survey in 1986 (69%).

- Americans are now walking longer distances when they walk for exercise.

- Walking attracts a solid core of long-term enthusiasts. More than 40% of adults who walk for exercise have been walking for "more than 5 years." The percentage of walkers increases with age.

- Older adults also walk more frequently. Over 54% of those over 65 years old walk "several times each week."

- One reason walking might be so popular is that it is a natural activity. Even a sedentary American worker will average 2 to 3 miles/day performing everyday tasks. Unfortunately, the walking that most people get as part of their everyday tasks is not continuous enough to contribute to the development of aerobic fitness.

Warm-up: The initial phase of the workout where you exercise at a low intensity. You increase your body temperature and the temperature of the muscles involved in the exercise in preparation for a more strenuous level of activity.

Cooldown: A process whereby you gradually slow down after a workout or exercise session rather than stopping abruptly.

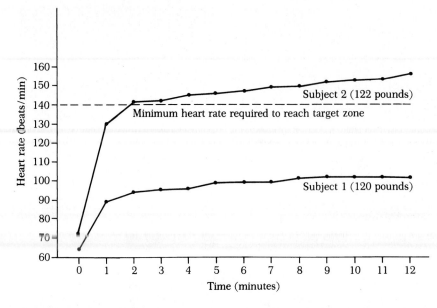

Figure 4-1 Heart rate response of two subjects walking 4 mph. *Subject 2* could use walking as her aerobic activity, whereas *subject 1* would need a running program to obtain the same results.

Fitness Flash

The correct ways to walk

To reduce your risk of injury while walking or jogging, you need to wear a pair of walking or jogging shoes and to learn how to walk correctly.[7]

- Walk with your back straight and be looking straight ahead, not at your feet.
- Always walk with the heel-to-toe method (Figure 4-2). The heel of the leading foot should always touch the ground before the ball of the foot and the toes.
- Land as softly as possible to absorb the shock.
- When pushing off, the knee is bent so that the heel is raised and the weight is shifted forward. The toes push off and the leg is accelerated forward to get in front of the body.

Fast walking and aerobic training

A question often asked is, "Is fast walking intense enough to sustain your heart rate within your target zone?" Several studies of fast walking have shown that it can be an effective exercise for most people for the development of aerobic fitness. In one study, for example, which involved 343 subjects, 91% of women and 83% of men were able to reach their target-zone heart rate while walking.[16] In a second study, even young men with a high level of aerobic fitness were able to achieve and maintain this target-zone heart rate during a 30-minute walk. For most adults, fast walking can be used as an adequate aerobic training stimulus.

Use of hand weights while walking

In recent years the use of light handheld weights while walking has become popular. Usually, weights ranging from 1 to 5 lb are held in each hand. The use of such weights while walking can produce a significant increase in both heart rate and caloric expenditure. However, this happens only if the arm movements are accentuated and more vigorous than they would normally be during regular walking. Simply carrying the weights with little or no arm movement results in only small increases of energy expenditure. Proper use of hand weights while walking provides the necessary stimulus for the development of aerobic fitness without the high-impact forces associated with running, which often result in injuries to the lower extremities.

Walking on a treadmill

Many people prefer walking on the treadmill to walking outside. It certainly has some advantages:

- There are no hills or wind to cope with, and neighborhood dogs will not attack you. Since the surface is flat and even, you will be less likely to twist your ankle.
- It is easier to maintain a constant pace. You simply set the treadmill at a specific speed and maintain your position on the treadmill.
- You can watch television or read a book while you walk. This helps the time pass more quickly.
- You can control the temperature, and it never rains indoors.

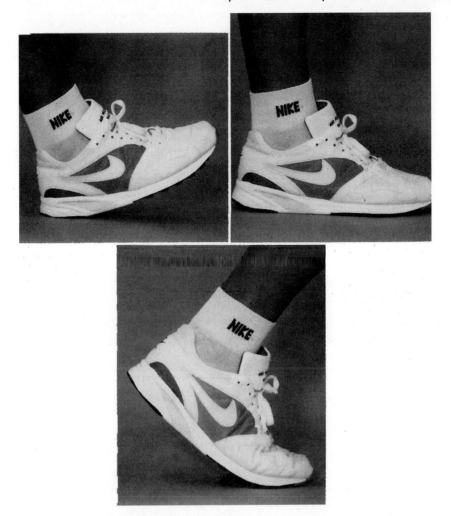

Figure 4-2 The correct way to run and walk is the heel-to-toe method.

- You can walk with a friend (if two or more treadmills are available) and be walking at different speeds so that you are both exercising at the right intensity (Figure 4-3).
- If you are walking as fast as you can and your heart rate is still not up to the desired level, you can continue to walk and increase the elevation until you reach your target-zone heart rate.

JOGGING AND RUNNING

It is not important to set arbitrary standards to distinguish between jogging and running. Jogging is a slow form of running that is done at a comfortable pace that can be maintained for a long time. Jogging and running are two of the most widely used methods of developing aerobic fitness, particularly for those who are less than 30 years of age. This might be because they require a low level of skill compared with other activities, and they give maximum benefits for a minimum investment of time (Figure 4-4).

The correct way to run

Although there is not *one* correct way to run, there are procedures that if followed can contribute to greater efficiency and possibly result in fewer muscular problems. Possibly the most important aspect is correct foot action. The recommended procedure is the same as described for walking—the heel-to-toe movement (Figure 4-2). The heel should touch the surface first as softly as possible. The jogger then rocks forward onto the ball of the foot and pushes off with the toes in preparation for the next stride. This procedure can reduce the stress placed on muscles in the leg and can significantly reduce the incidence of **shin splints** and other muscular problems.

> **Shin splints:** A catchall term that refers to a painful condition that occurs on the anterior portion of the lower leg. This condition often results from exercise performed on hard surfaces.

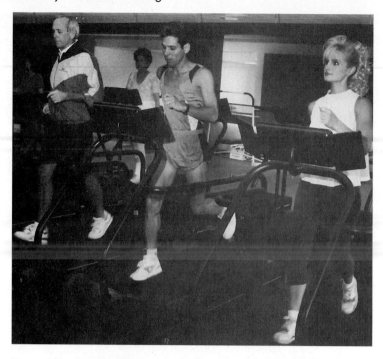

Figure 4-3   You can either run or walk on a treadmill and still be exercising with a friend at the right intensity.

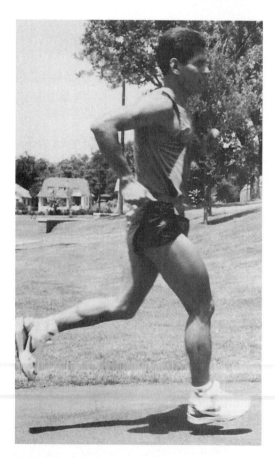

Figure 4-4   Jogging is a very popular form of aerobic exercise.

When a person lands on the balls of the feet or runs flat-footed, there is a constant jarring of the muscles. By wearing jogging shoes with padded heels and by landing softly on the heels and rocking onto the toes, this jarring can be reduced significantly.

If you have experienced shin splints in the past, or if you jog or run a lot, particularly on hard surfaces, you need to include an exercise in your program for strengthening the muscles in the front of your lower leg. Probably the best exercise for this is to sit with your legs straight in front of you and the bottom of your feet as close to the ground as possible. Now try to bring the top of your feet as close to your upper body as possible while a partner resists this movement by continuously pushing down on the top of your feet (Figure 4-5). Although no movement will take place, the muscles in the front of your lower legs will contract. Hold this contraction for at least 30 seconds. If this exercise becomes part of your regular exercise routine, over time this muscle group will become stronger.

Jogging should be a natural movement, not one that creates tension and stress. It is important to learn to relax while jogging and to eliminate extraneous movements that do not contribute to the forward momentum of your body. The length of the stride varies according to speed, and the knees should be lifted only high enough to obtain the desired stride length. The arms should be as relaxed as possible with the forearms about parallel to the ground. Arm action should be minimal and certainly not of such intensity that either hand crosses the midline of the body. The key to successful running, regardless of speed, is relaxation.

Jogging shoes

By far the most important piece of equipment for the jogger is shoes. In fact, shoes are the only equipment that make a difference in the type of jogging program suggested. Many beginners make the mistake of starting a serious jogging program with shoes designed for basketball, tennis, or racquetball. These may be expensive shoes, but they are not adequate for the serious jogger.

Running shoes usually have greater arch support than regular tennis shoes and a well-cushioned, padded sole raised slightly in the heel. This is particularly important because the heel must absorb most of the shock as the initial contact is made with the running surface. Jogging shoes should not fit quite as tightly as regular shoes, and a thick pair of socks can protect against blisters and sore feet (Figure 4-6).

Initiating a jogging program

Before starting a jogging program, it is important to make sure that your fitness level is such that when walking as fast as you can, your heart rate is below your desired target-zone level (see Laboratory Experience 4-1). Your starting speed will be influenced greatly by your initial level of aerobic fitness. The following suggestions are offered for those who have not participated regularly in a jogging program:

Step 1. Select a realistic distance to start your program. Recommended distances based on your aerobic fitness classification from either the 12-minute run test or the 1.5-mile run test are listed below. If your aerobic fitness classification is either "very poor" or

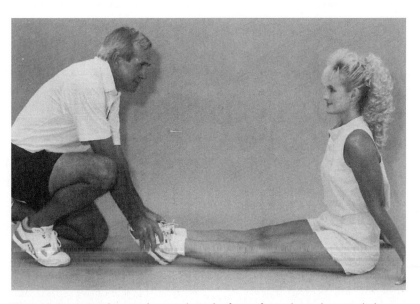

Figure 4-5 Strengthening the muscle in the front of your lower leg may help you to avoid shin splints.

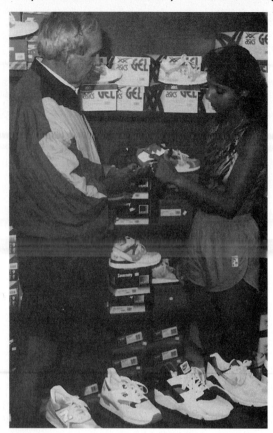

Figure 4-6 If you are going to walk or jog regularly, you need to purchase a good pair of walking or jogging shoes.

"poor," you will probably need to start out with a walking program.

Aerobic Fitness Classification	Suggested Distance for Step 1 (Miles)
Very poor	1
Poor	1
Average	2
Good	2
Excellent	3

Your initial objective is to jog continuously and cover the selected distance. If the initial distance selected is too easy or too difficult, make another selection so that you have a realistic objective. If you are unable to jog continuously and cover the entire distance, alternate periods of jogging and walking. You should gradually strive to reduce your walking time until you can run continuously at a constant speed and cover the entire distance. Exercise only 3 days per week at first, and progress slowly. This is the time when you are susceptible to muscular problems. Make sure that you warm up and cool down before and after each exercise session.

Step 2. After you have achieved the objective in step 1, check your heart rate to see if the intensity is correct. If your heart rate is within your specified target zone, your pace is good, and you should continue at that speed. If it is below the target zone, you must increase your speed slightly until it reaches the required level. If it is above the target zone, the intensity should be reduced slightly.

Step 3. When you are able to run the specified distance at the correct intensity, you should increase the number of jogging days from 3 to 5. This contributes to a gradual increase in your level of cardiovascular endurance and may help you to establish a regular habit of jogging. Continue for several weeks until you feel comfortable running this distance at this speed or until your heart rate drops below your target zone. Because of the anticipated decrease in your heart rate as your heart becomes more efficient, you should get into the habit of checking your heart rate periodically.

Step 4. Keeping the number of workouts between 3 and 5 per week, gradually increase your running distance until you accumulate approximately 15 miles each week. Remember, however, that the number of miles you accumulate is not as important as maintaining the correct intensity of exercise. You will experience little improvement if your level of intensity does not allow your heart rate to remain in the target zone.

SWIMMING

Swimming is one of the best aerobic exercises for the development of cardiovascular endurance. Following are several advantages it has over other activities:

- More musculature is involved in swimming than in jogging, and movement of the arms in each of the strokes occurs through a full range of motion. It should therefore contribute to the development of flexibility in addition to cardiovascular endurance.

- When swimming, people can achieve a complete workout with the body in a non–weight-bearing position. This means that less stress is placed on the joints, and fewer muscular problems result. Those who are unable to participate in other activities because of structural problems with the joints can usually participate in a swimming program.

The same principles that apply to jogging apply to swimming. Success depends on your ability to adjust the intensity of your workout so that you maintain your heart rate in the target zone for 20 to 30 minutes of continuous activity. Intensity of the work can be adjusted by the speed at which you swim or by the stroke used. Some strokes require much more vigorous activity than others. For example, except for competitive swimming, the crawl stroke almost always results in a higher heart rate than the breaststroke does. It is im-

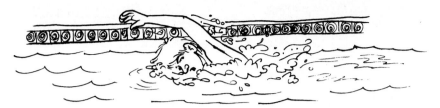

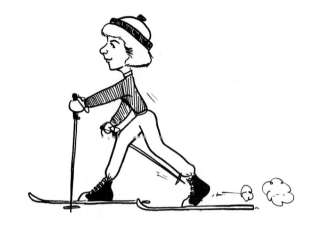

portant to know the intensity of strokes so that you can alternate a less vigorous stroke with a more vigorous one, which will enable you to swim continuously for 20 to 30 minutes. Few people can begin a program by swimming the crawl stroke continuously for 20 to 30 minutes.

Of course, swimming involves more skill than most other activities, and it is often difficult to find an uncrowded pool where you can swim continuously without interference. It is interesting to note that most individuals who can swim the crawl stroke continuously for 30 minutes or more had to develop their skill and endurance gradually; most started by swimming one lap at a time. Unless you are an experienced swimmer, start your program by swimming one or two laps using the crawl stroke at a comfortable pace. Stop and take your heart rate to determine if the intensity is correct.

You have several options to initially achieve a continuous workout:

- Walk in the pool back to the opposite end (when it is not too deep to walk the entire distance).
- Use a less vigorous stroke, such as the sidestroke, breaststroke or elementary backstroke, to return to the other end.

Gradually, you will increase the time spent swimming continuously using the crawl stroke. Make sure from time to time, however, that your heart rate remains in the target zone. Eventually, you will be able to swim continuously for 20 to 30 minutes and have an excellent aerobic program.

CROSS-COUNTRY SKIING

Many experts claim that cross-country skiing is the best aerobic activity. Certainly, it is *one* of the best for the development of cardiovascular endurance. As in swimming, the upper body is used extensively, and it is true that the highest maximum oxygen consumption figures for both men and women have been obtained from cross-country skiers. Many people who jog or run in the summer often turn to cross-country skiing for their aerobic workout in the winter. The same basic guidelines presented for walking and jogging can be used to develop a cross-country skiing program.

Cross-country skiing is one of the few sports in which the skill level of the participant is not an important consideration. Figure 4-7 shows that heart rate responses for those classified as skilled and beginners are similar. Each group of participants was able to keep the heart rate in the desired target zone regardless of skill.

BICYCLING

Bicycle riding is an excellent aerobic activity preferred by many over jogging and running. It certainly can be used for the development of cardiovascular fitness. Equipment is important. A good, lightweight bicycle or mountain bike is recommended. It is important that the height of the seat is adjusted correctly. If the seat is at the correct height, there will be a slight bend at the knee when the pedal is in the down position.

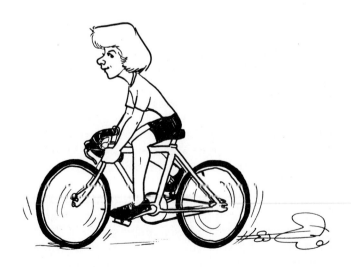

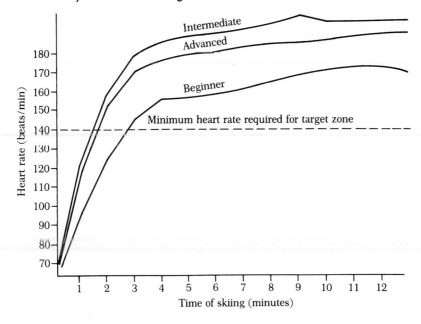

Figure 4-7   Comparison of heart rate responses for college-aged cross-country skiers according to skill level. Note that even for those classified as beginners, the activity was sufficient to elevate the heart rate above the level necessary to reach the target zone.

Intensity of the task depends on a number of factors. Probably the two most important ones are pedaling speed and gear ratio. All aerobic activities should be rhythmic, and bicycling is no exception. A steady rhythm should be maintained throughout with a constant rate of pedaling from 70 to 90 revolutions per minute (rpm). The highest gear ratio at which you can maintain this rate of pedaling should be selected. Of course, you should constantly check your heart rate to make sure it is maintained within the target zone. It has been estimated that to receive the same benefits as from jogging, you must cover about three to five times the distance. However, the distance covered and the speed vary with each person and are influenced by factors such as fitness level, age, and skill.

The 4-month beginning program described in Table 4-2 is designed for those with little or no experience. Those who have been involved in other aerobic programs and who find this program too easy should start with the program recommended for the second or third month.[19]

Most people who exercise regularly are interested in setting objectives and measuring progress. Both have been stressed in planning a good program. Realistic goals for different age-groups are presented in Table 4-3. These figures are different time goals to be achieved for distances of 10, 15, and 20 miles, either while you are participating in the program or after you have completed the recommended training program. To measure your progress, you might include a 10-, 15-, or 20-mile time trial once or twice each month. As your fitness level improves, you should see a decrease in the time it takes you to cover the designated distance.

Stationary bicycle riding

To some people, stationary bicycle riding seems to be the most boring form of exercise. It does, however, have advantages. You can work out in a comfortable environment; it is possible to read, watch television, or listen to a stereo while exercising; and you do not have to worry about traffic or hazards in the road while exercising. It is a safe and convenient way to get a good aerobic workout.

Many of the electronic bikes that are available have features to increase motivation. Several of these automatically adjust the intensity so that you appear to be riding up and down hills. Others present a digital display of your heart rate and caloric expenditure throughout the task. There are even bikes that have a color television and also those that allow you to race against one or more competitors while providing a graphic feedback of the race (Figure 4-8).

The secret to improving your aerobic fitness level while using a stationary bicycle is the same as for other forms of aerobic training. You must exercise at the right intensity. Intensity is determined by increasing the resistance or pedaling at a faster speed. If you use the correct resistance, one added advantage of stationary cycling is that you will increase the strength and tone of the muscles in your legs. With at least two types of stationary bikes it is also possible to exercise the arms at the same time (Figure 4-9).

Table 4-2	**Training Program for Beginning Bicycle Riders**				
	Weekday			**Weekend Day**	
Month	**Miles**	**Exercise Days**		**Miles**	**Exercise Days**
1	4-5	3		5-10	1
2	5-7	3		10-20	1
3	8-10	3		20-30	1
4	10-12	3		40-50	1

Table 4-3	**Objectives for 10, 15, and 20 Miles for Designated Age Groups**		
Age Range	**Time Goal for 10 Miles (min)**	**Time Goal for 15 Miles (min)**	**Time Goal for 20 Miles (min)**
20-30	36	55	75
31-40	40	60	84
41-50	44	65	93
51-60	48	70	102

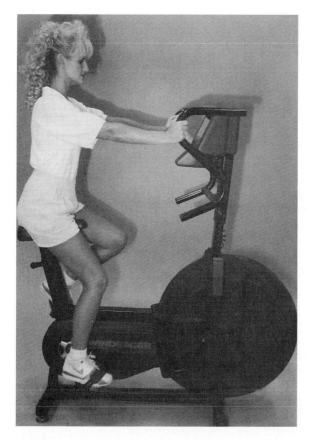

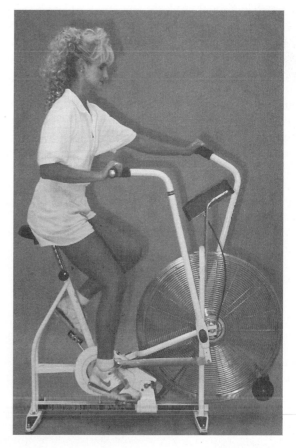

Figure 4-8 A stationary bicycle that allows you to "race" against one or more competitors.

Figure 4-9 A stationary bicycle designed so that you can use your upper body while pedaling.

AEROBICS TO MUSIC— AEROBIC DANCE

Exercises or dance routines performed to music have become popular. Such programs are often called **aerobic dance** or simply *aerobics* and are an excellent means of developing your aerobic fitness level. It is estimated that over 23 million Americans participate in aerobic dance.

There has been recent concern over the number of injuries associated with high-impact aerobics.[22] Research reports show a 10% to 55% injury rate among participants, depending on how injury is defined. Common types of injuries include shin splints, stress fractures, and tendinitis. It would appear that the number of injuries is dependent on the type of footwear used and the surface involved. It is also evident that many of the injuries are caused by overuse—exercising too frequently.

Because of concern relating to injuries, low-impact aerobics has emerged as an alternative.[13] With low-impact aerobics at least one foot must remain in contact with the floor at all times, and the stress placed on the feet, legs, and knees is reduced significantly. To compensate for this, the large upper body movements are accentuated, and the intensity level of the exercise can still remain high enough to produce aerobic benefits. Research has shown that the low-impact classes can be as much fun and demanding as the high-impact classes (Figure 4-10).

JUMPING ROPE

Jumping rope is a popular exercise that can effectively develop aerobic fitness.[1,3] The skill level of the participant and the type of jumping motion obviously affect the intensity of the exercise.[20]

REBOUND RUNNING

Rebound running (using a mini trampoline) is an exercise used by many individuals to develop aerobic capacity. Although conflicting results exist, it would appear that if the exercise is performed at the rate of 120 to 140 steps per minute, with an accentuated knee lift, this exercise can be used for the development of aerobic fitness.[11] Accentuated arm movement with handheld weights may be necessary for those who have a high level of aerobic fitness if they are to achieve the desired heart rate.

STATIONARY ROWING

Stationary rowing is at least as good a form of aerobic exercise as stationary bicycling. It is possibly better because it uses more musculature. The many benefits associated with stationary bicycle riding also apply to stationary rowing. It is easy to maintain your heart rate within your target zone while using such a machine. If it is not high enough, you simply row at a faster pace or increase the resistance. However, additional stress is

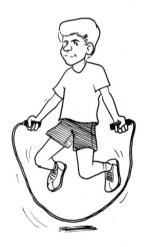

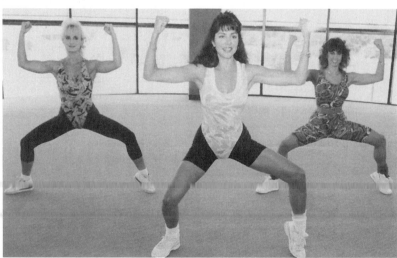

Figure 4-10 Aerobics to music is a very popular form of aerobic exercise.

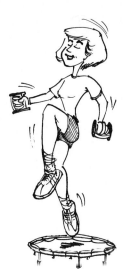

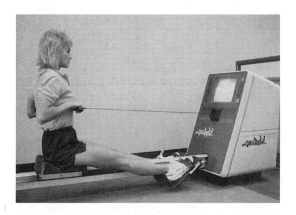

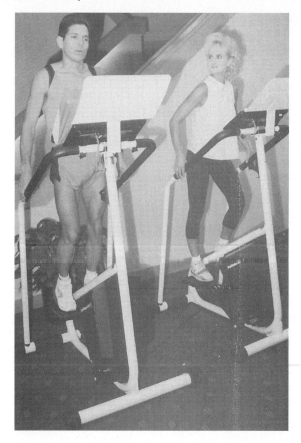

Figure 4-11 Stair climbers have become one of the most popular exercise machines at health clubs and exercise facilities.

placed on the lower back, and those with back problems should be cautious when performing this activity.

STAIR CLIMBING

At most exercise facilities across the country, stair climbers are fast becoming one of the most popular exercise machines. Since 1980 over 480,000 stair-stepping machines have been sold. The earliest models of stair-climbing machines, which were introduced in the early 1980s, featured stairs that continually rotated, similar to a treadmill.[5] Newer models soon evolved that were pedal-powered, where your feet stay in contact with the pedals, and you step up and down, keeping up with the pedals; your body weight acts as a resistance to the stepping motion (Figure 4-11). These machines are often referred to as steppers. The height of each step can be "set" in many of these machines so that you step a set distance each time. This usually ranges from 2 to 20 inches. In other machines, you can vary the height that you step. In most cases the faster you step, the shorter the range of motion.

Many people prefer stair steppers to treadmills. One advantage of the stair stepper is that individuals with a limited range of motion can take shorter steps to reduce stress on their joints. There is less stress on the lower legs because your feet stay in contact with the pedals. One study comparing treadmill running with stair stepping showed that the injury rate was much lower when the stair-stepping machines were used and that both these machines were equally effective in the development of aerobic fitness.

As with many of the stationary bicycles, computerized screens provide information to the user relating to calories burned, flights of stairs completed, and distance accumulated.

Aerobic dance: A series of exercises or dance routines performed to music. Also referred to as *aerobics to music* or simply *aerobics.*

Rebound running: Stepping or bouncing on a mini trampoline.

BENCH AEROBICS

A new trend in aerobic exercise is **bench aerobics.** It has been referred to as "the poor man's stair climber." This is a low-impact, high-intensity workout where participants step up to and down from a bench ranging in height from 4 to 12 inches. They use a variety of step combinations set to music[15] (Figure 4-12).

The following guidelines may be beneficial in helping you to get started[8,14]:

- Start out with a bench that is from 4 to 6 inches high.

- Unlike walking or jogging, step up with a flat foot, making sure that you place your entire foot on the bench.

- Do not land on the ball of your foot or bounce. Bouncing will cause you to remain on the ball of your foot.

- When you step down, step directly down and not back too far. Stepping too far back places extra stress on the lower back and on the back of the legs.

- Modify the intensity by varying the step height, increasing the range of motion at the joints, or by varying the footwork to maintain your heart rate in the desired target zone.

SLIDE AEROBICS

Slide aerobics is fast becoming a popular aerobic activity. It is a relatively inexpensive way to stay fit at home and has become so popular that many health clubs now offer slide aerobics classes. Apart from the aerobic benefits, slide aerobics also contribute to the development of strength and muscular endurance in the lower extremities, particularly the inner thigh muscles.[2]

WATER AEROBICS

Water aerobics is one of the fastest growing fitness activities in the United States, with the number of participants increasing from 200,000 in 1983 to over 2.2 million in 1988.[10] With this type of training, exercises involving the limbs are performed in the water with the water acting as a resistance.

When these exercises are performed in the shallow end of a pool, they are still weight-bearing activities, but because of the buoyancy, the stress on the joints, particularly the knee and hip joints, is reduced considerably. Therefore, water aerobics is a very popular form of exercise for those who are overweight or obese.

Research clearly indicates that the intensity of a water aerobics workout is sufficient to result in cardiovascular improvement and that those participating in an 8-week program also showed significant increases in strength, muscular endurance, and flexibility together with a decrease in their percentage of body fat.[10]

ROLLERBLADING

Rollerblading, or in-line skating as it is commonly called, is a fun recreational activity that can also be a good aer-

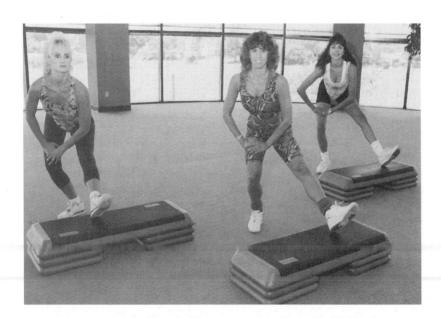

Figure 4-12   Bench aerobics is a new form of aerobic exercise.

Table 4-5	Point Values for Selected Activities in the Aerobics Program				
Running (time in minutes for 1 mile)	Running (time in minutes for 2 miles)	Handball or Basketball* (time in minutes)	Swimming (time in minutes for 400 yards)	Cycling (time in minutes for 3 miles)	Points
More than 20	—	Less than 8	—	18 or longer	0
14½-20	40 or longer	8	13½ or longer	12-17	1
12-14½	29-40	15	10-13½	—	2
10-12	—	20	7-9	9-11	3
8-10	24-28	28	—	—	4
6½-8	—	35	Less than 7	Less than 9	5
Less than 6½	20-24	40	—	—	6

*The times for handball or basketball are for continuous activity and do not include breaks; it must also be full-court basketball.

Table 4-6	Point Values for Additional Exercises in the Aerobics Program	
Activity	Amount of Activity	Points
Golf (no motorized carts)	18 holes	3
Hockey*	20 min	3
Rope skipping (continuous)	5 min	1.5
Skating*	15 min	1
Skiing*	30 min	3
Tennis	1 set	1.5
Volleyball*	15 min	1
Wrestling*	5 min	2

*Only the time that is spent actually participating is to be counted.

CIRCUIT TRAINING

Circuit training is a form of general fitness training designed to appeal to participants while increasing their level of fitness. The term **circuit** refers to a given number of exercises arranged and numbered consecutively in a given area. Each numbered exercise in the circuit is a *station*. The type of circuit that is set up depends on the time, space, facilities available, and objectives of the program. The stations are usually located at about equal distances from each other and are designated by signs on the walls or bleachers that might surround it. These signs state the sequence of activities and the prescribed number of repetitions at each station.

Objectives

In circuit training, you progress at your own rate from one station to the next, performing a prescribed amount of work at each, until the entire circuit has been completed. Usually, the single circuit is repeated several times, and the time for the total performance is recorded. Proceed from station to station without resting as you attempt to reduce the time taken for a given number of laps around the circuit. You can progress by decreasing the time required to complete a given number of laps of the circuit, by increasing the number of repetitions performed at each station, or a combination of both.

Advantages

The major advantage of circuit training over many other exercise programs is that circuit training stresses continuous activity. It has been shown that continuous activity is a prerequisite for developing the cardiovascular system. Unfortunately, many exercise programs stress only muscular endurance and flexibility and place little emphasis on developing cardiovascular endurance.

Following is a list of advantages of circuit training:

■ Each participant is able to start the program at an easy pace and experience success early.

■ Circuit training can be organized to involve a large number of participants in a relatively confined area.

■ Added motivation is provided by seeing progress from day to day.

■ Progression is ensured if the participant exercises regularly.

■ The exercise is continuous; thus stress is placed on the cardiovascular system.

Circuit training: A series of exercises arranged in a specific sequence so that participants can complete a predetermined number of repetitions as quickly as possible at each exercise station.

Circuit: A given number of exercises arranged and numbered consecutively.

■ Circuit training provides individualized self-competition. Each participant is competing only against himself or herself and works at his or her own rate.

Organization

Circuit training may be organized in a variety of ways. An example of the organization of a circuit consisting of eight stations designed to develop each of the components of physical fitness is presented. This circuit is for both men and women. A list of the activities and repetitions required for each are presented in Table 4-7. The specific activities are described later in this chapter.

Four progression levels have been established, although more may be added if needed. Your initial starting level can be determined by your performance on the 12-minute run test. Table 4-8 presents the criteria you can use to determine your starting level. If you have not taken this test, start at the lowest level and progress from there.

Description of activities in the circuit

Several of these activities are adapted from or are similar to those suggested by Robert Sorani in his book, *Circuit training.*[21] You can use these activities, or you can design your own circuit to include activities of your choice.

Lateral jump   Jump laterally across any line on the floor as fast as possible, keeping both feet together and parallel to the line. This activity develops muscular endurance of the legs and overall cardiovascular endurance.

Bent-leg curl-ups   Bent-leg curl-ups strengthen the abdominal muscles and increase their endurance. Lie down with your feet flat on the floor about shoulder width apart. Your knees should be flexed at a right angle. Your arms are folded across your chest with your chin held as close to your chest as possible. Curl up until your elbows touch the upper part of your thighs and then return until your lower back is in contact with the floor.

Rope jump   The rope jump is designed for development of cardiovascular endurance. A regular jump rope is used, and you must propel it in a counterclockwise direction so that it passes under your feet and over your head. Each time the rope passes under the feet is one repetition.

Lateral leg raise   Assume a position on the floor lying on either side with legs and lower arm completely extended, using the other arm to maintain your balance (see Figure 5-18). The upper leg is raised as high as possible, kept straight, and is then returned slowly to the start position. This is one repetition. This exercise is designed to develop the muscles responsible for abduction of the leg. If the circuit is completed more than one time, the sides should be reversed so that the leg that is raised is changed each time around the circuit.

Burpee   The burpee is also called the squat-thrust or the agility four-count exercise. Start in a standing position with the legs straight. Assume the squat position, extend the legs backward so that you are in the push-up position, then reverse this procedure back to the squat position and finally back to the upright position. This completes one repetition. Because this exercise involves many large muscle groups, it contributes to overall muscular endurance.

Table 4-7	**Circuit Training Activities**			
Activity	Level I	Level II	Level III	Level IV
Lateral jump	25	30	35	50
Bent-leg curl-ups	10	15	20	30
Rope jump	40	50	60	80
Lateral leg raise	8	10	20	30
Burpee	8	10	20	30
Push-ups	8	12	20	26
Bench jump (step)	10	16	20	26
Sprinter	20	30	40	50

Table 4-8	**Criteria for Determination of the Initial Starting Level for Circuit Training**		
Classification for 12-Minute Run Test	Distance Covered (miles)		Initial Circuit Level
	Men	Women	
Very poor or poor	<1.60	<1.26	Level I
Average	1.60-1.77	1.26-1.43	Level II
Good	1.78-1.94	1.44-1.60	Level III
Excellent	>1.95	>1.61	Level IV

Push-ups To perform the regular push-up, start from the front-leaning rest position with the head, back, hips, and legs in a straight alignment. The body is slowly lowered so that the chest lightly touches the floor. The body should remain straight throughout this exercise. The arms are then extended as the body is raised to the starting position. This exercise will develop muscular endurance and strength of the extensors of the forearm. Individuals should perform the modified push-up if they are unable to perform the regular push-up (Figure 4-13).

Bench step For the bench step, face a bench about 12 to 16 inches high. The lowest row of bleachers is usually satisfactory for this exercise. Step up to and down from the bench. This completes one repetition. This exercise is designed to develop strength and endurance of the leg extensors and cardiovascular endurance.

Sprinter Assume a position similar to a sprinter's starting position, with the weight on the hands and feet with one leg extended straight back and the other flexed with the knee pulled under the chest (Figure 4-14). The position of the feet is then reversed and reversed again as you return to the starting position. This completes one repetition. This exercise contributes to the development of strength and endurance of the shoulder and arm extensors and leg flexors and extensors.

Instructions for running a circuit
The following should be used as guidelines for beginning the circuit:

- Practice each exercise before starting the circuit.
- Fifteen minutes should be allowed for men and 18 minutes for women to complete two laps of the circuit.
- If two laps around the circuit are completed before the allocated time has elapsed, the remainder of the time can be spent jogging in place.
- If you complete the two laps of the circuit within the time limit, the next time you attempt the circuit, move up to the next level.
- If you fail to complete the two laps of the circuit in the prescribed time and are not working at the first level, move back one level.

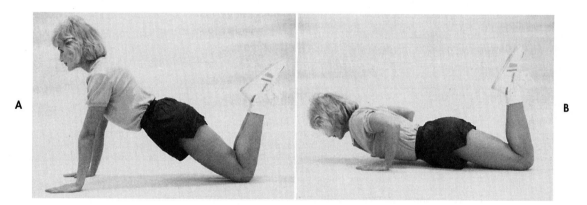

Figure 4-13 Start **(A)** and finish **(B)** positions for the modified push-up.

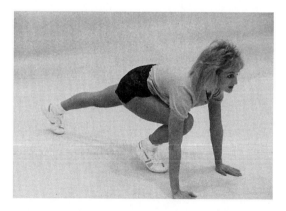

Figure 4-14 Start position for the sprinter exercise.

■ To measure progress each day, record the time taken to complete two laps of the circuit.

An alternative procedure for the organization of circuit training is to allow a specific time (usually 45 seconds or 1 minute) for each exercise. Perform as many repetitions as possible at each station. This is an effective way to show improvement.

CIRCUIT WEIGHT TRAINING

Development of strength and muscular endurance may be combined with development of cardiovascular endurance by using circuit training and weight training. Carefully selected weight-training exercises can be used in a predetermined sequence to provide a total workout for each major muscle group.

The following suggestions may be beneficial:

■ Exercises should be arranged so that you alternate between upper and lower body.

■ Perform 12 to 15 repetitions at each station, working at 40% to 60% of maximal capacity.

■ Each set of repetitions should be continuous and not take more than 30 seconds.

■ Fifteen to thirty seconds are allowed between each exercise, during which time you should move to the next station and select the resistance.

■ The objective is to work continuously for 30 minutes and to complete as many circuits as possible during this time.

THE SUPER CIRCUIT

The super circuit was developed to concentrate even more on the development of cardiovascular endurance while developing strength and muscular endurance. In the super circuit the 15- to 30-second rest period is replaced by a 30-second aerobic activity. Aerobic activities that might be used for each 30-second exercise are running, using an indoor jogger or stationary bicycle, jumping rope, or running in place. All other procedures as outlined previously for circuit weight training can be applied.

Results from a recent research study show dramatic changes after participation in circuit weight training and in the super circuit program.[9] The study involved 36 women and 41 men randomly assigned to one of the following three groups:

■ Circuit weight training group

■ Super circuit group

■ Control group

The two exercise groups did assigned activities for 30 minutes a day, 3 days a week, for 12 weeks. A summary of the improvements that occurred in each group for both men and women is presented in Table 4-9. The results indicate that when weight training exercises are organized into a continuous program with no rest between exercises, significant improvements will occur in cardiovascular endurance, strength, and body composition. These results compare favorably with those of other aerobic programs.

Table 4-9	**Percentage of Improvement in Designated Variables as a Result of Circuit Weight Training and Super Circuit Training**				
	Super Circuit Group		Circuit Weight Training Group		Control Group (men and women)
Variable	Men	Women	Men	Women	
Aerobic endurance	+12.0	+17.0	+12.0	+13.0	No change
Body fat	− 17.1	− 10.9	− 13.3	− 10.4	No change
Leg strength	+21.0	+26.0	+15.5	+17.7	No change
Bench press	+21.0	+21.0	+14.0	+20.0	No change

Chapter Summary

The following summary will help you to identify some of the important concepts covered in this chapter:

- Your overall objectives for your exercise program will determine how much exercise you really need.
- Most of the good aerobic activities are continuous and involve large muscle groups.
- Brisk walking can be an ideal aerobic activity for most adults.
- Jogging and running are two of the most popular forms of aerobic exercise for those who are less than 30 years of age.
- Swimming and cycling are excellent nonimpact aerobic activities.
- Low-impact aerobics can be as demanding as high-impact aerobics and is preferred by many because of the lower injury rate associated with it.
- Stair stepping has emerged as one of the most popular and effective forms of aerobic exercise.
- Despite the fact that racquetball and squash are not continuous activities, in most cases they are strenuous enough to raise and maintain the heart rate in the target zone.
- Continuous weight training, such as in circuit training, can be an excellent form of aerobic exercise.

References

1. *Aerobic Fitness Program Starter*, Chicago, 1988, Schwinn Air Dyne.
2. Allen TE et al: Metabolic and cardiorespiratory responses of young women to skipping and jogging, *The Physician and Sportsmedicine* 15(5):109-113, 1987.
3. Bishop JG: *Fitness through aerobics*, ed 3, Scottsdale, Ariz, 1995, Gorsuch Scarisbrick.
4. Buyze MT et al: Comparative training responses to rope skipping and jogging, *The Physician and Sportsmedicine* 14(11):65-69, 1986.
5. Cooper KH: *The aerobics program for total well-being*, New York, 1982, M Evans & Co.
6. De Benedette V: Stair machines: the truth about this fitness fad, *The Physician and Sportsmedicine* 18(6):131-134, 1990.
7. Duroe M: *Cardiovascular aspects of racquetball relative to skill level*, master's thesis, Marquette, Mich, 1979, Northern Michigan University.
8. Francis F: Injury prevention: physics of foot impact, *Consultant*, pp 107-126, March 1980.
9. Harste A: Bench aerobics: a step in the right direction? *The Physician and Sportsmedicine* 18(7):25-26, 1990.
10. Hempel LS, Wells CL: Cardiorespiratory cost of the Nautilus express circuit, *The Physician and Sportsmedicine* 13(4):82-97, 1985.
11. Hoeger WWK: Is water aerobics aerobic? *Fitness Management*, pp 29-30, April 1995.
12. Katch VL, Villanucci JF: Energy cost of rebound running, *Res Q Exerc Sport* 52(2):269, 1981.
13. Klug GA, Letternick J: *Exercise and physical fitness*, Guilford, Conn, 1992, Dushkin.
14. Koszuta LE: Low-impact aerobics: better than traditional aerobic dance? *The Physician and Sportsmedicine* 14(7):156-161, 1986.
15. Kravitz L, Deivert R: The safe way to step, *Idea Today*, p 59, March 1992.
16. LaForge R: Step exercise, *Idea Today*, p 32, Sept 1991.
17. Porcari J et al: Is fast walking an adequate aerobic training stimulus for 30- to 69-year-old men and women? *The Physician and Sportsmedicine* 15(2):119-129, 1987.
18. *Prevention Index '91*, Emmaus, Penn, 1992, Rodale Press.
19. *Prevention Index '86*, Emmaus, Penn, 1987, Rodale Press.
20. Solis K et al: Aerobic requirements for the heart rate responses to variations in rope jumping techniques, *The Physician and Sportsmedicine* 16(3):121-128, 1988.
21. Sorani R: *Circuit training*, Dubuque, Ia, 1966, Wm C Brown.
22. Wolf MD: Avoiding aerobic injuries, *Athletic Business*, pp 10-14, March 1985.

Determining Your Correct Pace for Walking or Jogging

Name	Section	Date

Purpose

To determine the pace at which you should be walking or jogging to maintain your heart rate in your target zone.

Procedures

You need to first calculate your target-zone heart rate according to the procedures outlined in Chapter 3.

Maximum heart rate = 220 − age

= 220 − ____

= ____ beats/min

Target-zone heart rate:

Upper limit = Maximum heart rate × 0.85

= ____ × 0.85

= ____ beats/min

Lower limit = Maximum heart rate × 0.7

= ____ × 0.7

= ____ beats/min

Target-zone heart rate ____ to ____ beats/min

You will need to measure a 1-mile course or use a measured track so that you know exactly what constitutes 1 mile. Start by walking as fast as you can, and try to cover the mile without stopping. Record the time it takes, and determine your heart rate immediately after completing the walk.

Results

Record your results in the spaces provided below.

Time to walk 1 mile: ____ minutes

Heart rate at completion of walk: ____ beats/min

Compare your heart rate at the end of the walk to your target-zone heart rate, which you calculated and recorded above and check the correct response below:

My heart rate at the end of the mile walk was:

____ Below my target zone

____ Within my target zone

____ Above my target zone

If your heart rate at the end of the walk was within your target zone, you know that the pace you were walking is the correct pace for you and that if you decide to include walking in your exercise program, this is the speed at which you need to walk.

If your heart rate was above your target zone at the end of the 1-mile walk, you need to walk the same distance again at a slower pace and repeat the above procedures until you find the correct pace to walk at so that your heart rate remains at the desired level.

At the end of the 1-mile walk, if your heart rate was below your target zone and you have no medical problems, you need to repeat the above procedures, jogging slowly rather than walking. By trial and error and making adjustments each time, it should not take you long to determine the speed at which you need to jog to achieve and maintain your desired heart rate.

Chapter Five **Strength and Muscular Endurance**

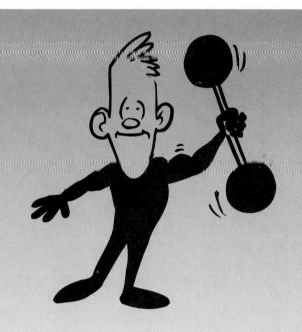

CHAPTER OBJECTIVES
Check off each objective you achieve.

- ❑ Differentiate clearly between strength and muscular endurance, and understand their importance.
- ❑ Identify and define the three types of muscle contraction.
- ❑ Evaluate the different procedures for development of strength and muscular endurance.
- ❑ Identify the major muscles and muscle groups in the body, and know which exercises can be used to develop each of these.
- ❑ Design and implement a strength/muscular endurance program based on your specific needs.
- ❑ Explain why "overload" is important in the development of strength and muscular endurance.
- ❑ Discuss muscle soreness, and know what steps you can take to avoid it.
- ❑ Evaluate your level of strength and muscular endurance for specific muscle groups.

In the past, strength was regarded as the symbol of physical fitness. Many fitness tests were simply strength tests. A person with a well-developed musculature and a good physique was considered to exhibit good physical fitness. However, fitness should not be based on physical appearance but instead on the body's functional capacity to perform work and its ability to supply energy.

Today many people believe that strength and muscular endurance are important only for athletes and for those doing heavy physical work. Certainly these people require a high level of strength and muscular endurance if they are to perform efficiently. However, these physical fitness components are also important to the average person.

Increasing strength and muscular endurance should make it easier to perform everyday tasks. Carrying a suitcase, moving furniture, pushing a stalled vehicle, or mowing the lawn will become easier if you develop the strength and endurance of the muscles involved in each task.

In addition, increased strength and muscular endurance should contribute to the following:

■ Maintenance of correct posture

■ Improved personal appearance

■ Decreased risk of muscle injuries

■ Prevention and alleviation of low back pain

■ Increased joint flexibility

DEFINITION OF TERMS

Strength and muscular endurance are important health-related physical fitness components that are often confused. It is important to clearly differentiate between them.

Strength is the amount of force a muscle or muscle group can exert against a resistance in one maximum contraction.

Muscular endurance is the ability of a muscle or muscle group to apply force repeatedly or to sustain a contraction for a period of time.

TYPES OF MUSCLE CONTRACTION

All body movements depend on the contraction of muscles. Your neurological system acts as a communication network between the muscular and skeletal systems. Messages are sent from the central nervous system to the muscles telling them to contract and how strongly they should contract to perform specific movements.

Skeletal muscles possess four unique properties:

■ *Excitability*—the ability to receive and respond to stimulation from the nervous system

■ *Contractibility*—the ability to develop internal force or tension

■ *Extensibility*—the muscle's ability to stretch past its normal resting length

■ *Elasticity*—the muscle's ability to return to its normal resting length

The force generated by a muscle or muscle group depends on gender and body weight and the number of active fibers recruited by the nervous system to perform a task.

When a muscle contracts, tension is created within the muscle and it may shorten, lengthen, or remain the same. There are two types of muscle contractions—isometric and isotonic.

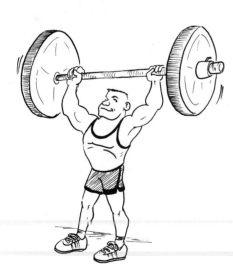

Strength of a muscle group can be determined by measuring the maximum weight that can be moved one time through a designated range of motion.

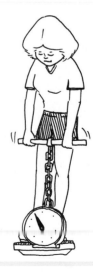

Strength can also be measured by applying a maximum force against a resistance. With this procedure, little or no movement takes place because the magnitude of the force is usually measured by using a dynamometer.

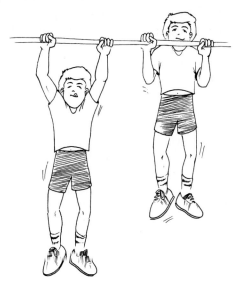

Muscular endurance of a muscle group can be determined by the number of repetitions performed by the muscle group.

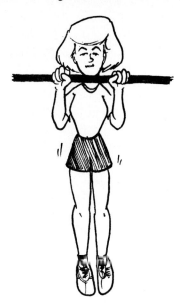

Muscular endurance can also be determined by measuring the time a contraction can be sustained. Body weight and gravity often act as the resistance.

Isometric contraction

Isometric contractions occur when the force exerted by the muscle as it contracts is equal to or less than the resistance. Tension develops in the muscles as an isometric contraction occurs. The muscles involved do not noticeably shorten or lengthen, and little or no movement takes place at the joint. This is often called a static contraction.

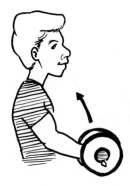

If sufficient force is generated by the biceps muscle as it contracts, the muscle will shorten and the forearm will move up as the weight is lifted. This then becomes an isotonic contraction.

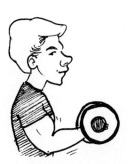

With this isometric contraction the force generated by the muscle is equal to the resistance. Since no movement occurs, the force necessary to sustain the resistance will depend on the angle of the joint.

Isotonic contraction

Isotonic contractions are often called dynamic contractions and occur when the force generated by the muscle as it contracts is greater than the resistance. Movement occurs at the joint, and the muscles involved shorten and lengthen (Figure 5-1).

> **Isometric contraction:** The application of force by a muscle or muscle group where no movement takes place at a joint. Also called a static contraction.
>
> **Isotonic contraction:** The application of force by a muscle or muscle group resulting in movement at a joint.

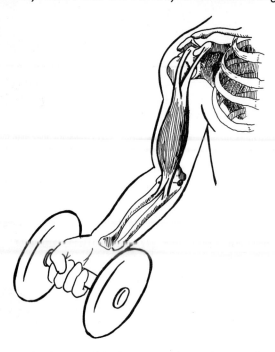

Figure 5-1 Position of the biceps muscle in relation to the elbow joint.

Each isotonic contraction consists of two contraction phases:

- **Concentric contraction** (positive work)—the muscle shortens and works against gravity.
- **Eccentric contraction** (negative work)—the muscle lengthens as it returns to its original position.

Force applied to the weight varies at different points throughout the range of motion. This happens because of gravity's effect against the rotary movement of the segment and because of the system of levers that exists in the body. For example, consider the two-arm curl. Once you have overcome the initial resistance, lifting the weight may be easy or difficult depending on the position of the weight in relation to your body (Figure 5-2).

The point where the force applied to the weight is weakest is often called the **sticking point.** The force necessary to move the weight is often insufficient at this point, and the task cannot be completed. If the weight can be moved past this point, the task gets easier again. It can then usually be completed because less force is needed for the remainder of the task.

During an isotonic task the muscles are not working at or near their capacity except at one point in the range of motion. For this reason, several companies have produced isotonic machines that vary the resistance throughout the range of motion to match the functional strength of the muscles. These are called variable resistance isotonic machines. These machines change the resistance by using a leverage system so that at the point where the muscle is weakest, the load is

the lightest and where the muscle is strongest, the load is the heaviest. Muscles therefore have to exert maximum effort throughout the range of motion if the correct resistance is used.

The most common equipment using this technique is the Nautilus brand (Figure 5-3). It is a system of chains and variable-shaped cams that provide a balanced resistance over a full range of movement.

With isotonic equipment, momentum can also influence the task's difficulty. It is important to perform isotonic contractions slowly to minimize the contribution that movement makes to task performance.

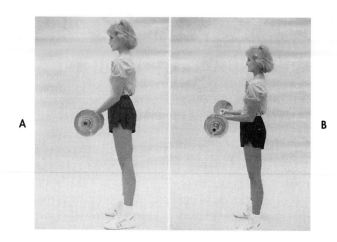

Figure 5-2 Relationship between joint angle and difficulty of a task. **A,** At an angle of about 120 degrees, the force that can be generated by the muscle group is the greatest and the task will appear to be easy. **B,** At an angle of 90 degrees, muscles involved in this movement are at a disadvantage and the task may appear to be difficult.

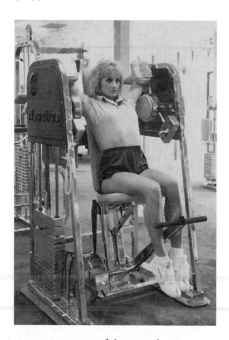

Figure 5-3 Use of the Nautilus Super Pullover machine for development of the upper body.

Isokinetic contraction

As noted in the previous section, in an isotonic contraction the muscle's functional strength varies at different angles and speed of movement can influence the task's difficulty. In an **isokinetic contraction,** speed of motion is controlled so that resistance is varied to match the force applied by the muscles. The most popular machines using this technique are the Cybex and Orthotron machines. You apply a maximum effort, and the isokinetic device automatically controls the speed at which you can move through the full range of motion. At the points at which muscular force and mechanical advantage are greatest, the resistance will also be greatest, resulting in a constant speed. This provides maximum resistance throughout the range of motion (Figure 5-4)

WEIGHT-TRAINING GUIDELINES AND SAFETY

These guidelines should be followed when you participate in weight training:

Warm-up: Each training session should be preceded by a 5- to 10-minute warm-up. The warm-up should include stretching exercises for each muscle group involved.

Breathing: While executing each exercise, make sure that you breathe correctly. You should breathe out while performing the lift and breathe in while returning to the starting position.

Range of motion: Make sure that each exercise is performed correctly through the full range of motion. Exercises performed incorrectly or with too much resistance are likely to reduce flexibility and could cause muscle injury.

Spotting: When using free weights, it is important to work out with a partner who can be a spotter when you are performing exercises. This is particularly important when working with heavy weights in such exercises as the bench press.

Weights and collars: When using free weights, make sure that the collars are tight and fastened securely so that weights do not fall off.

Speed: Each exercise should be performed slowly with a steady application of force. This is important with the lowering phase (negative work). It is recommended that the lowering phase take about twice as long (4 seconds) as the lifting phase (2 seconds).

Sequence: The order in which major muscle groups should be exercised is important. The largest muscle groups should be exercised first, and the same muscle groups should not be exercised successively.

Symmetry: Muscles are usually grouped in sets that oppose one another. In many cases, because of what we do, the body favors specific muscle groups, and quite frequently, one muscle group will be naturally strong and the opposing group will be much weaker. For example, because we constantly lift and carry various items, the biceps muscle in the front of the arm will usually be well developed. However, because we seldom do much to develop the muscles at the back of the arm, the triceps will usually be much weaker.

To maintain balance and symmetry, when muscles on one side of a joint are exercised, then the opposing muscle group should also be exercised. When an imbalance occurs between muscle groups, it can negatively affect your posture, reduce the flexibility of the joint, and possibly increase the risk of injury.

A good example of increased risk of injury relates to shin splints, which are often caused by muscle im-

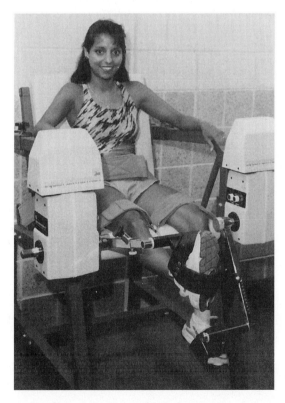

Figure 5-4 An Orthotron machine, which controls the speed of motion.

Concentric contraction: An isotonic contraction where the muscle shortens and works against gravity.

Eccentric contraction: An isotonic contraction where the muscle lengthens and returns to its original position.

Sticking point: The point in a range of motion in an isotonic contraction where force applied by the muscle is weakest.

Isokinetic contraction: An isotonic contraction where the speed of motion is controlled.

balance. The large muscle in the back of the leg—the gastrocnemius—is usually well developed, whereas the muscle in the front of the lower leg—the tibialis anterior—is usually not well developed and in most cases needs to be strengthened.

The major muscle groups in the body are identified in Figures 5-5 and 5-6.

Opposing muscles or muscle groups that often create problems are listed below[8]:

Quadriceps (front of thigh)	Hamstrings (back of thigh)
Adductors (inner thigh)	Abductors (outer thigh)
Pectorals (chest)	Rhomboids (upper back)
Abdominals (stomach)	Erector spinae (lower back)
Gastrocnemius (back of lower leg)	Tibialis anterior (front of lower leg)
Biceps (front of upper arm)	Triceps (back of upper arm)

If a particular muscle or muscle group is stronger than what it should be, it often needs to be stretched. If it is weaker than its opposing muscle or muscle group, it needs to be strengthened. Exercises for the development of the major muscle groups in the body are included later in this chapter. Stretching exercises for each of the major muscle groups in the body are included in Chapter 6.

BASIC TERMINOLOGY

Repetition: A repetition is the completion of a designated movement through a full range of motion.
Set: A set is a designated number of repetitions attempted without a rest.
Resistance: Resistance is the workload you are attempting to move.

PRINCIPLES FOR WEIGHT TRAINING USING NAUTILUS EQUIPMENT

These guidelines are recommended when using Nautilus equipment:

- Select a resistance for each exercise that allows performance of between 8 and 12 repetitions.

- Perform only one set for each exercise during each exercise session.

- Use this equipment no more than three times each week.

- Continue each exercise until no more repetitions can be performed, up to a maximum of 12. When

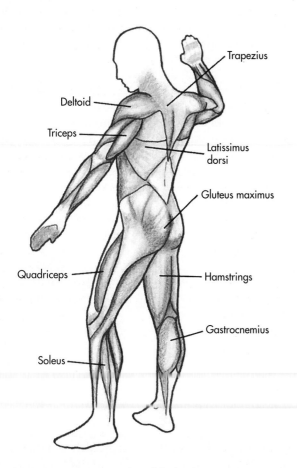

Figure 5-5 Major muscles of the body—a posterior view.

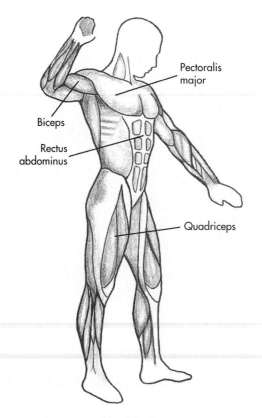

Figure 5-6 Major muscles of the body—an anterior view.

this number can be performed, add one additional weight.

- For maximum results the position of the body in relation to the machine is important. For all single-joint rotary machines the axis of the cam must line up with the joint that is being exercised (Figure 5-7).
- The first two or three repetitions of each exercise should be performed at a slightly slower pace than the rest as you concentrate on moving through the entire range of motion.
- The lowering portion of each exercise should be accentuated. It should take about 2 seconds to lift the weight and about 4 seconds to lower it.
- On machines that have two-part exercises, it is important to move quickly from the first to the second task.

BASIC PRINCIPLES OF WEIGHT-TRAINING PROGRAMS

When you participate regularly in a good weight-training program, you will increase the strength and endurance of muscles involved. There may also be a corresponding increase in muscle size. This is called **muscle hypertrophy** and results from an increase in size of the cross-sectional area of fibers that make up the muscle.

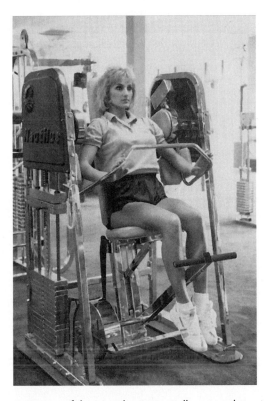

Figure 5-7 Use of the Nautilus Super Pullover machine. Note how the axis of the cams lines up with the shoulder joint.

A basic principle involved in weight-training programs is the **overload principle.** This states that muscular strength, endurance, and size will increase only if muscles are systematically subjected to workloads greater than those to which they are accustomed. As your muscle group becomes stronger, your body will adapt to the increased resistance. If further improvement is to occur, the workload must be progressively increased. For each exercise, each muscle must perform at or near its strength and endurance capacity if maximum gains are to occur.

Overload may be achieved by any combination of the following:

- Increasing the amount of weight lifted
- Increasing the repetitions in a set
- Increasing the number of sets
- Increasing the speed with which repetitions are performed
- Decreasing the time for rest between sets (if more than one set is attempted)

Note that if the speed of movement is increased, you must perform the exercise correctly and move through the full range of motion.

Many resistance training programs are available. They manipulate the training variables to maximize strength, endurance, or size. The best procedures have not been clearly established. For this reason, only general guidelines are presented.

DEVELOPMENT OF STRENGTH AND MUSCULAR ENDURANCE

The same criteria that apply to the development of cardiovascular endurance also apply to the development of strength and muscular endurance. These relate to intensity, duration, and frequency.

Intensity

In weight training, intensity of the workout relates to the extent that muscles are overloaded. Programs can be specifically designed for the development of either strength or muscular endurance. Differences between these programs relate to the number of repetitions and the amount of resistance. As a general rule, a strength

Muscle hypertrophy: An increase in the size of the muscle.

Overload principle: Subjecting a muscle or muscle group to a workload greater than that to which it is accustomed.

program will involve a low number of repetitions (usually 8 or less) with a heavy resistance. For those wishing to develop muscular endurance, a greater number of repetitions must be performed (usually 12 to 20) with less resistance.

Most people involved in a weight-training program are interested in both strength and endurance. Performing between 8 and 12 repetitions is probably ideal for this. These concepts are summarized in Figure 5-8. The amount of weight that will create an adequate resistance for each of these programs will vary among people and programs. The suggested percentages in Figure 5-8 can be used as a starting point to determine what might be best for you. Additional procedures for planning such a program are presented in a later section in this chapter.

Duration

The duration of each training session will vary depending on the person's level of strength and muscular endurance and his or her objectives. Several weight-training programs are available using different procedures and pieces of equipment. Your program will depend on the equipment available and how much time you have. If the weight-training program is to supplement an aerobic program, the exercises may need to be selected so that they can be completed in 15 to 20 minutes. Procedures for circuit weight training and the super circuit have been set up so that each of these programs can be completed in about 30 minutes. Information on these programs is presented in Chapter 4. Research indicates that each of these programs can be used to combine weight training and aerobic workout.

Frequency

When the muscular system has been stressed, it must be allowed to rest. It needs time for recovery and to adapt to a higher physiological level. It is not wise to perform exercises for the same muscle groups on successive days. A good weight-training program should be performed 3 or 4 days per week on every other day.

GUIDELINES FOR DEVELOPMENT OF STRENGTH AND MUSCULAR ENDURANCE

The following procedures can be followed for setting up a basic weight-training program.

- Select the muscle groups you wish to develop. There are several major muscle groups that you may want to include in a training program. These include the following:

    The anterior muscles in the upper legs
    The muscles in the chest and upper arms
    The posterior muscles in the upper legs
    The muscles in the shoulders and upper back
    The posterior muscles in the lower legs
    The abdominal muscles

- Select exercises for each of the muscle groups you wish to develop. Exercises for development of each of these muscle groups are described in later sections in this chapter.

- Determine the maximum weight you can lift one time for each of these exercises. It is necessary to determine your absolute strength for each of these exercises. This is called **1 RM (repetition maximum).** This allows you to measure your progress.

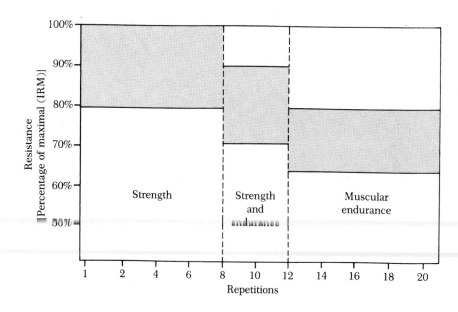

Figure 5-8   Guidelines for developing strength and muscular endurance.

Table 5-1	**Sample Weekly Recording Sheet for Individualized Weight-Training Program**

Name _____

Week Number __1__

Body Weight

Day 1 ____ lb

Day 2 ____ lb

Day 3 ____ lb

		Day 1		Day 2		Day 3	
		Date _____		Date _____		Date _____	
Exercise	1 Rm	Resistance	Reps/sets	Resistance	Reps/sets	Resistance	Reps/sets
Two-arm curl	_____	_____	__/__	_____	__/__	_____	__/__
Bench press	_____	_____	__/__	_____	__/__	_____	__/__
Quadriceps lift	_____	_____	__/__	_____	__/__	_____	__/__
Leg curl	_____	_____	__/__	_____	__/__	_____	__/__
Lateral pull-down	_____	_____	__/		__/	_____	__/__
Upright rowing	_____	_____	__/__	_____	__/__	_____	__/__

It may also be used to determine the initial resistance for each exercise.

- Start with a resistance equal to 70% of your maximum strength for each of the exercises selected, and determine how many repetitions you can perform using this weight. If you cannot perform 8 repetitions continuously, the weight is too heavy and should be reduced.

- The objective of the program is to increase your strength to where you can perform three sets of 12 repetitions with a short period of rest between each set. When you can do this, you need to increase the resistance.

- If you want a program directed more toward either strength or muscular endurance, adjust the number of repetitions and the resistance to incorporate the information previously presented.

- Perform each exercise three times per week. Make sure that you alternate exercise and rest days.

- Retest every 2 to 4 weeks to measure your progress.

A sample weekly recording sheet that can be used for weight training is included in Table 5-1.

ISOTONIC EXERCISES FOR THE DEVELOPMENT OF STRENGTH AND MUSCULAR ENDURANCE

The following procedures may be helpful in organizing and implementing an isotonic exercise program without the use of weights.

- Select the exercises you wish to incorporate in your program. Some test items included in this chapter are excellent exercises that can be included. Other good exercises are described in the section on circuit training in Chapter 4, or you may include exercises of your own.

- Determine the maximum number of repetitions you can perform in 1 minute for each exercise so that you can measure improvement.

- For the first week, use half of the maximum number of repetitions for each exercise and perform two sets on each of 3 nonconsecutive days. Make sure that you complete the first set for all the exercises before starting the second set.

- For the second and third weeks, use half the maximum number of repetitions for each exercise and perform three sets on each of 3 nonconsecutive days.

- For the fourth week, do one set using the maximum number of repetitions on each exercise day.

- Starting the fifth week, add one to three repetitions per week to each exercise.

- Retest every 4 to 8 weeks and determine the maximum number of repetitions that you can perform for each exercise. By doing this, you will be able to measure improvement.

A sample recording sheet is in Table 5-2.

WEIGHT-TRAINING EXERCISES FOR THE DEVELOPMENT OF STRENGTH AND MUSCULAR ENDURANCE

Six major muscle groups have previously been listed. In this section the major muscles in each of these groups are identified, and exercises that you can use for their development are explained. Most exercises use free

One repetition maximum (1RM): The maximum force that can be exerted once and only once by a muscle or group of muscles.

Table 5-2	**Sample Weekly Recording Sheet for Isotonic Exercise Program Without the Use of Weights**					

Name _____   Body Weight
Week Number _____   Day 1 ____ lb
                                  Day 2 ____ lb
                                  Day 3 ____ lb

		Day 1	Day 2	Day 3
		Date _____	Date _____	Date _____
Exercise	**Max Number of Repetitions/Minute**	**Reps/sets**	**Reps/sets**	**Reps/sets**
_____	_____	__/__	__/__	__/__
_____	_____	__/__	__/__	__/__
_____	_____	__/__	__/__	__/__
_____	_____	__/__	__/__	__/__
_____	_____	__/__	__/__	__/__
_____	_____	__/__	__/__	__/__
_____	_____	__/__	__/__	__/__
_____	_____	__/__	__/__	__/__
_____	_____	__/__	__/__	__/__

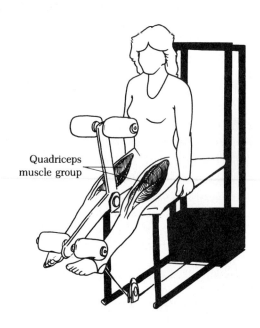

Quadriceps muscle group

Figure 5-9   Location of the quadriceps muscle group.

weights or equipment such as the Universal or Nautilus, which are available at many institutions and health clubs. The equipment you have available may not be quite the same, and you may need to adapt the procedures slightly for the exercises described.

Anterior muscles in the upper legs

The four main muscles located in front of the upper legs are collectively called the quadriceps group (Figure 5-9). The muscles that make up this group are the rectus femoris, vastus intermedius, vastus lateralis, and vastus medialis. Weight-training exercises for their development include the quadriceps lift and leg press.

Quadriceps lift   Sit with your lower leg at right angles to your thighs and the front of your ankles against the bar (Figure 5-10). Extend your legs until they are parallel with the floor, and then return to the starting position. The upper body must remain in an upright posi-

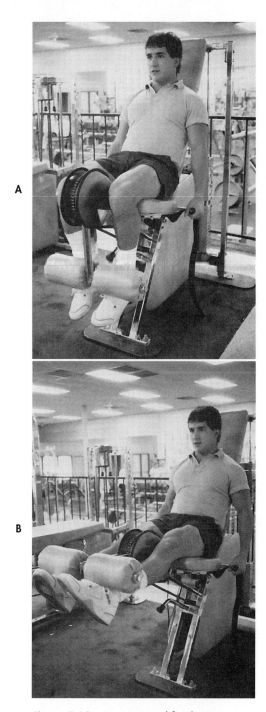

Figure 5-10 Start **(A)** and finish **(B)** positions for quadriceps lift exercise.

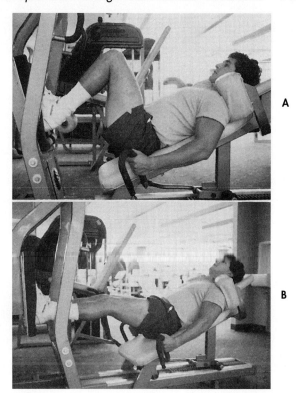

Figure 5-11 Start **(A)** and finish **(B)** positions for the leg press exercise.

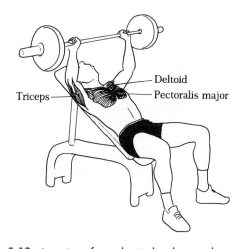

Figure 5-12 Location of muscles in the chest and upper arms.

tion, and the back of the knees should remain in contact with the end of the bench.

Leg press Sit at the leg press machine with legs bent at 90 degrees or less at the knee joint. Place feet firmly on the pedals, and grasp the seat handles. Press the feet forward until the legs are straight, then bend them slowly back to the starting position (Figure 5-11).

Muscles in chest and upper arms

The main muscles that are located in front of the chest and the upper arms are the pectoralis major and minor, the anterior deltoid, and the biceps and triceps (Figure 5-12). Exercises for the development of these muscles include the following: the bench press, military press, parallel dips, biceps curl, shoulder flexion, and shoulder adduction.

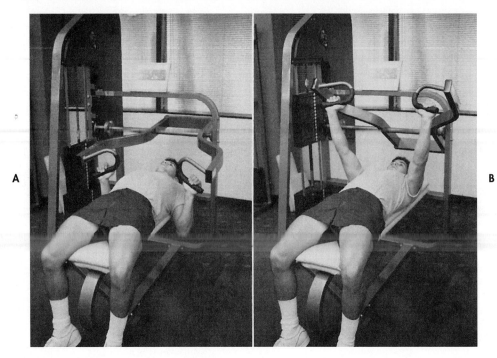

Figure 5-13   Start **(A)** and finish **(B)** positions for the bench press.

Bench press   Lie flat on a bench with knees bent and feet flat on the floor (Figure 5-13). Hold handles with the palms-forward grip at about shoulder width. Press weights directly upward until arms are fully extended; return to the starting position. Your back should remain straight throughout.

Military press   This exercise may be performed while sitting or standing upright. The palms-forward grip should be used with the hands slightly more than shoulder-width apart. Push the bar overhead until the arms are fully extended, and then lower it slowly until it touches the chest (Figure 5-14).

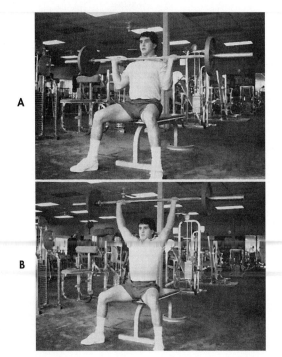

Figure 5-14   Start **(A)** and finish **(B)** positions for the military press.

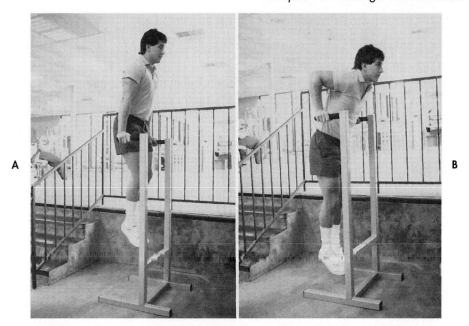

Figure 5-15   Start **(A)** and finish **(B)** positions for the parallel dip exercise.

Parallel dips   Support your body in an upright position with your arms straight and with your feet off the floor. Bend your arms and lower your body until there is a right angle or less at the elbow joint. Push up with your upper arms until you return to the start position (Figure 5-15).

Two-arm curl   Stand with your feet shoulder-width apart in an upright position. A barbell is held with the palms-forward grip and your arms extended. With elbows close to your body, the bar is curled to the shoulder/neck area and then returned to the starting position. This constitutes one repetition (Figure 5-16). This

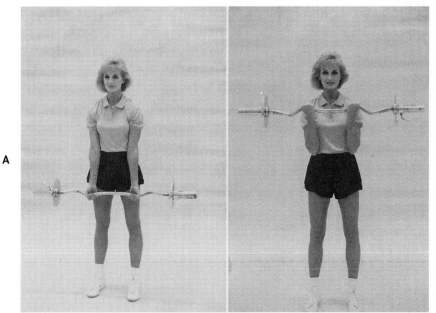

Figure 5-16   Start **(A)** and finish **(B)** positions for the two-arm curl exercise.

exercise may also be performed using a machine (Figure 5-17).

Shoulder flexion   Stand with your feet together and legs straight. Hold a hand weight with the right hand, with the overhand grip in front of the thigh. Keeping the arm straight, lift the arm up until it is at the height of the shoulder. Hold this position momentarily, and then return to the starting position in front of the thigh. This constitutes one repetition. Repeat this exercise as described using the weight in the left hand (Figure 5-18).

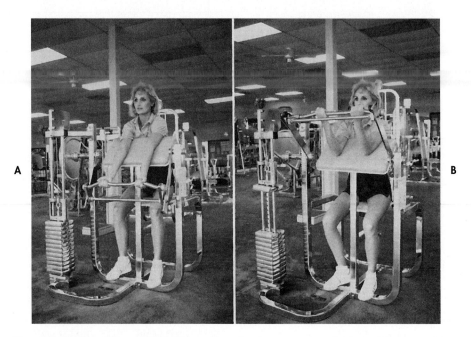

Figure 5-17 Start **(A)** and finish **(B)** positions for the two-arm curl using a biceps machine.

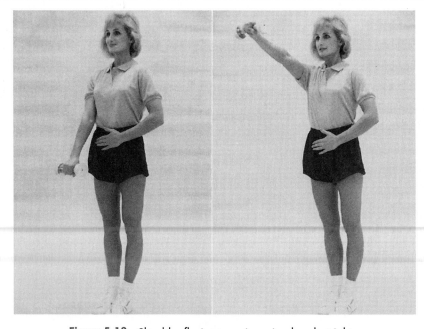

Figure 5-18 Shoulder flexion exercise using hand weights.

Shoulder adduction This exercise is often referred to as horizontal adduction. Sit with your forearms and palms placed against the pads in the machine. Your elbows should be positioned at about the height of the shoulder. Slowly push the pads together until they meet, and then return to the starting position (Figure 5-19).

Posterior muscles in upper legs

The large muscle group at the back of the legs that crosses both the hip and knee joints is the hamstring muscle group. It consists of three muscles—the semimembranosus, semitendinosus, and the biceps femoris (Figure 5-20). Exercises for development of the hamstring muscles are leg curls and hip extension.

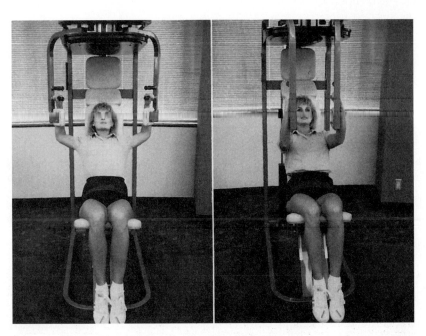

Figure 5-19   The shoulder adduction exercise.

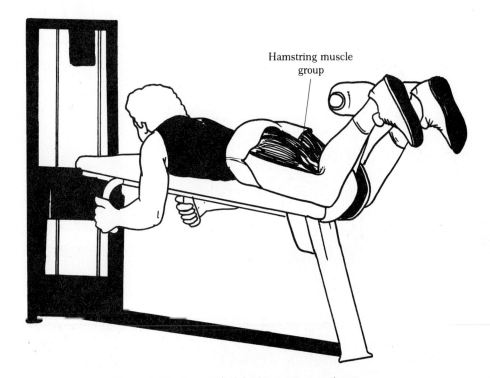

Hamstring muscle group

Figure 5-20   Location of the hamstring muscle group.

Leg curls   Lie face down with legs extended and the back of your heels against the bar. Your feet are then lifted upward until they touch your buttocks. They are then returned to the starting position (Figure 5-21).

Hip extension   Stand sideways to the machine, placing the roller behind the bent knee and holding the bar for support. Press the roller back until both knees are together, making sure that you do not lean forward or arch your back. Return to the start position (Figure 5-22).

Muscles in the shoulders and upper back

The major muscles associated with the shoulders and the posterior aspect of the upper arms are the rhomboids, triceps, trapezius, latissimus dorsi, and deltoid (posterior head) (Figure 5-23). Exercises for development of these muscles are the lateral pull-down, bent-over rowing, triceps curl, seated rowing, shoulder elevation, and shoulder abduction.

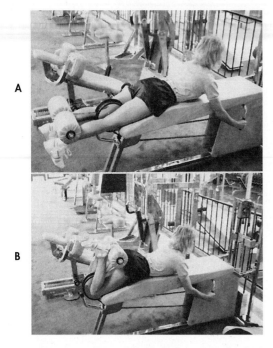

Figure 5-21   Start **(A)** and finish **(B)** positions for the leg curl exercise.

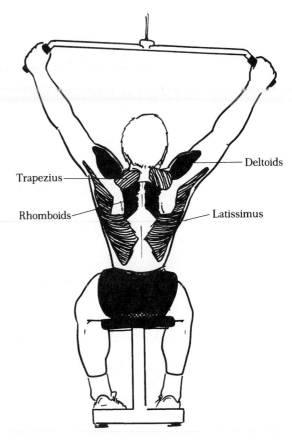

Figure 5-23   Muscles associated with the shoulders and the upper back.

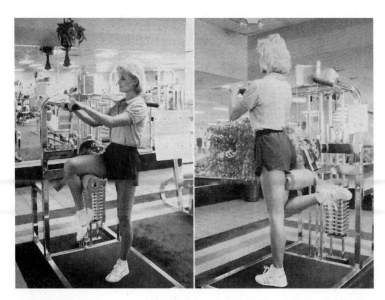

Figure 5-22   Exercise positions for the hip extension exercise.

Lateral pull-down Kneel and grasp the bar with the palms-forward grip or sit on a bench as shown in Figure 5-24. The bar is pulled down until it touches the base of your neck and then returned to the starting position to complete one repetition. Your body must be kept straight throughout. If the weight lifts you off the floor, the effectiveness of this exercise is reduced. If this happens, you must be held down by another person.

Bent-over rowing Stand in the bent-over position with your back straight and slightly above parallel to the floor. Your feet should be shoulder-width apart, with your knees comfortably bent. The bar should be grasped with the overhand grip, with the hands slightly wider apart than the shoulders. Pull the bar up slowly until it touches the chest, and lower it to the start position with the arms completely extended (Figure 5-25).

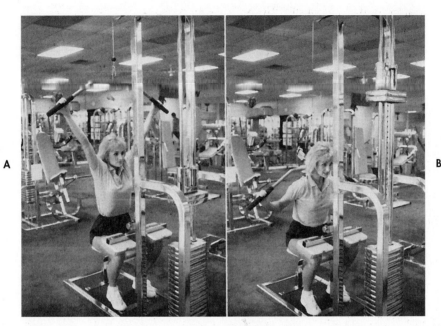

Figure 5-24 Start **(A)** and finish **(B)** positions for the lateral machine pull-down exercise.

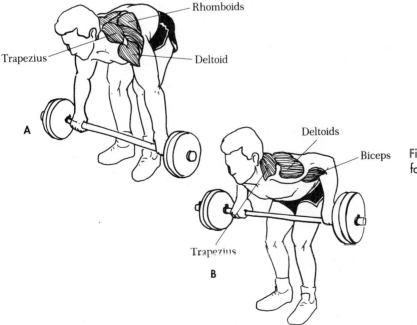

Figure 5-25 Start **(A)** and finish **(B)** positions for bent-over rowing.

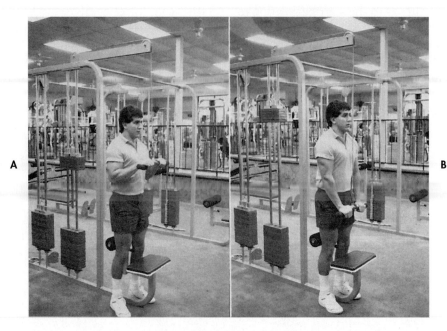

Figure 5-26   Start **(A)** and finish **(B)** positions for the triceps curl.

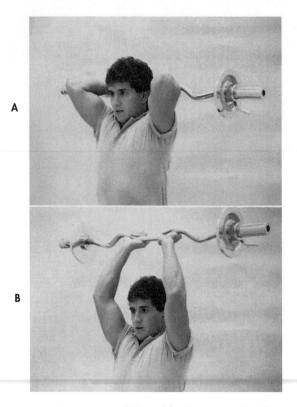

Figure 5-27   Start **(A)** and finish **(B)** positions for
the triceps curl using free weights.

Triceps curl   Grip the bar with the overhand grip. Keeping your upper arms and elbows motionless and close to your sides, push the bar down in front of your thighs until your arms are straight. Return to the start position (Figure 5-26). This exercise can also be performed using free weights (Figure 5-27).

Seated rowing   Use the overhand grip with the hands about shoulder-width apart. Pull the bar to the chest, extend the arms, and lower the weight (Figure 5-28).

Shoulder elevation   This is commonly called the shoulder shrug. Start with the bar at the rest position in front of the thigh. Use the overhand grip, and keeping the arms straight, elevate the bar by contracting the trapezius and then lower the bar to the rest position (Figure 5-29).

Shoulder abduction   Sit in the machine with your elbows by your sides and with your forearms resting against the arm pads. Press up against the pads until

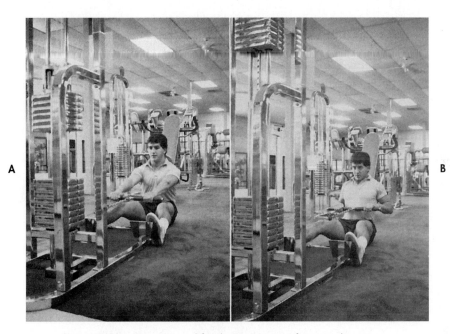

Figure 5-28   Start **(A)** and finish **(B)** positions for seated rowing.

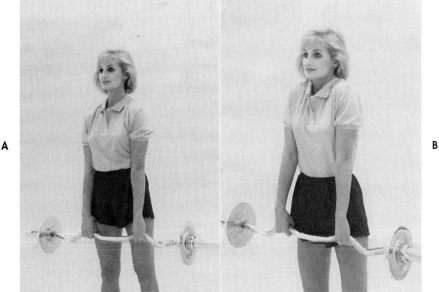

Figure 5-29   Start **(A)** and finish **(B)** positions for the shoulder elevation exercise.

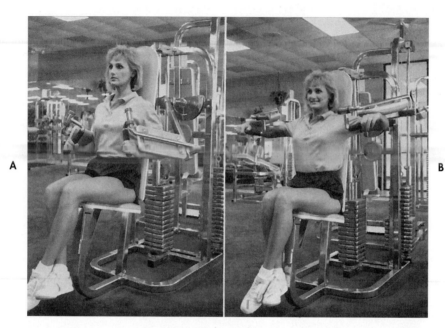

Figure 5-30   Start **(A)** and finish **(B)** positions for the shoulder abduction exercise.

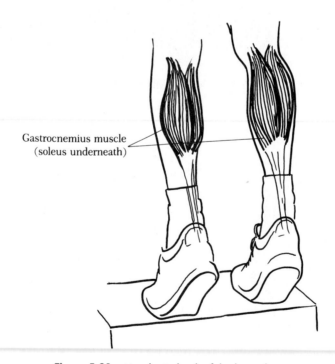

Gastrocnemius muscle
(soleus underneath)

Figure 5-31   Muscles in back of the lower leg.

they are at shoulder height and then slowly lower them to the start position (Figure 5-30).

Posterior muscles in lower legs

The two major muscles in back of the lower legs are the gastrocnemius and the soleus, which is beneath the gastrocnemius (Figure 5-31). The calf raise exercise develops these muscles.

Calf raise   Stand on your toes on a 2-inch by 4-inch board with the bar on your shoulders behind your neck. Raise to full extension, lifting your heels as high as pos-sible while keeping your toes in contact with the board, and then lower your heels so that they are as close as possible to the ground (Figure 5-32).

Abdominal muscles

There are three major muscles in the abdominal muscle group. These are the rectus abdominous and the internal and external oblique muscles (Figure 5-33). Two exercises are given for their development.

Curl-ups with weights   The arms are folded across the abdominal area, and a weight is held there. Use a sit-up

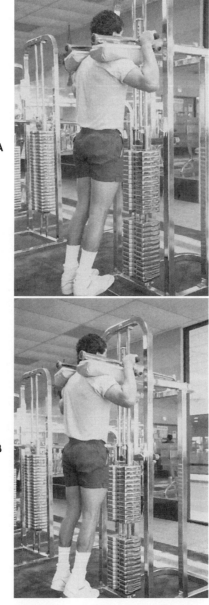

Figure 5-32   Start **(A)** and finish **(B)** positions for the calf raise exercise.

bench with the feet tucked under the support and the head tilted forward with the chin close to the chest. Curl up slowly, touching the elbows to the upper leg (Figure 5-34). This exercise can be made more difficult by moving the weight farther away from the abdominal area toward the head or by increasing the amount of weight that is being used.

Hip flexion   For this exercise, support yourself on your forearms so that you hang vertically, making sure that you keep your shoulders parallel to the floor. With your legs held together, bend your knees and raise them until they are perpendicular to the waist. Hold this position for 2 seconds, and then lower them slowly back to the start position (Figure 5-35).

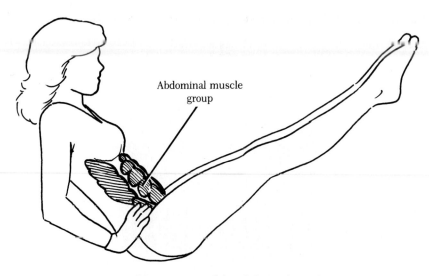

Figure 5-33   Position of the abdominal muscles.

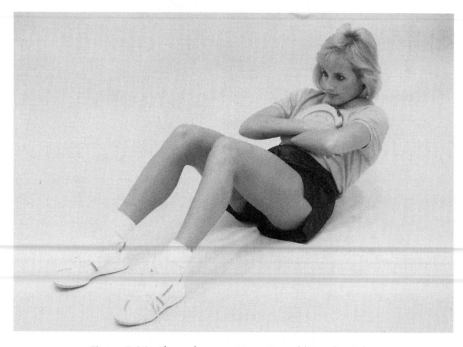

Figure 5-34   The curl-up exercise using additional weight.

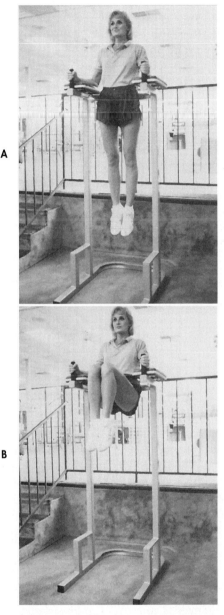

Figure 5-35 Start **(A)** and finish **(B)** positions for the hip flexion exercise.

MUSCLE SORENESS

Muscle soreness often occurs as a result of participation in an exercise program. It may occur during, immediately after, or 24 to 48 hours after the exercise session. The cause of this pain is not fully understood. However, it is believed that the acute pain that occurs during exercise is caused by accumulation of metabolic by-products created by insufficient blood flow. This type of pain usually disappears soon after exercise stops.[3]

Delayed muscle soreness is usually the result of repetitive strenuous muscle contractions, such as in isotonic programs involving weight training or calisthenics. The cause is unknown, although it is believed that microscopic tears may occur where muscles attach to bones. Delayed muscle soreness is usually felt at the start of an exercise program or during an exercise program when you increase the intensity of the workload. The following suggestions might help you to avoid it:

- Warming up properly
- Starting an exercise program at a low level of intensity
- Increasing the workload gradually throughout the program
- Cooling down correctly after each exercise session

If delayed muscle soreness does occur, static stretching combined with the use of heat may help to alleviate the pain.

USE OF ANABOLIC STEROIDS

An anabolic steroid is a synthetic drug that functions similar to the male hormone testosterone. It was developed for use by physicians in the treatment of disorders in which protein synthesis was important.[10] Unfortunately, in recent years, considerable interest has arisen among athletes concerning its use for increasing their athletic performance and also among high-school students who may use it to enhance physical appearance. Anabolic steroids are taken most frequently in conjunction with a high-intensity strength/weight-training program. Evidence suggests that this combination can result in rapid gains in muscle size and strength. However, it would appear that such a practice is potentially dangerous and can create a health hazard.[4]

The American College of Sports Medicine has conducted a comprehensive survey of the literature and carefully evaluated the claims made for and against the use of anabolic steroids for improving human physical performance. Following is a summary of some of their conclusions[2]:

- Anabolic steroids in the presence of an adequate diet can contribute to an increase in body weight.
- An increase in muscle strength achieved through high-intensity exercise and proper diet can be enhanced by the use of anabolic steroids in some individuals.
- The use of anabolic steroids does not increase aerobic power or capacity.
- The use of anabolic steroids has been associated with adverse effects on the liver, cardiovascular system, reproductive system, and psychological status in limited research with athletes.
- The use of anabolic steroids is contrary to the rules and ethical procedures of athletic competition as set forth by most sports-governing bodies. The American College of Sports Medicine supports these ethical procedures and deplores the use of anabolic steroids by athletes.

It should be noted that anabolic steroids are not just used by athletes. A recent study estimated that approximately 1 in 15 high-school students have used steroids, and although the most common reason given for their use was improved athletic performance, 25% used steroids simply for enhanced appearance.[4]

Of particular concern is recent evidence that shows that the use of steroids[5,7]:

- Significantly lowers high-density lipoprotein (HDL) levels
- Elevates low-density lipoprotein (LDL) levels
- Increases total cholesterol levels

These three changes are associated with an increased risk of coronary artery disease and are explained in detail in Chapter 11.

In Summary

The use of anabolic steroids is unethical, unhealthy, and—in most cases—illegal. The possibility of developing severe and harmful side effects would appear to far outweigh any potential gains in athletic performance.

MEASUREMENT OF STRENGTH AND MUSCULAR ENDURANCE

Principle of specificity

Cardiovascular endurance is a general component and can be measured by one test. However, this is not the case with either strength or muscular endurance. Each of these is likely to vary considerably for each of the muscle groups. Because one muscle group has a high degree of strength and muscular endurance does not necessarily mean that other groups will be similarly developed. This is the principle of specificity. A good example is a gymnast who works on the parallel bars. If he or she is to be successful, a high degree of strength and muscular endurance in the upper body must be developed. Because the legs are used much less, strength and muscular endurance in the lower body will be considerably less than in the arms and shoulders.

Because of the principle of specificity, it is necessary to administer many different strength and muscular endurance tests so that different muscle groups can be evaluated.

Strength tests

Strength is measured by determining the maximum force that a muscle or muscle group can exert once and only once. This is referred to as 1 RM. Strength may be measured by either the isometric or isotonic method. Regardless of which is used, some equipment is necessary.

To measure strength isometrically, a dynamometer or tensiometer is used. A muscle or muscle group contracts, and this force is transmitted by springs or cables to the face of the instrument. The score can be read there. Little or no movement takes place with isometric tests. It is therefore important to standardize the angle for each test so that consistent results are obtained.

Strength may also be determined isotonically by determining the maximum amount of weight that can be moved once and only once through the designated range of motion. For example, if a person can perform one two-arm curl using 100 lb but cannot move 110 lb through the full range of motion, then the strength of the muscle group being tested (the flexors of the forearm) is approximately 100 lb. A trial and error system must be used with this method, and weights must be added or subtracted with adequate rest between trials in an attempt to determine the maximum weight that can be moved once. It should be emphasized that performing a number of repetitions with the same weight or sustaining a contraction over time measures muscular endurance rather than strength. Procedures for four strength tests are presented in Laboratory Experience 5-1 at the end of this chapter. However, the isotonic method just described can be used with any weight-training exercises to determine the strength of the muscle group involved. You may want to use the specific weight-training equipment that you have available to determine your strength for each muscle group that you exercise. In this way, you will be able to measure your progress.

Muscular endurance tests

For each group of muscles, muscular endurance can be measured by how many repetitions are performed continuously or in a designated period of time (isotonic), or by how long a contraction can be sustained (isometric). Procedures for the muscular endurance tests for men and women are included in Laboratory Experience 5-2 at the end of this chapter.

An alternate procedure for measuring muscular endurance is included in Laboratory Experience 5-3. The results from seven tests are combined to give you an "overall" measurement of muscular endurance.

Chapter Summary

The following summary will help you to identify some of the important concepts covered in this chapter:

- The level of strength and muscular endurance that you have will determine the efficiency with which you perform everyday tasks.
- All movements that occur in the body depend on the contraction of muscles.
- Because strength and muscular endurance are specific to each muscle group, you need to include specific exercises for each of the muscle groups that you wish to develop.
- The intensity of a weight-training workout relates to the extent that muscles are overloaded.
- To avoid muscle soreness, you need to warm up, start out at a low level of activity, and gradually increase the amount of work that you do.
- To measure strength, determine the maximum force that you can exert one time, whereas to measure muscular endurance, determine how many repetitions you can perform or how long you can sustain a specific contraction.

References

1. Allsen PE, Harrison JM, Vance B: *Fitness for life: an individualized approach*, ed 5, Dubuque, Ia, 1993, Brown & Benchmark.
2. American College of Sports Medicine: The use of anabolic-androgenic steroids in sports, *Sports Medicine Bulletin* 19:13, 1984.
3. Armstrong RB: Mechanisms of exercise-induced delayed onset muscle soreness: a brief review, *Med Sci Sports Exerc* 16:6-36, 1984.
4. Buckley W et al: Estimated prevalence of anabolic steroid use among male high school seniors, *JAMA* 260:3441, 1988.

5. Costill D et al: Anabolic steroid use among athletes: changes in HDL-C levels, *The Physician and Sportsmedicine* 12:112, 1984.

6. DiGennario J: *The new physical fitness: exercise for everybody,* Englewood, Colo, 1984, Morton.

7. Hurley BF et al: HDL cholesterol in body builders vs. power lifters. Negative effects of androgen use, *JAMA* 252:4, 1984.

8. Institute for Aerobic Research: *Common muscle imbalances,* Dallas, Tex, 1988, the Institute.

9. Manz RL: *The hydrafitness manual for omnikinetic training,* Belton, Tex, 1983, Hydra-Fitness Industries.

10. Prentice W: *Fitness for college and life,* ed 4, St Louis, 1994, Mosby.

11. Shields CL et al: Comparison of leg strength training equipment, *The Physician and Sportsmedicine* 13(2):49-56, 1985.

12. Stamford B: Building bigger muscles, *The Physician and Sports Medicine* 15(6):266, 1987.

13. Stone WJ, Kroll WA: *Sports conditioning and weight training. Programs for athletic competitors,* Newton, Me, 1986, Allyn & Bacon.

14. Westcott WL: *Strength fitness: physiological principles and training techniques,* ed 2, Boston, 1987, Allyn & Bacon.

Laboratory Experience 5-1

Measurement of Strength

Name _____   Section _____   Date _____

The following tests can be used to measure strength:
- Grip strength
- Back strength
- Bench press
- Leg strength

Grip Strength

Grip strength is probably the most common measurement, possibly because the hand dynamometer is available at many universities, health clubs, and schools. Squeeze the dynamometer as tightly as possible, using the musculature of the hand. No part of your upper or lower arm or your hand may push against any object or against any other part of your body. The force exerted may be read from the dial of the dynamometer and should be recorded to the nearest pound (Figure 5-36).

Results

Record results in the space provided.
Grip strength ____ lb

Back Strength

For testing back strength (Figure 5-37), use a back dynamometer. Stand upright on the base of the dynamometer with your feet shoulder-width apart, your arms straight, and your fingers extended downward as far as possible on the fronts of your thighs. The bar is then attached to the chain so that it is 1 to 2 inches below your fingertips. Then bend forward slightly and grasp the bar. The correct position to lift is with your back bent forward slightly at the hips and keeping your legs straight. Your head should be held upright, and you should look straight ahead. Lift steadily, keeping legs straight and feet flat on the base of the dynamometer. At the completion of the test, your back should be almost straight. If it is perfectly straight, the test should be repeated with the bar slightly lower.

Results

Record results in the space provided.
Back strength ____ lb

Bench Press

Either free weights or a bench press machine may be used for this test (Figure 5-13). Lie flat on the bench with your knees bent and feet flat on the floor. Determine by trial and error the maximum weight that can be lifted once. When lifting the weight, hold the barbell with the palms-forward grip at about the width of the shoulders. Press the bar directly upward until your arms are fully extended. Your back must not be arched during this test; it must remain in contact with the bench. If the bench is wide enough, it will be beneficial to bend your legs so that you have about a 90-degree angle at the knee joint and place your feet flat on the bench rather than on the floor.

Results

Record results in the space provided.
Bench press ____ lb

Leg Strength

The bar should be held in the center, with both hands together and with the palms facing toward the body. It should be at a level where the thighs and trunk meet (Figure 5-38). Your back must be kept straight as you pull as hard as possible on the chain and try to straighten your legs. Maximum performance will result when your legs are almost straight at the end of the lift. This will usually occur if the bar is attached to the dynamometer when the knees are bent at about 120 degrees.

Results

Record results in the space provided.
Leg strength ____ lb

Classification of Strength Scores

To evaluate the scores for each of the strength tests, refer to Table 5-3 (men) or Table 5-4 (women).

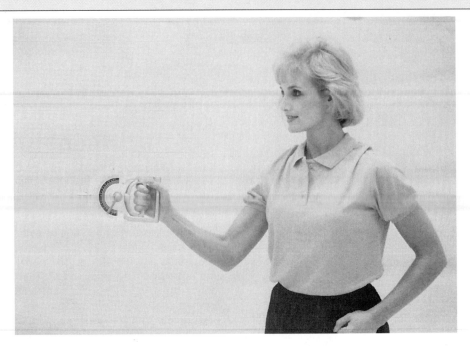

Figure 5-36   Measurement of grip strength.

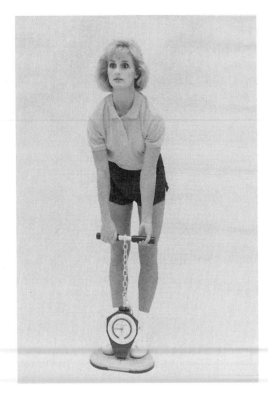

Figure 5-37   Measurement of back strength: an example of an isometric contraction.

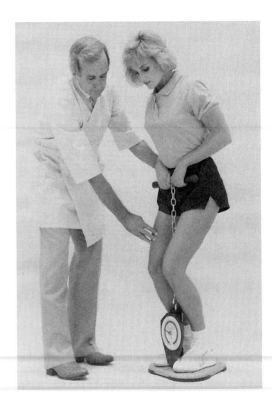

Figure 5-38   Position for the leg strength test.

Table 5-3 Strength Profile Chart (Men)

Percentile Rank	Grip Strength (lb)			Back Strength (lb)			Bench Press (lb)			Leg Strength (lb)			Fitness Category
	<30	30-50	>50	<30	30-50	>50	<30	30-50	>50	<30	30-50	>50	
95	150	135	118	451	406	358	203	183	161	504	454	400	Excellent
90	144	129	114	422	380	335	191	172	151	474	426	326	
80	136	123	108	387	348	307	175	158	139	436	393	346	Good
70	131	118	104	362	325	286	164	148	130	409	369	325	
60	126	114	100	340	306	269	155	139	122	386	348	307	Average
50	122	110	97	320	288	263	146	131	115	365	329	290	
40	118	106	94	300	270	237	137	123	108	344	310	273	
30	113	102	90	278	251	220	128	114	100	321	289	255	Fair
20	108	97	86	253	228	199	117	104	91	294	265	234	
10	100	91	80	218	196	171	101	90	79	256	232	204	Poor
5	94	85	76	189	170	148	89	79	69	226	204	180	
Mean	122	110	97	320	288	253	146	131	115	365	329	290	
Standard deviation	17	15	13	80	72	64	35	32	28	85	76	67	

Table 5-4 Strength Profile Chart (Women)

Percentile Rank	Grip Strength (lb)			Back Strength (lb)			Bench Press (lb)			Leg Strength (lb)			Fitness Category
	<30	30-50	>50	<30	30-50	>50	<30	30-50	>50	<30	30-50	>50	
95	84	76	67	266	239	210	105	95	84	301	271	238	Excellent
90	81	73	64	251	226	199	100	91	81	285	257	226	
80	76	69	61	234	210	185	95	86	76	266	240	211	Good
70	73	66	58	221	199	175	91	83	73	252	227	200	
60	71	63	56	210	189	166	88	80	71	241	217	191	Average
50	68	61	54	200	180	158	85	77	68	230	207	182	
40	66	59	52	190	171	150	82	74	66	219	197	174	
30	63	56	50	179	161	141	79	71	63	208	187	164	Fair
20	60	53	47	166	150	131	75	68	60	194	174	153	
10	55	46	44	149	134	117	70	63	55	175	157	138	Poor
5	52	46	41	134	121	106	65	59	52	159	143	126	
Mean	68	61	54	200	180	158	85	77	68	230	207	182	
Standard deviation	10	9	8	40	36	32	12	11	10	43	39	34	

Laboratory Experience 5-2

Measurement of Muscular Endurance

Name _____   Section _____   Date _____

Tests recommended for the measurement of muscular endurance for men and women are given in Table 5-5. Note that for women it may be necessary to modify the push-up and pull-up tests. The reason for this is the difference in upper body strength between men and women. Many college-aged women lack sufficient strength to do one regular pull-up and/or are unable to perform one regular push-up. The static push-up is offered as an alternate for the push-up or modified push-up because of the ease of administering the test.

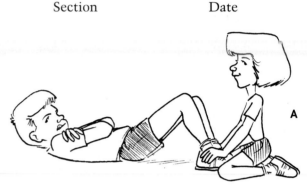

Table 5-5	Muscular Endurance Tests	
Test	**Suggested for Men**	**Suggested for Women**
Bent-leg curl-up	Yes	Yes
Push-up	Yes	No
Modified push-up	No	Yes
Static push-up	Yes	Yes
Pull-up	Yes	No
Flexed arm hang	No	Yes
Modified pull-up	No	Yes
Bench jump	Yes	Yes

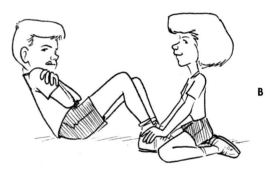

Figure 5-39 Start **(A)** and finish **(B)** positions for the bent-leg curl-up test.

Bent-leg Curl-up

The bent-leg curl-up measures muscular endurance of the abdominal muscles. These muscles are important in maintaining good posture. Poorly developed abdominal muscles also contribute to low back pain. To begin this test, lie on your back on the floor with your feet flat on the floor about shoulder-width apart and held by a partner. Knees should be flexed, approximately forming a right angle (Figure 5-39). Fold your arms across your chest, and move the top of your head as far forward as possible while pressing your chin against your chest. This is the start position for this test. Curl up until your elbows touch the upper part of your thighs, and then return until your lower back is in contact with the floor. Perform as many curl-ups as possible in 1 minute.

Results

Record results in the space provided.
Number of curl-ups in 1 minute ____

Push-up (Men Only)

The push-up measures endurance of the muscle group responsible for extension of the forearm. The largest muscle of this group is the triceps. Assume a prone position on the floor with hands directly under your shoulder joints, legs straight and together, and toes tucked under in contact with the floor. Then push with your arms until they are fully extended. The body is then lowered until your chin or chest touches the floor. At this point there should be a straight line from your head to your toes. All of this movement must be performed by the arms and shoulders, and not by any other part of the body. Perform as many push-ups as possible in 1 minute. You may rest in the up position if desired.

Results

Record results in the space provided.
Number of push-ups ____

Modified Push-up (Women Only)

To start this exercise, assume the regular push-up position but support your weight on your knees and not your feet. Your legs should be bent upward at the knees (Figure 5-40). Keeping your body in a straight line from the top of your head to your knees, lower your upper body until your chest just touches the floor and then push back up to the fully extended position. Perform as many repetitions as possible in 1 minute.

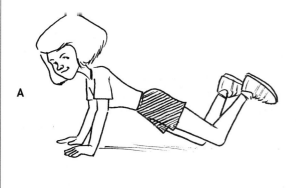

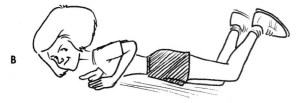

Figure 5-40 Start (**A**) and finish (**B**) positions for the modified push-up.

Results

Record results in the space provided.
Number of modified push-ups ____

Static Push-up

The static push-up (Figure 5-41) is an alternate test for the push-up or modified push-up test. It may be preferred because it is easier to administer and much easier to standardize the procedures. From a straight-arm front-leaning position with your hands directly under your shoulders, lower your body until your elbows are at 90 degrees. Hold this position for as long as possible. The test is terminated when any part of your body other than your hands or toes touches the floor or when you can no longer maintain your body in a straight line parallel to the floor.

Results

Record results in the space provided.
Time for static push-up ____ seconds

Bench Jump

The bench jump determines muscular endurance of the lower extremity. A 16-inch bench is used, and you jump up to the bench as many times as possible in 1 minute. If you are unable to jump, you may step up; however, this takes more time. Your arms may swing freely, but you are not permitted to push down on your thighs with your hands. One repetition is counted each time both feet are planted on the bench and then returned to the floor.

Results

Record results in the space provided.
Number of bench jumps in 1 minute ____

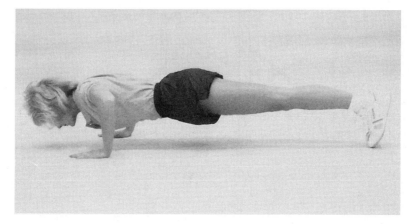

Figure 5-41 The position to be maintained in the static push-up. Note that the back must be straight, and the elbow joint must be at an angle of 90 degrees or less.

Pull-up (Men Only)

The pull-up primarily measures endurance of the muscle group responsible for flexion of the forearm. The major muscle of this group is the biceps brachii or, as it is commonly called, the biceps. Grasp the horizontal bar with both hands, palms forward. The "dead hang" position is assumed, with arms fully extended and feet off the ground. Raise your body until your chin is above the top of the bar, and then lower yourself until your arms are fully extended. The pull-up is repeated until you can no longer raise your chin above the bar. The knees may not be raised nor is kicking permitted to perform more pull-ups.

Results

Record results in the space provided.
Number of pull-ups ____

Flexed-arm Hang (Women Only)

The flexed-arm hang measures endurance of the flexors of the forearm. You must use the overhand grip with palms facing forward. Then raise your body off the floor until the chin is level with the bar. This position is maintained for as long as possible. Time is stopped when the chin cannot be maintained level with the bar.

Results

Record results in the space provided.
Time for flexed-arm hang
____ minutes ____ seconds

Modified Pull-up (Women Only)

For the modified pull-up, the chinning bar is adjusted to the height of the sternum and the feet remain in contact with the floor throughout. Grip the bar with palms forward, and slide your feet under the bar until your arms form a right angle with your body. Your weight must rest on your heels as you attempt to pull up, so that your chin or forehead touches the bar with the body held straight. This is repeated as many times as possible (Figure 5-42).

Results

Record results in the space provided.
Number of modified pull-ups ____

Evaluation of Muscular Endurance Test Scores

To evaluate your score for each of the muscular endurance tests, refer to Table 5-6 (men) or Table 5-7 (women).

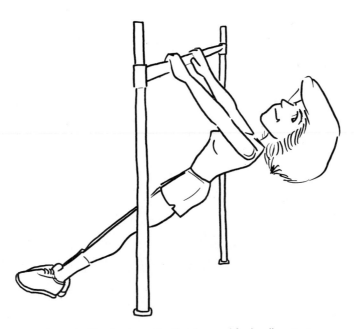

Figure 5-42 Start position for the modified pull-up test.

Table 5-6 Muscular Endurance Profile Chart (Men)

Percentile Rank	Bent-Leg Curl-Ups (1 minute) Age (years)			Static Push-Up (Time—seconds) Age (years)			Push-Ups (Repetitions) Age (years)			Pull-Ups (Repetitions) Age (years)			Bench Jump (Repetitions) Age (years)			Fitness Category
	<30	30-50	>50	<30	30-50	>50	<30	30-50	>50	<30	30-50	>50	<30	30-50	>50	
95	62	57	49	77	69	60	53	47	41	14	13	11	38	35	31	Excellent
90	59	54	46	72	65	57	50	44	39	12	11	10	36	33	29	
80	54	50	43	67	60	53	46	41	36	10	9	9	34	31	27	Good
70	51	47	40	63	57	50	43	38	34	9	8	8	33	30	26	
60	49	44	38	60	54	47	40	36	32	8	7	7	31	28	25	Average
50	46	42	36	57	51	45	38	34	30	7	6	6	30	27	24	
40	44	40	34	54	48	43	36	32	28	6	5	5	29	26	23	
30	41	37	32	51	45	40	33	30	26	5	4	4	27	24	22	Fair
20	38	34	29	47	42	37	30	27	24	4	3	3	26	23	21	
10	33	30	26	42	37	33	26	24	21	2	1	1	24	21	19	Poor
5	30	27	23	37	33	30	23	21	19	0	0	0	22	19	17	
Mean	46	42	36	57	51	45	38	34	30	7	6	6	30	27	24	
Standard deviation	10	9	8	12	11	9	9	8	7	4	4	3	5	5	4	

Table 5-7 **Muscular Endurance Profile Chart (Women)**

Percentile Rank	Bent-Leg Curl-Ups 1 minute Age (years)			Modified Push-Up (Repetitions) Age (years)			Static Push-Ups (Time—seconds) Age (years)			Flexed-Arm Hang (Time—seconds) Age (years)			Modified Pull-Ups (Repetitions) Age (years)			Bench Jump (1-minute) Age (years)			Fitness Category
	<30	30-50	>50	<30	30-50	>50	<30	30-50	>50	<30	30-50	>50	<30	30-50	>50	<30	30-50	>50	
95	50	45	39	45	41	35	39	34	31	19	18	14	41	36	32	28	25	23	Excellent
90	47	42	37	40	37	32	36	32	29	17	16	13	38	33	30	26	24	21	
80	43	39	34	35	32	28	33	29	26	15	14	12	34	30	27	24	22	19	Good
70	40	36	32	31	29	25	30	27	24	14	13	11	31	27	25	23	21	18	
60	37	34	30	28	26	22	28	25	23	13	12	10	28	25	23	21	19	17	Average
50	35	32	28	25	23	20	26	23	21	12	11	9	26	23	21	20	18	16	
40	33	30	26	22	20	18	24	21	20	11	10	8	24	21	19	19	17	15	
30	30	28	24	19	17	15	22	19	18	10	9	7	21	19	17	17	15	14	Fair
20	27	25	22	15	14	12	19	17	16	9	8	6	18	16	15	16	14	13	
10	23	22	19	10	9	8	16	14	13	7	6	5	14	13	12	14	12	11	Poor
5	20	19	17	5	5	5	13	12	11	5	4	4	11	10	10	12	10	9	
Mean	35	32	28	25	23	20	26	23	21	12	11	9	26	23	21	20	13	16	
Standard deviation	9	8	7	12	11	9	8	7	6	4	4	3	9	8	7	5	5	4	

Evaluating Muscular Endurance Using Weights or Weight Machine

Name _____ Section _____ Date _____

An alternate method of evaluating muscular endurance is adapted from Allsen, Harrison, and Vance[1] and is based on the earlier work of DiGennario.[6] Seven exercises are done to evaluate muscular endurance. These are identified in Table 5-8 and are described in detail previously in this chapter.

The resistance to be used in each exercise is a percentage of your body weight. These percentages are identified in Table 5-8. The resistance should be calculated by multiplying this percentage by your body weight and recorded in Table 5-8.

For each exercise, try to perform the maximum number of repetitions possible consecutively using the designated resistance. A maximum of 17 repetitions is allowed for men and 15 for women. Points are earned for each exercise based on the number of repetitions completed. These points may be determined by consulting Table 5-9. Points for each exercise should be recorded in Table 5-8, and the total number of points for all seven exercises is then determined. This is your overall score for muscular endurance. This score may be interpreted by consulting Table 5-10.

Table 5-8	Muscular Endurance Tests Using Weights				
Exercise	Body Weight	Percentage of Body Weight	Resistance To Be Used	Repetitions Completed	Points Earned
Two-arm curl	_____	× 0.33 =	_____	_____	_____
Bench press	_____	× 0.67 =	_____	_____	_____
Lateral machine pull-down	_____	× 0.67 =	_____	_____	_____
Upright rowing	_____	× 0.33 =	_____	_____	_____
Quadriceps lift	_____	× 0.67 =	_____	_____	_____
Leg curl	_____	× 0.33 =	_____	_____	_____
Curl-up	_____	× 0.14 =	_____	_____	_____

Table 5-9	Evaluation of Muscular Endurance Tests		
Repetitions			Muscular
Men	Women	Points	Endurance Category
0-3	0.2	5	Very poor
4	3	7	Poor
5-8	4-7	9	Fair
9-11	8-10	11	Good
12-16	11-14	13	Very good
17	15	15	Excellent

Table 5-10	Overall Muscular Endurance Classification (Total Points for All Seven Tests)
Points	Category
35-48	Very poor
49-62	Poor
63-76	Fair
77-90	Good
91-104	Very good
105	Excellent

Results

Record results in the space provided.

Total points earned: _____

Muscular endurance category: _____

Chapter Six **Flexibility**

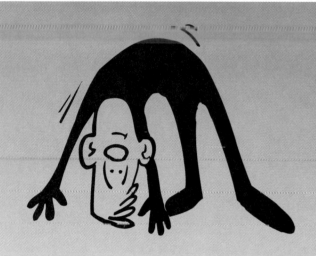

CHAPTER OBJECTIVES

Check off each objective you achieve:

- ❑ Define flexibility, and explain why it is important.
- ❑ Identify and discuss the factors that limit flexibility.
- ❑ Evaluate the different procedures used for the development of flexibility.
- ❑ Develop a flexibility program designed to meet your individual needs.
- ❑ Discuss the causes of low back pain, and know how to avoid and/or alleviate this problem.
- ❑ Measure your level of flexibility, and know how to interpret the results.
- ❑ Define each of the important terms.

Flexibility is one of the most important health-related components of physical fitness. It is often overlooked and misunderstood. It can be defined as the maximum range of motion possible at a **joint.**

The ability to move each joint through a full range of motion without undue strain is essential for the efficient execution of many everyday tasks. With limited flexibility, you may experience "tightness" or "stiffness" at joints and have difficulty performing some movements. Such simple tasks as pulling a shirt or blouse over your head, putting on slacks, tying shoelaces, or getting into or out of the back seat of a two-door car are often difficult for those with a limited range of motion at certain joints. Increased flexibility allows freer and more efficient movement with less resistance.

JOINT STRUCTURE AS IT RELATES TO MOVEMENT

Minimal information about joint structure and the role of muscles is necessary for a basic understanding of flexibility.

A joint is a junction of two or more bones where movement takes place. The joint's structure is important because it will determine what movements can take place at the joint and in some cases will limit the range of motion. For example, the elbow and knee joints are **hinge joints** that allow movement in only one direction. The only movements possible are flexion and extension. When the forearm and lower leg are fully extended, the bones "lock" into position and the structure of these joints permits no further movement in that direction.

In contrast, joints such as the shoulder and hip are **ball-and-socket joints.** The rounded head of one bone fits into a hollow cavity of another. This allows movement in many directions and will usually allow a greater range of motion than does a hinge joint.

Flexibility, however, it not limited just by the structure of joints. If it were, we could not improve flexibility because we are unable to change the structure of joints. Soft tissues play an important role and greatly influence the amount of movement possible at a joint. These tissues include muscles, **tendons,** and **ligaments.**

Muscles pass across joints and are attached to bones by a tendon. The force exerted by a muscle as it contracts is applied to a bone, and movement will take place at a joint if the force is sufficient to overcome the resistance. In Figure 6-1, if the force exerted by the biceps brachii is greater than the resistance caused by the weight and the forearm, then movement will take place at the elbow joint.

Muscles are arranged strategically in sets so that when one set contracts and shortens, another set lengthens and must relax. This is demonstrated in Figure 6-2.

Muscles are protected from overstretching by the **stretch reflex.** If you try to overstretch a muscle, it will actually contract to prevent this muscle from overstretching.

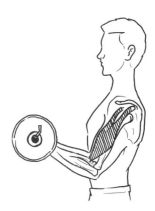

Figure 6-1   Contraction of the biceps brachii, resulting in flexion at the elbow point.

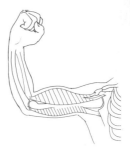

Figure 6-2   Contraction of the biceps muscle to cause flexion at the elbow joint will result in maximum range of motion only if the triceps muscle relaxes.

Flexibility: The maximal range of motion possible at a joint.

Joint: A junction of two or more bones.

Hinge joint: A joint that allows movement to take place in one direction where the only movements are flexion and extension.

Ball-and-socket joint: A joint where the rounded head of one bone fits into the hollow cavity of another.

Tendon: Fibrous tissue that connects muscles to bones.

Ligament: A tough band of tissue that holds joints together.

Stretch reflex: A mechanism that prevents overstretching of a muscle by forcing the muscle to contract.

BASIC FACTS ABOUT FLEXIBILITY

Following are some basic facts concerning flexibility. As you become more knowledgeable about flexibility, you will realize how important it is to maintain an adequate level of flexibility and you will be much more likely to take time to include flexibility exercises in your regular exercise program.

Inactivity contributes to poor flexibility

People who are active tend to be more flexible than those who are not because flexibility depends on movement. With little or no movement, muscles and other soft tissues tend to become shorter and tighter. They lose elasticity, and flexibility is decreased. This can clearly be seen by observing what happens when, because of an injury, an arm or a leg is placed in a cast. The reason for the cast is to immobilize the limb so that little or no movement takes place. When the cast is removed, the first thing you notice is that the muscles have lost both size and strength and that very little movement is now possible at the joint. Physical therapy is usually prescribed in an attempt to restore normal movement.

When you sit for extended periods, very little movement takes place and muscles can become weaker and joints less flexible. The hamstring muscle group is a good example. This is the large muscle group that crosses both the hip and knee joints at the back of your thighs. When you are sitting for long periods and there is flexion at both of these joints, these muscles are in a shortened position and they become accustomed to that position. The end result is that these muscles become shorter than what they should be, resulting in loss of flexibility at the hip joint, unless time is taken to stretch these muscles.

Decreased flexibility with age is usually caused by physical inactivity

Most people become less flexible as they get older. They have greater difficulty in performing basic skills and also have more aches and pains after physical activity. The reason for this is that most people become less active as they get older. This has some negative implications as far as flexibility is concerned.

The muscles become weaker, fatigue more easily, and function less efficiently. In some instances, this results in poor body alignment with a corresponding loss of flexibility. Also, lack of activity can contribute to loss of bone density, which contributes to osteoporosis. As joints become weaker, there is a significant loss of flexibility. A good flexibility program is important to decrease the loss of flexibility that occurs as you get older.

Women are usually more flexible than are men of the same age

During adolescence, when flexibility reaches its highest level, the difference between males and females is most pronounced. Girls have a much greater range of motion than do boys. The norms for college students and adults indicate that women have slightly higher scores than do men. The reason may be that they tend to participate more in activities that promote flexibility, such as dance and gymnastics (Figure 6-3).

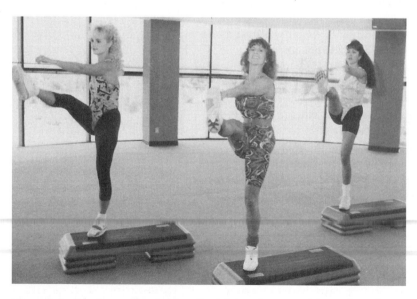

Figure 6-3   Bench aerobics develops flexibility and is a good form of aerobic exercise.

Excessive body fat usually limits flexibility

Obese people usually have difficulty moving efficiently, and their range of motion at certain joints is often restricted. Fat deposits act as a wedge between moving parts of the body, thus restricting movement.

Participation in some activities improves flexibility

Regular participation in physical activities that involve a full range of movement at a joint will help to prevent loss of movement and increase flexibility. A good example is the crawl stroke in swimming. The elbow joint moves through a full range of motion, and flexibility will be developed (Figure 6-4).

Some activities use a limited range of motion and will possibly decrease flexibility. For example, with jogging there is slight flexion at the hip and knee joints most of the time. This can result in a shortening of muscles in the back of the leg. Unless they are stretched, particularly after each exercise session, decreased flexibility can occur (Figure 6-5).

Flexibility is specific to each joint

Flexibility is not a general component of physical fitness. Instead, it is specific to each joint. This means that you may have a good range of motion in some joints and a poor range of motion in others. Flexibility is not a single characteristic because it is not uniformly present in each joint. Because of this, you must include specific exercises for each movement at each joint for which you want to increase flexibility.

Poor flexibility can contribute to poor posture

Poor flexibility is often caused by muscles that are shorter and tighter than they should be. It may also be a result of an imbalance of development of opposing pairs of muscles. These conditions often contribute to poor posture.

Poor flexibility is often associated with increased tension and pain

It has been known for a long time that stretching is beneficial for alleviation of stress and tension. Those who are under prolonged stress often have pain in the neck, shoulders, and back. One reason is that with constant tension and stress, muscles are tighter than they should be. We have already seen that this can contribute to poor flexibility.

Too much flexibility may be harmful

It is important to stretch within the normal limits of your body and not exceed this range of motion. When joints are overstretched, ligaments and muscles tend to lose elasticity and may remain lengthened rather than returning to their original size. If this happens, a joint may become less stable and more prone to injury. This condition often occurs with basketball players who fre-

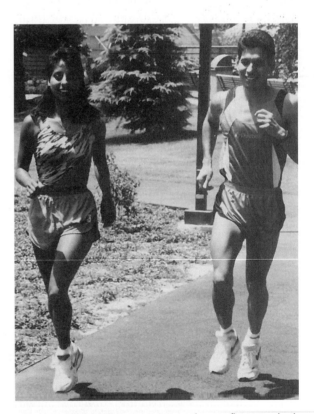

Figure 6-5 With walking or jogging, there is flexion at both the hip and knee joints. For this reason, it is important to stretch the hamstring muscle group at the end of each exercise session.

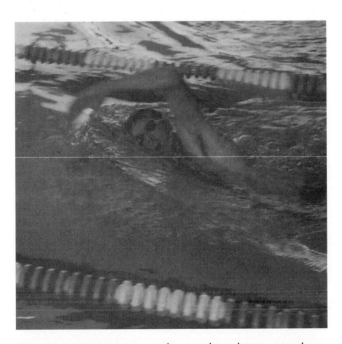

Figure 6-4 Swimming is another good aerobic exercise that develops flexibility.

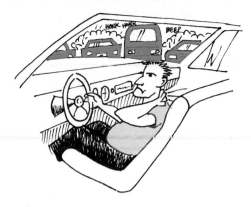

Stress often creates tension in the neck and shoulders.

quently land off balance on the side of their feet after jumping. Ligaments holding the ankle joint in place become stretched and lose their elasticity.

Muscle imbalance may reduce flexibility

We have seen that muscles are arranged in pairs and that as one muscle shortens and contracts, another will lengthen and relax (Figure 6-2). It is important to maintain a strength and flexibility "balance" between opposing pairs of muscles. For example, if weight training strengthens one group of muscles and neglects the opposing group, a loss of flexibility at that joint will occur.

Skill often depends on a high level of flexibility

Participants in sports recognize the importance of flexibility and are aware that good performance depends on adequate flexibility. A flexible joint increases your ability to reach and stretch during performance and allows you to move more easily and efficiently from one position to another. The importance of this can be seen in such sports as racquetball, tennis, and soccer. In other sports and activities, an extremely high level of flexibility is essential for success. These include dancing, gymnastics, figure skating, diving, sprinting, and cheerleading. Participants in these activities need to work at maximum development of flexibility (Figure 6-6).

Increased flexibility helps to prevent muscle related injuries

Joints are constantly stressed during activities when muscles contract repeatedly. Injuries often occur when a short, tight muscle contracts vigorously. Increased flexibility can reduce injuries by allowing body parts to move more freely. This is particularly true in activities involving agility or speed.

Increased flexibility helps to reduce muscle soreness

A good stretching program, particularly after an exercise session, can reduce the muscle stiffness and soreness that often result from a vigorous workout.

DEVELOPMENT OF FLEXIBILITY

Flexibility may be developed using several techniques. The three most common are the ballistic, static, and contract-relaxation methods.

Ballistic stretching technique

Although the **ballistic stretching** technique is successful in the development of flexibility, most authorities no longer recommend its use, particularly for those simply interested in the development of an adequate level of flexibility. In addition, it is not recommended for those who are suspect to frequent muscle injuries.

This method uses momentum generated from bouncing and jerking movements to produce the force necessary to stretch muscles. The alternate toe-touch exercise is an example of a ballistic stretching exercise. With this exercise, you assume a standing position with the legs straight, feet shoulder-width apart, and arms extended above your head. Keeping your legs straight, reach down to touch the left foot with your right hand, then return to the starting position before reaching down again to touch the right foot with your left hand (Figure 6-7).

The major concern relative to this method of stretching is that the force generated by the body's mo-

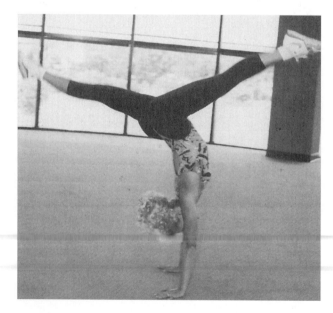

Figure 6-6   Skill in gymnastics requires a high degree of flexibility.

Stretching exercises are important but should not substitute for the warm-up. The reason is that each stretching exercise is designed to increase the range of motion at a specific joint. They do little to increase the circulation of the blood or to raise the body temperature or temperature of muscles.

Warming up first before performing flexibility exercises will result in the following:

- A greater range of motion at the joint
- Reduced likelihood of injury and soreness
- Maximum increase in the elasticity of the muscle

Flexibility and weight training

It is a common misconception that weight training reduces flexibility and will contribute to a decrease in the range of motion possible at joints. This will not occur in a weight-training program where each exercise is performed correctly through a full range of motion and where exercises for opposing muscle groups are included. A good weight-training program should supplement a good flexibility program. Not only will it increase flexibility, but it will also strengthen the muscles that cause movement at each of the joints. This additional strength should assist in avoiding injury during any activity, but particularly in those such as football, soccer, basketball, and racquetball, which involve contact or sudden vigorous bursts of movement.

EXERCISES FOR DEVELOPMENT OF FLEXIBILITY

The following exercises can be used to develop the range of motion at specific joints.

Forward lunge stretch

Step forward with the right leg flexing your knee and keeping your knee directly above your ankle. Your left leg is stretched back behind you as you thrust your hips forward and down until your left knee comes close to the floor. Hold this position. Repeat this movement with the opposite leg (Figure 6-8).

Sitting hamstring stretch

Start this exercise by sitting on a bench with one leg extended and the other leg flexed at the knee joint with the foot resting comfortably on the floor (Figure 6-9). Bend slowly from the waist, making sure that you keep

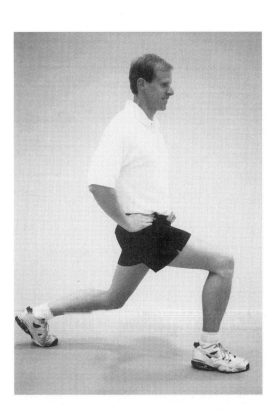

Figure 6-8 Forward lunge stretch.

your lower back straight, and slide both your hands slowly down the extended leg until you feel tightness in the back of your leg. If you can reach your toes, grasp them and pull them toward you to exert a stretch in the calf and hamstring muscles. Hold this position. Repeat the movement with the opposite leg.

Lying hamstring stretch

Start this exercise by lying on your back with your left leg straight. Grasp behind the right thigh and, with your right leg flexed at the knee joint, pull your right leg gently toward your chest until you feel tension in the hamstrings. Hold this position (Figure 6-10).

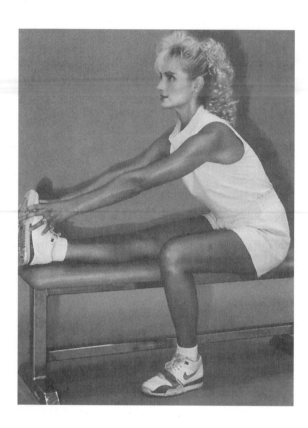

Figure 6-9   Sitting hamstring stretch performed while sitting on a bench. Care should be taken to make sure your back remains straight.

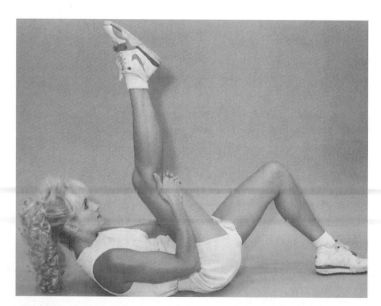

Figure 6-10   Lying hamstring stretch.

Achilles tendon and calf stretcher

Stand facing the wall with your feet about 12 inches apart, 2 to 3 feet from the wall (Figure 6-11). Lean forward and place the palms of your hands flat against the wall. Slowly bend forward, bringing the elbows closer to the wall, making sure that your body and legs remain straight and your heels remain in contact with the floor. Bend forward until you feel tightness in the calf and in the tendons that attach to your heel. Hold this position.

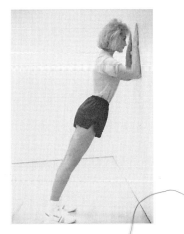

Figure 6-11 Achilles tendon and calf stretcher.

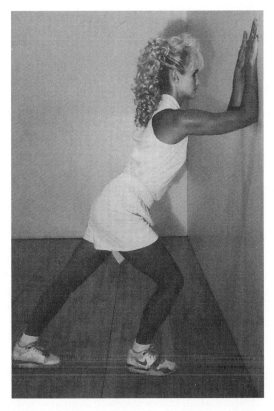

Figure 6-12 Achilles tendon and calf stretcher. Stretch one leg at a time.

This exercise may also be performed by stretching one leg at a time. If this is preferred, place one foot in front of the other foot, with the front foot approximately 9 inches from the wall, and follow the same procedures as outlined previously. If this stretch is to be effective, the heel of the back foot must remain in contact with the floor (Figure 6-12).

Low back stretcher

Start the low back stretcher (Figure 6-13) by lying on your back with your left leg bent at the knee and your left foot flat on the floor. Your right leg should be straight, and your arms should be by your sides. Slowly flex your right leg, and, grasping it just below the knee, pull your knee toward your chest. At the same time, tuck your chin in and bring your forehead as close to your knee as possible. Hold this position. This stretch should be felt in the lower back. Care must be taken to keep the flat of your back in contact with the floor at all times. This exercise may also be performed by pulling both knees toward your chest at the same time (Figure 6-14).

Lateral bend

The lateral bend (Figure 6-15) is designed to stretch the lateral muscles of the trunk and upper body. Start in the front standing position, with the feet shoulder-width apart and the left arm extended upward and the right arm down with the palm touching the outer right thigh. Bend your trunk to the right by sliding the right hand down the side of the right thigh as far as possible. At the same time, lift the left side of your body toward the ceiling so that the stretch is felt in the left side above your waist. Hold this position.

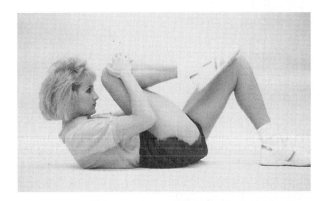

Figure 6-13 Low back stretcher.

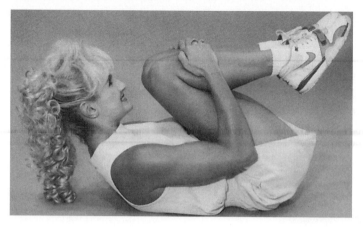

Figure 6-14   Low back stretcher, pulling knees toward your chest.

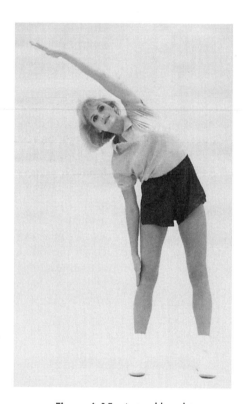

Figure 6-15   Lateral bend.

Quadriceps stretch

The quadriceps stretch (Figure 6-16) is designed to stretch the quadriceps muscle group—the large set of muscles located in the front of the thigh. Start by standing 2 to 3 feet away from a wall, and support yourself by placing your left hand against the wall. Supporting your weight on your left foot, flex your right knee, lift it up in front of you, and grasp the front of your right ankle with your right hand. Slowly move your bent right knee downward and backward, and at the same time push your right foot slowly away from your buttocks while resisting this movement with your hand. You should feel tension in your right front thigh. Hold this position.

Groin stretch

The groin stretch (Figure 6-17) is designed to stretch the muscles in the inner thighs. Start by sitting on the floor with the knees flexed, with the bottoms of your feet touching each other, and attempt to reach a position in which your heels are no more than 9 inches from your buttocks. Grasp your ankles with both hands, and pull your head and chest forward and downward as you push your knees toward the floor, until the stretch is felt in the upper thigh area. Make sure that you keep your back straight at all times. Hold this position. The elbows may be used to press on the inside of the thighs to add to the stretch.

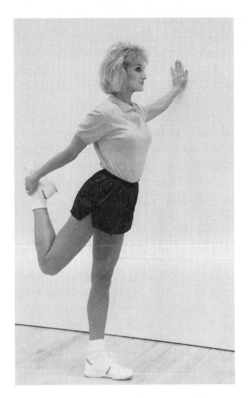

Figure 6-16   Quadriceps stretch.

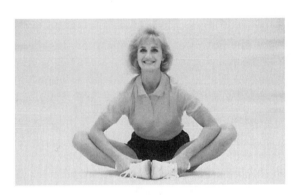

Figure 6-17   Groin stretch.

Lateral leg raises

Lateral leg raises (Figure 6-18) are designed to contract the lateral hip muscles and stretch the adductor muscles on the medial side of the leg. Start by lying on your right side with your left leg bent slightly at the knee and in contact with the floor. Your left leg should remain straight. Your right arm should be extended above your head and in contact with the floor, and your head should rest comfortably on your right arm. Your left arm should be positioned so that your left hand rests on the floor in front of your chest to maintain balance. Move your left leg upward slowly as far as possible with the leg straight and the knee facing frontward. Your foot should be extended with your toes as far away from the ankle as possible. Hold this position.

Arm circles

Arm circles (Figure 6-19) increase the flexibility of the shoulder joint. Start this exercise by standing with your feet shoulder-width apart. Let your arm describe a circle from front to back, initiating the movement at the shoulder joint and making sure it moves through a full range of motion. This exercise may be performed with one arm at a time or with both arms at the same time and may be done by moving the arm(s) front to back or back to front. If it is performed with one arm, the body should give slightly with it; there will be a slight body rotation. If it is performed with both arms together, the circles will come closer to the front of your body, and there will be no body rotation.

Hip circles

Hip circles (Figure 6-20) develop flexibility of the hip joint. Start this exercise by standing 2 to 3 feet away from a wall, and place your right hand against the wall

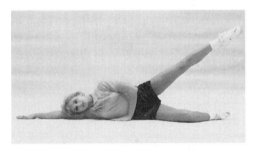

Figure 6-18   Lateral leg raise.

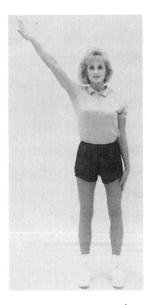

Figure 6-19   Arm circles.

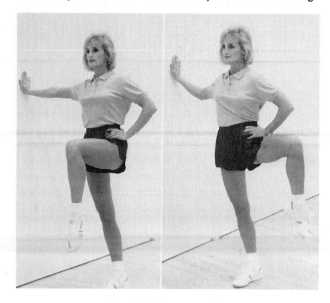

Figure 6-20   Hip circles.

to maintain balance. Support your weight on the right leg. Bend the left knee comfortably and describe a circle, starting with the thigh in front of the body and moving it through the full range of motion to where it is level with or even slightly behind the hips. This movement may also be performed in the opposite direction.

LOW BACK PAIN

Low back pain is one of the most common complaints among adults in the United States. If you have difficulty in straightening up after sitting all morning, if you feel pain in your back when you bend over to pick something up, or if you have difficulty bending to tie your shoelaces, there is a strong possibility that you are a prime candidate for low back pain.

Facts and Figures

Low back pain

- An estimated 80% of all Americans will experience low back pain at least once during their lives.
- More than 85 million Americans suffer from low back pain each year.
- Low back pain frequently occurs between the ages of 25 and 50 when many people become less active.
- It is estimated that 80% or more of all low back pain problems are caused by improper muscular development.

Causes of low back pain

For most people, low back pain is a hypokinetic disease caused by lack of activity that results in inadequate muscular development. Development and maintenance of muscle function depend on its use. The strength of a muscle is directly related to the amount of work it does. As a muscle works against a resistance, the strength of that muscle will increase. If the muscle does not perform well, a loss of strength will result. In an inactive person, many of the large muscle groups are not used often enough. They therefore lack enough strength to maintain correct body alignment, which is one of their specific tasks.

Poor abdominal development is one of the most common causes of low back pain. The pelvis should be tipped up in the front, but if the abdominal muscles are weak, they are unable to exert enough pressure to keep the pelvis in place and it drops down in the front, causing a forward pelvis tilt. This in turn causes the vertebrae in the low back region to be slightly displaced, and their articular processes press against one another, causing the ache in the lower area of the back.

Another group of muscles associated with low back pain is commonly referred to as the hamstring muscle group. This group consists of three large muscles that are located at the back of the thigh, and all are associated with movement at both the hip and the knee joints.

Most people experience difficulty in touching their toes with the fingertips without bending the knees because the hamstring muscles often are not long enough to permit such extreme stretching. This shortening of the hamstring muscle group often occurs in those who spend a lot of time sitting (Figure 6-21, *A*). If these muscles are not given stretching exercises, and if they are constantly held in positions that tend to shorten them, they become adjusted to this position. When a person stands, both the knee and hip joints are fully extended (Figure 6-21, *B*). If the hamstring muscles are shorter than they should be, this will cause both direct pain in the immediate area of the muscles and referred pain in the low back region.

LOW BACK PAIN AND PERFORMANCE OF EVERYDAY TASKS

If you have already experienced low back pain or if you want to reduce your chances of suffering from it in the future, it may be necessary to change the way you perform everyday activities. How you sit, stand, rest, or sleep can be extremely important. The following suggestions may help:

- When sitting, if possible, have your knees slightly higher than your hips and sit upright rather than with your shoulders forward.

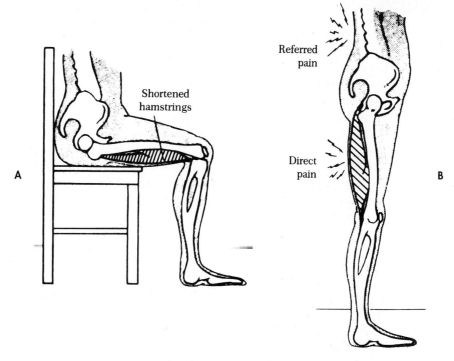

Figure 6-21 **A,** Position of the hamstring muscle group in relation to the bone structure when sitting. If much of the time is spent sitting, this muscle group may become much shorter than it should be. **B,** Effect that a shortening of the hamstring muscles has on the pelvis when you assume an upright standing position.

- When sitting at a desk, move the chair in as close as possible so that you are more upright rather than bent over your work.

- When standing, try to keep your knees slightly bent and one foot slightly in front of the other.

- When lifting objects, bend at the knees and hips and make sure the object is as close to your body as possible when both lifting and carrying it.

- At least once a day, try to lie flat on the floor or other flat surface with your knees bent at right angles and legs resting on the top of a chair or coffee table.

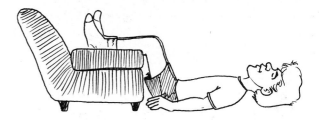

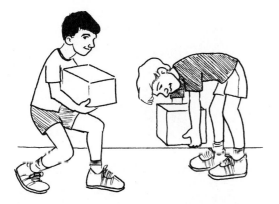

The correct and incorrect ways to lift objects.

- When sleeping on your back, place a pillow under your knees so that they are raised slightly.

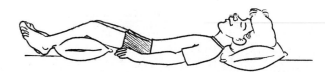

EXERCISES FOR ALLEVIATING LOW BACK PAIN

Most of those who suffer from low back pain can relieve the problem if they perform a few simple exercises each day. These can also be done for prevention of low back pain. Exercises need to be selected that will place a minimal amount of stress on the lower back and that will strengthen the abdominal muscles and stretch the hamstring muscles. The following six exercises can be used for these purposes. It is suggested that two sets of each be performed each day, starting with five repetitions per set and gradually increasing to 10.

Pelvic tilt

Lie on your back on the floor with your knees bent, your feet on the floor, and your arms resting comfortably by your sides (Figure 6-22). Tighten your stomach muscles, and consciously tilt your pelvis so that your lower back is flat against the floor. Hold this position for a minimum of 10 seconds, then relax.

Partial curl-up

Lie on your back with your knees bent at 90 degrees, with your feet flat on the floor and your arms crossed comfortably across your chest (Figure 6-23). Slowly curl your head, shoulders, and trunk toward your knees without jerking, until you can feel the contraction of your abdominal muscles. Your lower back should remain in contact with the floor. Hold for a minimum of 10 seconds, and return to the floor.

Partial wall slide

Stand with your back toward a wall and your feet shoulder-width apart, about 3 to 6 inches from the wall (Figure 6-24). Lean against the wall, and slide your buttocks down slowly until you can feel your lower back flat against it. Hold this position for 10 seconds. (NOTE: For those wishing to develop the quadriceps at the same time, the buttocks should be moved farther down until the thighs are positioned parallel to the floor, and this position should be held.)

The following three additional exercises can be used for relief or prevention of low back pain:

- Lying hamstring stretch (see Figure 6-10)
- Low back stretcher (see Figure 6-13)
- Sitting hamstring stretch (see Figure 6-9)

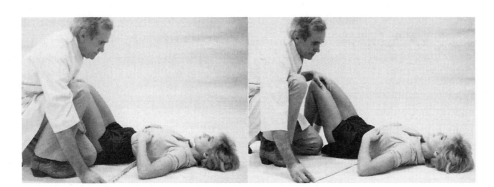

Figure 6-22 Pelvic tilt.

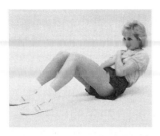

Figure 6-23 Partial curl-up.

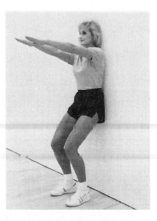

Figure 6-24 Partial wall slide.

MEASUREMENT OF FLEXIBILITY

Because flexibility is specific to each joint, it is not possible to measure it with one test. Each movement possible at a joint must be measured if all aspects of flexibility are to be evaluated (Figure 6-25).

A number of indirect tests requiring little or no equipment have been developed for classroom use that measure movement at certain joints. The three most common tests are the following:

- Trunk flexion—sit and reach
- Trunk extension
- Shoulder lift

The procedures for these tests are included in Laboratory Experiences 6.1 to 6.3 at the end of this chapter. Norms are also included so that you can evaluate your results.

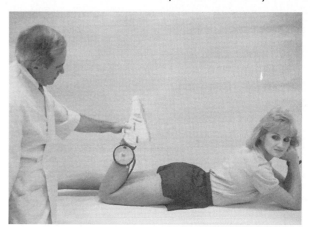

Figure 6-25 An instrument such as a flexometer can measure joint flexibility.

Let's Get Started

Preventing Low Back Pain

Because of the increase in the incidence of low back pain and the rising cost associated with its treatment, it would appear as if prevention is the best solution. The following suggestions may help you to get started:

- Regularly perform exercises to strengthen the abdominal muscles.
- Regularly perform exercises to stretch your hamstring muscles at the back of your legs.
- Reduce your percent of body fat, if necessary, to decrease the amount of stress on the back. This is particularly important if you accumulate excessive body fat in the abdominal area.
- Maintain a correct posture as frequently as possible. Do not "slump" when sitting at your desk or when driving your car.
- Avoid sitting or standing in any one position for long periods of time.
- Warm up and stretch before participating in vigorous exercise, particularly those forms of exercise that involve stop-start motion, such as racquetball, tennis, etc.

Chapter Summary

The following summary will help you to identify some of the important concepts covered in this chapter:

- Your level of flexibility will be reflected by the range of movement that is possible at each of the joints.
- If you do not exercise and/or you sit for long periods, your flexibility at certain joints is likely to be less than adequate.
- Poor flexibility is often associated with poor posture, muscle soreness, and increased incidence of muscle-related injuries, tension, and pain.
- The two best methods for the development of flexibility appear to be static stretching and the contract-relaxation method. The ballistic method is not recommended.
- Flexibility exercises need to be included in each exercise session, in addition to warm-up activities and your aerobic workout.
- Possibly 80% of low back pain problems are directly related to improper muscular development.
- Flexibility exercises are designed to reduce pain and muscle soreness, not to create them.

References

1. Alter JM: *Stretch and strengthen*, Boston, 1986, Houghton Mifflin.
2. Alter JM: *The science of stretching*, Champaign, Ill, 1988, Human Kinetics.
3. Anderson B: *Stretching for everyday fitness*, Bolinas, Calif, 1980, Shelter Publications.
4. Brehm BA: How to warm up and why, *Fitness Management*, p 18, Nov/Dec 1987.
5. Brehm BA: Stretching, *Fitness Management*, p 15, Sept/Oct 1987.
6. Brehm BA: The warm-up: its physiological contribution to safe and effective exercise, *Fitness Management*, pp 19-20, Nov/Dec 1987.
7. Corbin CB: *Concepts of physical fitness*, ed 8, 1994, Dubuque, Ia., Brown & Benchmark.
8. Eller D: Flextime, *Am Health* 12(3):68-73, 1993.
9. Leighton JR: Instrument and technic for measurement of range of joint motion, *Arch Phys Med Rehabil* 36:571, 1955.
10. Low back pain, *Mayo Clinic Health Letter*, 7:4, 1989.
11. Nieman DC. *Fitness and sports medicine: an introduction*, ed 2, Palo Alto, Calif, 1995, Bull Publishing.
12. Prentice WE: *Fitness for college and life*, ed 4, St Louis, 1994, Mosby.
13. Rushing S: *Exercises for people who hate to exercise: exercises for flexibility, muscle tone and relaxation*, San Antonio, Tex, 1982, Rushing Productions.
14. Shellock FG: Physiological benefits of warm-up, *The Physician and Sportsmedicine* 11(10):134, 1983.

Measurement of Flexibility: Trunk Flexion— Sit and Reach Test

Name   Section   Date

Purpose

The purpose of this test is to measure trunk flexion. This will be determined by your ability to stretch the lower back and hamstring muscles.

Equipment

Equipment needed is a flex box with a measuring scale marked in inches or centimeters. (NOTE: A yardstick taped to either the lowest row of bleachers or to a bench turned on its side can be used.)

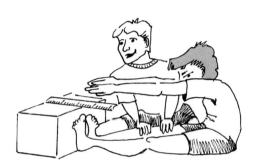

Procedure

1. Remove your shoes and sit with your knees fully extended and the bottom of your feet flat against the surface of the flex box.
2. Your arms are extended forward, with one hand placed on the top of the other.
3. With the instructor or partner holding your knees straight, steadily reach as far forward as possible and maintain this position for 3 seconds. (NOTE: No bouncing or jerking movements are allowed, and it is important that the knees remain absolutely straight. Slight flexion at the knee joint will greatly influence the results.)

Scoring

The distance in front of or beyond the edge of the board that can be sustained is measured and recorded. Measurements in front of the board are negative, whereas those beyond are positive. Record your score in the space provided below.

Trunk flexion—sit and reach

____ inches

(Be sure to indicate + or −.)

Classification of Scores

To evaluate your score, refer to Table 6-1.

Table 6-1	**Trunk Flexion: Sit and Reach Test**		
Classification	**Percentile Rank**	**Men**	**Women**
Excellent	95	9.5	10.5
	90	8.0	9.0
Good	80	6.5	7.5
	70	5.0	6.0
Average	60	4.0	5.0
	50	3.0	4.0
	40	2.0	3.0
Fair	30	1.0	2.0
	20	−0.5	0.5
Poor	10	−2.0	0.0
	5	−3.5	−2.5

Measurement of Flexibility: Trunk Extension

Name   Section   Date

Purpose

The purpose of this test is to determine the range of motion when the back is arched from the prone position.

Procedures

1. Lie face down on the floor, with a partner applying pressure on the back of the thighs.
2. With fingers interlocked behind your neck, gently raise your head and shoulders as far as possible from the floor.
3. This position must be held for 3 seconds (Figure 6-26).

Scoring

The distance from the floor to the chin is measured to the nearest ½ inch. Record your score in the space provided below.

Trunk extension _____ inches

Classification of Scores

To evaluate your score, refer to Table 6-2.

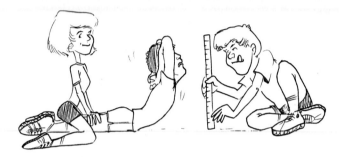

Figure 6-26 Trunk extension test of flexibility.

Table 6-2	**Trunk Extension Flexibility Test**		
Classification	**Percentile Rank**	**Men**	**Women**
Excellent	95	23.5	26.0
	90	22.0	24.0
Good	80	20.0	22.0
	70	19.0	20.5
Average	60	18.0	19.0
	50	17.0	18.0
	40	16.0	17.0
Fair	30	15.0	15.5
	20	14.0	14.0
Poor	10	12.0	12.0
	5	10.5	10.0

Laboratory Experience 6-3

Measurement of Flexibility: Shoulder Lift Test

Name _____   Section _____   Date _____

Purpose

The purpose of this test is to measure flexion at the shoulder joint.

Procedure

1. Lie face down with your chin on the floor and your arms fully extended and parallel.
2. Hold a stick or ruler horizontally with both hands. Keep elbows and wrists straight.
3. Raise your arms upward as far as possible, with your chin remaining in contact with the floor. (NOTE: Make sure your chin remains in contact with the floor and that you do not extend the wrists to increase your score.) (Figure 6-27)

Scoring

The distance is measured from the bottom of the stick or ruler to the floor. Record your score in the space provided below.

Shoulder lift ____ inches

Classification of Scores

To evaluate your score, refer to Table 6-3.

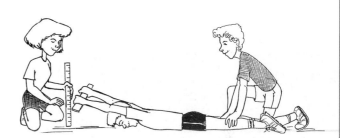

Figure 6-27   Shoulder lift test of flexibility.

Table 6-3	**Shoulder Flexion Test**		
Classification	**Percentile Rank**	**Men**	**Women**
Excellent	95	28.0	29.0
	90	26.0	27.0
Good	80	24.0	25.0
	70	22.0	23.0
Average	60	21.0	21.5
	50	19.0	20.0
	40	17.0	18.5
Fair	30	16.0	17.0
	20	14.0	15.0
Poor	10	12.0	10.0
	5	10.0	11.0

Chapter Seven   Nutrition and Fitness

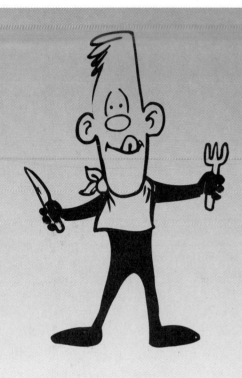

CHAPTER OBJECTIVES

Check off each objective you achieve:

☐ Describe what it means to eat well and be able to analyze and evaluate your eating habits.

☐ Identify the six major categories of nutrients that you need to be healthy, and know how to plan a nutritionally balanced diet to include appropriate amounts of each of them.

☐ Differentiate between simple and complex carbohydrates and know how to increase your intake of complex carbohydrates without getting an excessive amount of fat.

☐ Differentiate between complete and incomplete protein and know how to select foods to ensure an adequate protein intake.

☐ Explain why an excessive amount of fat is more fattening than is the same amount of protein and carbohydrates and be able to identify foods low in fat.

☐ Analyze your food intake using the exchange lists or other appropriate techniques, evaluate your obtained scores, and know how to incorporate necessary changes.

Many students who are fighting to control their weight and/or body fat seldom find time to exercise and have constantly been on one diet or another. While most of these students are aware of the importance of regular exercise and good nutrition, they either do not know what to do or else they lack the motivation to do it.

The 1988 Surgeon General's Report on Nutrition and Health states that for people who do not smoke or drink excessively, one personal choice influences their long-term health more than any other and that is what they eat. The results from a recent national survey substantiate this. More than 85% of the American population agreed with the following two statements:

"I can do more for my health by what I do and what I eat than anything doctors or medicine can do."

"If I exercise and eat right I am almost certain to stay healthy."

The average person in today's world is confused about what constitutes a healthy diet and has a hard time establishing a consistent healthful eating pattern.

In America our nutritional habits have changed during recent years

The average American now eats out four times each week, with fast-food restaurants accounting for almost 50% of the business. There are too many choices, and the everyday decisions that we must make are not as easy as they used to be.

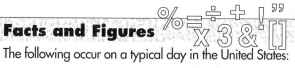

Facts and Figures

- The average American adult eats almost half of his or her meals away from home.
- Only 39% of adults eat the traditional three meals each day.
- Less than 50% of the entire population eats breakfast each day.
- Over 40% of the people who eat out eat at fast-food restaurants.

In Summary

Skipping meals and eating out make it difficult to develop good, consistent eating habits.

The large variety of foods now available makes it difficult to make good choices

With over 15,000 different food items now available in supermarkets, a person may have a difficult time deciding which ones to purchase. Advertising claims such as cholesterol free, reduced calorie, fat free, low fat, all natural, and high fiber contribute to the confusion about what is truly healthy and what is not. The advertising claims made by many of the health food stores regarding their foods and supplements are also misleading. Although there are many healthy foods available, they are often outnumbered by less nutritious foods that are advertised more frequently and made to look more attractive. A recent survey showed that despite the fact that 75% of shoppers cited nutrition as their primary reason for selecting certain foods, 90% of them actually made their selections on the basis of taste.

Facts and Figures

The following occur on a typical day in the United States:

- The average person will drink more soft drinks than milk. (Note: Coca-Cola spends $500,000 per day on advertising.)
- Half of the food consumed each day is processed rather than fresh.
- Almost two thirds of the total calories consumed each day comes from fat and sugar.
- One quarter of the vegetables eaten each day are potatoes, with the majority of these being in the form of French fries or potato chips.

Case Study

JILL and JANE

Jill and Jane work in the same office. Jill carefully plans her schedule for the day so that she has 10 minutes before going to work in the morning to eat a healthy breakfast at home. She usually has a bowl of cereal with a glass of milk and a piece of fruit. Jane on the other hand, rushes out the door each morning without eating and either stops at McDonald's, where she gets an Egg McMuffin and eats in her car while driving to work, or she stops at the local Dunkin Donut store where she picks up a bran muffin. The following comparison of these three meals shows that when you eat out it is often more difficult to limit your fat consumption because of the choices available and how the food is prepared.

Food	Cereal, Skim Milk, and Fruit	McDonald's Egg McMuffin	Dunkin Donut Bran Muffin
Calories	315	327	353
Fat grams	2	15	13

The many different food choices now available create confusion about which ones are best (Figure 7-1).

The nutritional information that is available is often confusing and contradictory

We are exposed to different diets, different health foods and supplements, and conflicting research reports daily. These add to the confusion, and the average person has a hard time knowing what to believe and deciding what is best. Even the information on food labels is very confusing. This has forced the Federal Drug Administration to initiate new standards for food labeling. Although the new labels are much better than the old ones, there is still a lot of confusing information.

Some of the everyday questions that people have are the following:

- "Do I need vitamin and mineral supplements?"
- "Do I have to eliminate red meat from my diet?"
- "Are fast foods really that bad for me?"
- "Is it important to eat breakfast?"
- "Do I have to limit my calories?"
- "How much fat should I eat?"

Because of the confusion and conflicting information available, it is not surprising that in a recent national survey, almost 80% of the American adult population admitted that they would need help if they were to make a commitment to permanently change their eating habits.

By understanding the material in this chapter and the next two chapters, you will become more knowledgeable about nutrition and exercise and understand their roles in relation to weight management. In addition to learning how to change your lifestyle, you must be willing to implement these changes. Eleven important guidelines are listed in Chapter 9. These should help you to identify which changes you need to make. A simple self-evaluation form is included with these guidelines so that you can evaluate the consistency of your eating and exercise habits. It will take motivation and dedication if you are to be successful.

EATING WELL

In theory, eating well is not difficult. All you need to do is to eat a sufficient portion of the foods that supply adequate amounts of all the essential nutrients, and learn how you can eat all these foods without gaining weight or getting fat. If you eat well, you should not always feel hungry, be consistently lacking in energy, or constantly be craving certain foods. Because no one food contains all the essential nutrients, it is important to eat well-balanced meals consisting of a variety of different foods. You must also learn how to limit the foods that are high in calories and provide very few of the essential nutrients.

What we eat can significantly affect our health, how we develop and grow, and how efficiently we can perform our everyday tasks. Specifically, by eating well you can achieve the following:

- Reduce your body weight
- Have less body fat
- Have more energy throughout the day
- Look and feel better
- Lower your cholesterol level
- Reduce your chances of cardiovascular disease, certain types of cancer, and osteoporosis
- Enhance your performance of everyday tasks

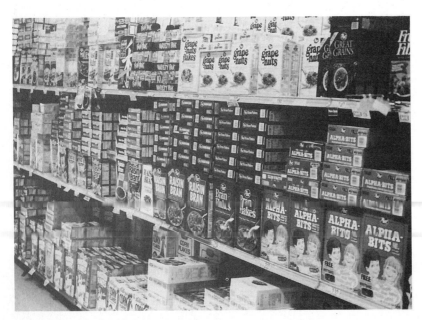

Figure 7-1 So many breakfast cereals are now available that the average person has a hard time deciding which one is best.

NUTRIENTS

A **nutrient** is defined as a basic substance the body uses for a variety of important functions. In simpler terms, it is anything you eat for which your body has a use. Nutrients are needed by the body for a variety of reasons:

- For normal growth and development of the body
- To supply energy for the performance of everyday tasks
- For resistance to infection and disease
- To regulate the functions of the body's cells

The six major categories of nutrients are as follows:

- Carbohydrates
- Fats
- Proteins
- Vitamins
- Minerals
- Water

Most plants and animals that we use for food, as well as our own bodies, consist primarily of these six nutrients. All nutrients are composed of elements or atoms bonded together by energy. The composition of the six classes of nutrients is shown in Figure 7-2.

Note that all of the nutrients, except minerals, contain hydrogen and oxygen, the elements of which water is made. Four of the nutrients contain carbon and are therefore classified as **organic.** This means that they can be oxidized, or burned, to produce energy. However, only three of these—carbohydrates, fats, and protein—can be oxidized in the human body to yield energy. Vitamins help in the oxidation process, but they do not yield energy for human use.

Unlike minerals, vitamins are organic and can be easily destroyed by heat and light. To maintain the maximum level of vitamins, be careful not to overcook the foods that contain them.

Energy nutrients

The energy derived from foods is measured in kilocalories, or as they are more commonly known, **calories.** Calories can be used to express the potential energy in food and the amount of energy used by the body in performing everyday activities. The energy equivalent of 1 lb of fat is 3500 calories. If a person takes in 3000 calories per day from the food he or she eats and uses only 2500 calories each day, he or she will accumulate 500 excess calories per day. This adds up to 3500 calories per week, which is equivalent to 1 lb of fat.

Energy can be derived from only three of the nutrients—carbohydrates, fats, and proteins. Vitamins, minerals, and water have no calories. It is also important not to forget one other organic compound—alcohol. Alcohol is not a nutrient because it is not essential to the functioning of the body, but it does contain calories. Alcohol basically contains no nutrients, so the calories obtained from it are often referred to as "empty" calories. Because of this, you must be careful to limit your intake of calories from alcohol.

The four sources of calories are as follows:	
Fat	9 cal/g
Protein	4 cal/g
Carbohydrate	4 cal/g
Alcohol	7 cal/g

Note: There are approximately 28 g in 1 oz.

Practically all foods contain mixtures of fats, proteins, and carbohydrates. If you know how many grams of each are contained in the food you eat, you can determine the numbers of calories. In any nutritional plan, these percentages are very important. The recommended percentages for each of these nutrients are discussed later in this chapter. To calculate these percentages for an entire day, you need to record the amounts of each of the foods consumed. The total number of grams for each of these nutrients can then be obtained by consulting a table showing the nutritional content of foods (see Appendix B), getting this information from food labels, or using the food exchange lists (see Appendix A). The following examples should help you to understand how this is done.

	Hydrogen	Oxygen	Carbon	Nitrogen
Carbohydrate	X	X	X	
Fat	X	X	X	
Protein	X	X	X	X
Vitamins	X	X	X	
Minerals				X
Water	X	X		

Figure 7-2 Composition of six nutrients.

Nutrient: A basic substance needed by the body for a variety of functions.

Organic: A nutrient containing carbon that can usually be oxidized or burned to produce energy.

Energy nutrient: A nutrient that provides energy in the form of calories (carbohydrates, fat, and protein).

Calorie: A unit for measuring energy; calories in food represent the energy value of foods.

Example:

Following is the nutritional information given by McDonalds Corporation for their McLean Deluxe hamburger with cheese:

Protein	24 g
Carbohydrates	35 g
Fat	14 g

The energy equivalent is calculated as follows:

Protein	24 g × 4	= 96
Carbohydrates	35 g × 4	= 140
Fat	14 g × 9	= 126
	TOTAL CALORIES	= 362

The percentage of calories derived from each of the energy nutrients can now be calculated as follows:

Protein	96/362	= 26%
Carbohydrates	140/362	= 39%
Fat	126/362	= 35%

Example:

Suppose that your caloric consumption for the day was as follows:

Protein	75 g
Carbohydrates	400 g
Fat	100 g

You must now convert these figures to calories.

Protein	75 g × 4	= 300 cal
Carbohydrates	400 g × 4	= 1600 cal
Fat	100 g × 9	= 900 cal
	TOTAL CALORIES	= 2800

The percentages for each of the nutrients can now be obtained as follows:

Protein	= 300/2800	= 11%
Carbohydrates	= 1600/2800	= 57%
Fats	= 900/2800	= 32%

Do not forget that if alcohol is consumed, it must be figured into the calculations. Each gram of alcohol contributes 7 cal.

Essential nutrients

Your body is capable of making some of the specific nutrients from others. However, certain nutrients are absolutely indispensable to your body's functioning and cannot be made by your body. These are termed **essential nutrients.** Note that the term *essential* means more than necessary, because many of the nutrients that the body makes for itself are necessary. For example, cholesterol is necessary for the efficient functioning of the body, but it is not an essential nutrient because sufficient amounts can be manufactured within the body. An essential nutrient is a necessary nutrient that can be obtained only from the food you eat. There are at least 42 nutrients that are considered essential. These are identified in Table 7-1.

This might seem like a lot to worry about to ensure that you take in all of these in the appropriate amounts. However, the use of the eating right pyramid and the exchange lists makes it possible to plan a balanced diet from a variety of foods that usually will meet all your nutritional needs.

RECOMMENDED DIETARY ALLOWANCES

If you choose to think in terms of nutrients, it will be necessary to use a standard such as the **Recommended Dietary Allowances** (RDA) to evaluate your nutritional intake. These are determined by a committee funded by the U.S. government. They represent the amounts of essential nutrients that are considered adequate to meet the known nutritional needs of most healthy persons in the United States. It should be noted that they are recommendations, not requirements, and certainly not minimal requirements. They are based on the concept that there is a range within which a healthy person's intake of nutrients probably should fall. Different people have different requirements, so these recommended allowances are set at a reasonably high point so that the majority of the population can be included. It is probably wise to aim at getting 100% or more of each nutrient. The adult RDA values for each of the essential nutrients are included in appropriate places throughout this chapter.

In addition to an RDA for each of the essential nutrients, there is also a recommendation for total caloric intake. In setting this recommendation, the committee took a different approach. In establishing the RDA for the nutrients, it was agreed that it would be sensible to set generous allowances to provide insurance against deficiencies. However, extra calories will eventually lead to obesity or being overweight. Thus the RDA for caloric intake was set at the mean, not at the upper end of the curve as it was for the individual nutrients. The recommended energy intakes for males and females are presented in Table 7-2.

It should be noted that these are the recommendations for healthy individuals who are trying to maintain their body weight. Those trying to lose weight will need to take in considerably fewer calories. Males require more calories than females because the average male weighs more than the average female. Your body weight significantly affects how many calories you will use each day in performing your everyday tasks (see Chapter 8).

How many calories you *use* each day will obviously determine the number of calories you can consume if you are trying to maintain your body weight. Note that for a 20-year-old male, the recommendation is 2900 cal per day. For a 20-year-old female it is 2100 cal per day.

Table 7-1	**Identification of Essential Nutrients**					
Fat (2 essential fatty acids)	Protein (9 essential amino acids)	Carbohydrate (2)	Vitamins (13)		Minerals (15)	Water
Linoleic acid	Leucine	Glucose	**Fat-soluble**		Calcium	
Linolenic acid	Isoleucine	Fiber	VItamin A		Chlorine	
	Lysine		Vitamin D		Chromium	
	Methionine		Vitamin E		Cobalt	
	Phenylalanine		Vitamin K		Copper	
	Threonine				Iodide	
	Tryptophan		**Water-soluble**		Iron	
	Valine		Vitamin C (Ascorbic		Magnesium	
	Histidine		acid)		Manganese	
			B Complex		Phosphorus	
			B1 (Thiamin)		Potassium	
			B2 (Riboflavin)		Sodium	
			Niacin		Sulphur	
			B6 (Pyridoxine)		Selenium	
			Pantothenic acid		Zinc	
			Folacin			
			B12			
			Biotin			

Table 7-2	**Recommended Daily Energy Intake**				
	Men			Women	
Age (years)	Recommendation (calories)	Range (calories)	Recommendation (calories)	Range (calories)	
11-14	2700	2000-3700	2200	1500-3000	
15-18	2800	3100-3900	2100	1200-3000	
19-22	2900	2500-3300	2100	1700-2500	
23-50	2700	2300-3100	1800	1400-2200	
51-75	2400	2000-2800	1600	1200-2000	
>75	2050	1050-2450	1600	1200-2000	

CARBOHYDRATES

As the name implies, **carbohydrates** are compounds composed of carbon, hydrogen, and oxygen. The most basic form is glucose, which is produced by green leafy plants through a complex process known as photosynthesis. Carbohydrates have traditionally been categorized in two groups—simple and complex. However, this classification is misleading. A further breakdown is presented in Figure 7-3. Note that the simple carbohydrates are often referred to as *sugars,* and the complex carbohydrates are referred to as *starches* and *fiber.*

Simple sugars

It is important to distinguish between **simple sugars** that occur naturally in fruits and concentrated **refined sugar.** This further classification of the simple sugars is

Essential nutrient: A necessary nutrient that cannot be manufactured by the body and therefore must be obtained from the food you eat.

Recommended Dietary Allowance (RDA): The amounts of essential nutrients considered adequate to meet the known nutritional needs of most healthy persons.

Carbohydrate: An organic nutrient derived from a plant source; a major source of energy in the body.

Simple sugar: A form of carbohydrate that contains either one or two sugar units linked together.

Refined sugar: A term used to describe sweeteners, such as table sugar, that are created by processing.

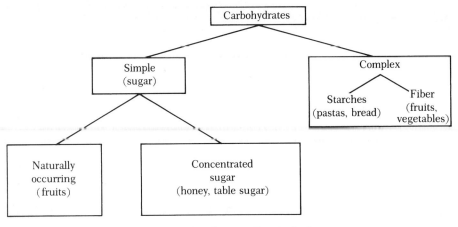

Figure 7-3 Classification of carbohydrates.

very important. The naturally occurring simple carbohydrates in fruits usually come packaged with vitamins, minerals, and possibly fiber. The concentrated sugar in cakes and cookies is considered empty calories and is of limited nutritional value. It is also important to note that sugar has been added to many other products. Canned fruits and vegetables, soft drinks, and many breakfast cereals contain large amounts of simple sugars. The following comparison of nutritional information for two different breakfast cereals clearly shows this.

Table 7-3 shows the sugar content of selected foods. The equivalent teaspoon measurement of sugar is given for each of the foods listed. Each teaspoon of sugar is equivalent to 4 to 5 g of carbohydrates and is equal to 16 to 20 calories.

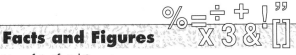

Facts and Figures

Use of Artificial Sweeteners

Despite the widespread use of artificial sweeteners, the consumption of simple refined sugar has continued to rise. In 1992 the average American consumed 148 lb of simple refined sugar as compared with 124 lb in 1975.

Simple refined sugars now contribute approximately 19% of the total calories consumed by the average person. Because sugar is of little nutritional value, this means that you must rely on 81% of the total calories consumed to provide 100% of the essential nutrients needed each day. The recommendation is that we get no more than 10% of our calories from simple refined sugar. For a person eating 2000 cal per day, this would mean that no more than 200 cal should come from simple refined sugar. This is the equivalent to approximately 10 tsp of sugar per day. The average American consumes approximately 36 tsp of sugar per day.

Extra sugar also means that we get extra calories. For example, for a person eating 2000 cal per day with 19% of these calories from simple refined sugar, he or she will be getting 180 extra cal per day from sugar, compared with a person who limits his or her intake of sugar to 10%. This occurring each day over a period of 1 year is the equivalent of approximately 18 lb of fat, which this person is likely to accumulate as a result of the extra sugar intake.

Starches

Starches are made of long chains of glucose molecules that are linked together. They are found in the following:

	Total Raisin Bran	Nabisco Shredded Wheat
Serving size	1 oz	1 oz
Calories	86	90
Carbohydrates	22 g	23 g
Fiber	3 g	3 g
Simple sugars	10 g	0 g
Complex carbohydrates	9 g	20 g

NOTE: There are 10 g of simple sugar in Total Raisin Bran, whereas Nabisco Shredded Wheat does not contain any. Of the 23 g of carbohydrates in Nabisco Shredded Wheat, 20 g come from complex carbohydrates. From a nutritional standpoint, Nabisco Shredded Wheat is clearly the better choice.

Table 7-3   Sugar Content for Selected Foods

Food	Portion Size	Teaspoons of Added Sugar
Beverages		
Wine	3.5 oz	3.0
Gatorade	8 oz	3.5
Lemonade (Country Time)	8 oz	6.0
Tonic Water	8 oz	8.4
Sprite	12 oz	9.0
Most other soda	12 oz	8.0
Dairy products		
Ice cream—vanilla	1 cup	6.0
Lowfat yogurt (Dannon)	1 cup	6.0
Sherbet ice cream	1 cup	11.0
Yogurt—fruit flavored	1 cup	8.0
Chocolate milkshake	1 cup	6.0
Hot-fudge sundae	1 dish	16.0
Cakes, pies, desserts, snacks		
Apple pie	1 slice (6 oz)	6.5
Strawberry shortcake	1 serving	12.0
Popsicle	1	4.5
Cupcake (with icing)	1 (2½″ diam.)	3.2
Twinkies	2	9.6
Chocolate cake	1 piece (2.3 oz)	5.3
Cookies and doughnuts		
Doughnut—plain	1 large	3.0
Doughnut—glazed	1 large	6.0
Brownie	1 (2 oz)	4.6
Sugar cookie	1 (2 oz)	6.0
Candy		
M&M Peanuts	14	3.0
Milk chocolate with almonds	1 oz	3.2
Peanut butter cup	1	4.8
Breads/grains		
Hot dog bun	1	3.0
Hamburger bun	1	3.0
Bread—white	1 slice	2.5
Cinnamon bun	1 medium	10.5
Breakfast cereals		
Sugar Frosted Flakes	1 oz	2.8
Fruitful Bran—Kelloggs	1 oz	1.8
Fruit & Fiber—Post	1 oz	1.6
Grape Nuts—Post	1 oz	.6
Raisin Bran—Total	1 oz	2.0
Fruit Loops	1 oz	3.3

Modified from *How sweet is it?* Center for Science in Public Interest, Washington, DC, 1985, and *Hidden sugar in familiar foods*, Texas Agricultural Extension Services, College Station, Texas, 1985.

Grain products	Starchy vegetables
Rice	Corn
Pasta	Potatoes
Bread	Peas
Cereals	Beans

Other vegetables and fruits contain lesser amounts of **complex carbohydrates.**

Complex carbohydrate: A compound consisting of many sugar molecules linked together including starches and fiber.

Starch: The most familiar form of carbohydrates; found in plants, seeds, and grain from which bread, cereal, spaghetti, and pasta are made.

Table 7-4	**Wendy's Baked Potato with Toppings**		
Item	Calories	Fat (g)	Percent of Calories from Fat
Baked potato with sour cream and chives	460	24	47
Baked potato with cheese	590	34	52
Baked potato with chili and cheese	510	20	35
Baked potato with bacon and cheese	570	30	47
Baked potato with broccoli and cheese	500	25	45

Many people mistakenly think that carbohydrates are fattening. The reason they think this is that they frequently combined carbohydrates with large amounts of fat. For example, we often add whole milk to breakfast cereal, large amounts of butter to foods such as bread, baked potatoes, and corn, and rich, high-fat sauces or dressings to pasta. When this happens, you frequently finish up getting more calories from the fat than you get from the carbohydrates. For example, a large baked potato usually contains approximately 200 cal, with almost all of these calories coming from carbohydrates. Toppings such as butter, margarine, cheese, and chili can often increase the caloric value to 500 or 600 cal. Table 7-4 contains information pertaining to some of the baked potatoes available at one of the leading fast-food restaurants.

In Summary

The secret to eating well is to learn how to eat lots of complex carbohydrates without adding large amounts of fat.

Fiber

The term **fiber** is used by most people as if it represented a single entity. Actually there are many compounds, mostly carbohydrates, that make up fiber. Fiber is defined as any part of a food plant that cannot be broken down and digested by the human body. It includes the parts that give the plant shape, structure, and strength. It has been referred to as *roughage* or *bulk*. Fiber is contained in vegetables, fruits, legumes, grains, and seeds. There are two different types of fiber—insoluble and soluble.

Insoluble fiber This type of fiber does not dissolve in water. It is the fiber that gives plants their firm structure. It is found in the cell walls of many grains, vegetables, and fruits. Insoluble fiber helps to prevent constipation, hemorrhoids, and diverticulosis and may also help to prevent certain types of cancer.

Soluble fiber This is the second type of fiber. It is soluble in water and forms a gel from the water that it absorbs. It is the nonstructural materials in plant cells such as pectins and gums. It is found in oats, barley, kidney beans, and most vegetables. Soluble fiber has been shown to lower cholesterol levels in some people and can be used by diabetics to help stabilize their blood glucose levels. Foods that contain soluble fiber are also more likely to satisfy your appetite. When fiber combines with water it swells and expands, creating a feeling of fullness.

How much fiber should you eat? The average fiber intake in the United States is 15 g per day. This is much less than what you need. Although there is no RDA value for fiber, the American Dietetic Association recommends that we increase our fiber intake to 25 to 35 g per day to ensure the maximum health benefits. Many well-known nutritionists are suggesting that you need 30 to 40 g or more each day.

A listing of the fiber content for selected foods is included in Laboratory Experience 7-1. You can evaluate your fiber intake and determine whether it is adequate.

Fitness Flash

Foods high in fiber are usually good for those trying to control their weight. They are foods that are typically low in fat; they generally take longer to chew, therefore slowing down your food intake, and they often promote a feeling of fullness.

Functions of carbohydrates

Carbohydrates perform a number of important functions in the body:

- They are the primary source of energy for the body, because they can provide energy more efficiently than do the other energy nutrients.
- Glucose is the simplest form of carbohydrates. The body must maintain a normal level of glucose in the blood, because the brain and central nervous system constantly require glucose.

Carbohydrate Intake

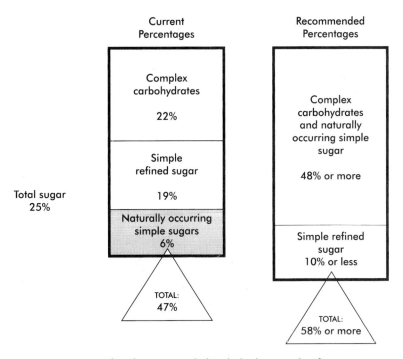

Figure 7-4   Actual and recommended carbohydrate intakes for Americans.

■ An adequate intake of carbohydrates is necessary for the complete metabolism of fat.

■ Carbohydrates are stored in the body in the muscles and the liver in the form of glycogen. An adequate intake of carbohydrates is necessary if these stores are to be replenished. The more glycogen you have stored, the more you will have available as fuel for the body. This is particularly important for those who participate regularly in endurance-type activities such as jogging, running, cycling, and swimming.

Carbohydrate intake: how much do you need?

It is apparent that Americans need to change their eating habits in relation to their carbohydrate intake. A comparison of the current habits and the recommended values is shown in Figure 7-4.

The material presented in this section indicates that we need to double our intake of complex carbohydrates, reduce our intake of simple refined sugar by almost 50%, and significantly increase our fiber intake.

FATS

Fats, which are often referred to as *lipids* or *oils,* are a secondary source of energy and currently make up approximately 37% of the calories consumed in the average American diet. They appear in a variety of ways in

various foods. They may appear as visible fats and oils in the form of butter or oil; they may also occur in the form of fat attached to a steak, ham, or bacon. They may also be less obvious in food such as nuts, cheese, and avocados.

In recent years, fats have fallen into disrepute. The federal government, American Heart Association, American Cancer Society, and National Academy of Sciences are all urging us to eat less fat. There are several reasons for this recommendation:

Fiber: Any part of a food plant that cannot be broken down and digested by the human body—usually found in the stems, leaves, and seeds of plants.

Insoluble fiber: The type of fiber that does not dissolve in water—it is found in the cell walls of many grains, vegetables, and fruits.

Soluble fiber: Fiber that dissolves in water to form a gel—it is the nonstructural material in plant cells, such as pectins and gums.

Fat: A nutrient that is a secondary source of energy in the body and can be stored in the body—also referred to as a *lipid* or an *oil.*

- Each gram of fat provides you with more than twice as many calories as each gram of carbohydrate or protein.

- Excess fat is easily stored in the body, whereas excess proteins and carbohydrates must be converted to fat to be stored. For this reason, excess calories from protein and carbohydrates will affect your metabolism differently from excess calories obtained from fat. It has been shown that the metabolic cost associated with an excess of 100 cal of fat is only 3%; thus 97% of these calories will be stored as fat. With an excess of 100 cal of carbohydrates the metabolic cost is 23%, and only 77% of these calories will be stored as fat.

- Excess calories from fat can be used as energy or else stored as fat. These are the only options. However, we have seen that excess calories from carbohydrates can be stored as glycogen in the body and can be used to replace the glucose in the blood that constantly must be replenished. Only after the body has made these adjustments will the excess carbohydrates be stored as fat. Fat calories are thus more fattening (Figure 7-5).

- Dietary fat is thought to be a contributing factor in the development of certain diseases, including cardiovascular disease, diabetes, and certain forms of cancer.

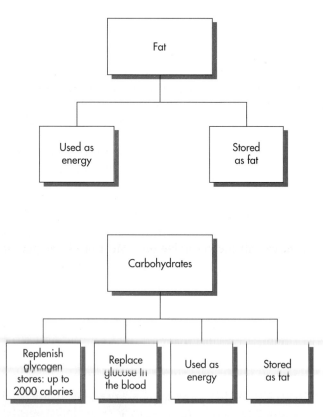

Figure 7-5 Excess carbohydrate calories are unlikely to be stored as fat in the body.

Functions of fats

It should be stressed that fat is an important dietary component and that the problems associated with dietary fats are related to *excessive* fat intake. In addition to providing energy, fat enhances the flavor of food, and because it takes twice as long to digest, fat makes a meal seem more filling. Fat also contains two fatty acids that are essential, and it provides transportation for certain fat-soluble vitamins. Moderate deposits of fat serve as support and protection for several of the vital organs and aid in the regulation of body temperature. However, excessive fat deposits create serious health problems.

Saturated and unsaturated fat

Fats contained in food are primarily in the form of triglycerides. Triglycerides are made up of a simple three-carbon alcohol called *glycerol*, which serves as a backbone for the attachment of three fatty acids (Figure 7-6).

A fatty acid is basically a chain of carbon atoms linked to hydrogen atoms. If the hydrogen atoms fill each available spot on the chain, then the fatty acid is said to be **saturated.** An **unsaturated** fatty acid contains two or more empty spots on the carbon chain (Figure 7-7).

Each food that contains fat basically has a certain amount of saturated and unsaturated fat. The saturated and unsaturated fat content for select foods is presented in Table 7-5. By dividing the saturated fat grams by the total fat grams, the percentage of saturated fat in a particular food can easily be determined. For example, with olive oil, 1.9 of its 14 g of fat come from saturated fat. This represents 14% of the total fat.

In general, fats found in animal foods tend to be high in saturated fat, whereas those found in plant foods tend to be low in saturated fat. Exceptions are the tropical oils—palm and coconut oil—which are predominantly saturated. It should be noted that all fats, whether they contain mainly saturated or unsaturated fat, provide the same number of calories—9 cal per gram.

From a health standpoint, it is good to reduce your intake of saturated fat. It is now well established that increased levels of saturated fats in your diet will in-

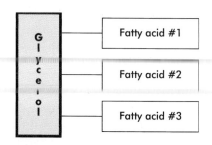

Figure 7-6 Structure of a triglyceride.

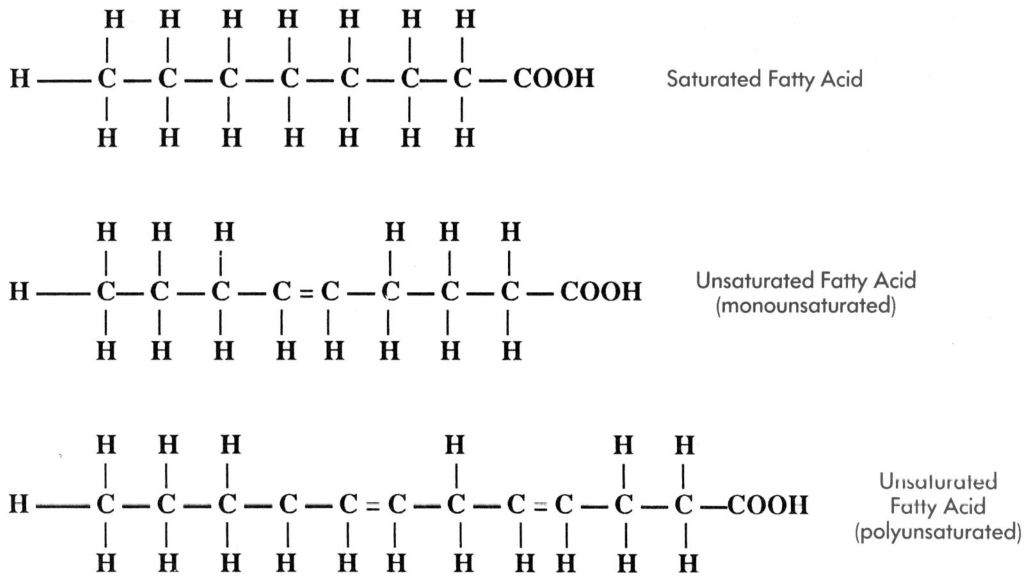

Figure 7-7 Example of the differences between saturated and unsaturated fatty acids.

Table 7-5	Saturated Fat and Unsaturated Fat in Select Foods				
Food	Serving Size	Calories	Total Fat (g)	Saturated Fat (g)	Saturated Fat (%)
Olive oil	1 tbsp	125	14.0	1.9	14
Peanuts	3 oz	495	42.0	5.7	14
Chicken—white meat	3.5 oz	133	4.5	1.4	30
Sirloin steak	3.5 oz	280	17.5	7.4	42
Butter	1 tbsp	100	11.0	7.0	65

crease your blood cholesterol level, which increases the incidence of atherosclerosis and this increases your risk of other cardiovascular diseases. There is also some evidence that polyunsaturated fats may lower your blood cholesterol level (see Chapter 11).

Classification of some of the common sources of fat, according to whether they are predominantly saturated or unsaturated, is presented in the box below.

Classification of Some Common Sources of Fat

Saturated	Monounsaturated	Polyunsaturated
Beef	Almonds	Corn oil
Butter	Avocadoes	Cottonseed oil
Cheese	Olives	Mayonnaise
Chocolate	Olive oil	Safflower oil
Coconut	Peanuts	Soybeans
Coconut oil	Peanut butter	Soybean oil
Cream	Peanut oil	Sunflower oil
Ice cream		Vegetable oil
Lamb		
Milk		
Palm oil		
Veal		

Essential fatty acids

There are two polyunsaturated fatty acids the body cannot produce that perform important functions in the body and are therefore considered as essential. These are linoleic acid and linolenic acid. These fatty acids play an important role in the immune system, help form cell membranes, and aid in the production of certain hormones. In addition, linolenic acid has been shown to play an important role in reducing the incidence of certain forms of cardiovascular disease.

Linoleic acid is readily available in large quantities in nearly all the vegetable oils. Most of us can get all the linoleic acid we need each day in 1 to 2 tsp of prac-

Saturated fat: Fat found mainly in animal products that carries the maximum number of hydrogen atoms.

Unsaturated fat: Fat found mainly in plant products that is usually liquid at room temperature. It contains less than the maximum number of hydrogen atoms.

tically any vegetable oil. However, linolenic acid is much less readily available. It only occurs in significant amounts in canola and soybean oil. If these oils are not consumed regularly, a related form of this can be obtained in large quantities in most of the fatty cold-water fish, such as salmon and tuna, and in small quantities in most other fish. Because of the relationship of this fatty acid to cardiovascular disease, the American Heart Association recommends that we eat at least two servings of fish each week.

Recommendations for fat intake

The actual and recommended fat intakes for Americans are presented in Figure 7-8. The average American now gets approximately 37% of his or her calories from fat, compared with 42% in 1988. However, this figure is still considerably higher than the recommended 30%.

The recommended percentage is now much easier to achieve than it was several years ago, because there are now so many fat-free products available. We now have fat-free salad dressings, ice cream, yogurt, cheese, tortilla chips, cookies, and so on. In addition, many of the other products are much lower in fat than they were several years ago. For example, Healthy Choice now has a very lean ground beef that has less fat than does chicken (4 g of fat per 4 oz). Also, the fat content of most cuts of pork is now 35% less than it was in 1985.

There are many successful weight-loss programs that no longer focus on total calories consumed but instead concentrate on the number of fat grams consumed. Certainly there is a growing body of research to support this concept.

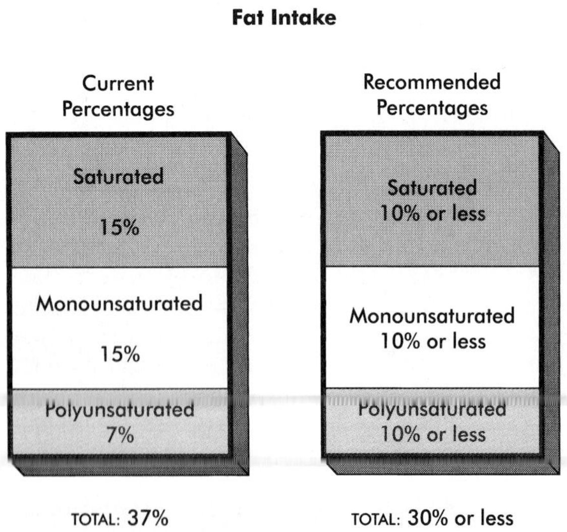

Fat Intake

Figure 7-8   Actual and recommended fat intakes for Americans.

If you are overweight and have fat to lose, you will probably be more successful in losing this weight and fat if you try to lower your total fat intake to 20% or less, rather than the recommended 30%. Table 7-6 contains information that will help you determine how much fat you should be eating. Table 7-6 shows the grams of fat you can eat each day for a wide range of calories when 20%, 25%, or 30% of these calories are obtained from fat.

Fat content of foods

Most people are confused when it comes to reading labels, particularly information pertaining to fat. One of the problems is that many labels contain numbers or percentages with little or no explanation as to what these numbers represent. Consider the following three examples:

> Extra-lean ham—96% fat free
> Milk—2% fat
> Extra-lean ground beef—16% fat

The average person would assume that the ham contains 4% fat, milk 2%, and extra-lean ground beef 16%. You will see that this is not so if you are considering calories.

Figures such as these, which usually appear in large print on the labels, in most cases refer to the fat content by weight. For example, the extra-lean ham serving size is 1 oz (28 g), and only 1 of the 28 g comes from fat. This means that 1/28 or 4% of the product by weight comes from fat; hence the term 96% fat free.

You need to be more concerned with the percentage of calories in food that comes from fat. To determine this, you need to look at the nutritional information for the product—usually given in small print—and figure this out as follows:

1. Each gram of fat contains 9 cal, so you need to multiply the number of grams of fat by 9 to determine the number of calories coming from fat.
2. Divide this number by the total number of calories from the food to determine the percentage of the calories from fat.

Reducing your fat intake

A large percentage of people fail to realize how much fat they eat. They are constantly making poor choices. The case study on p. 152 will emphasize this point.

Table 7-6	**Desired Caloric Intake: Fat Grams**		
Daily Caloric Intake (calories)	Fat Grams for Selected Percentages of Calories From Fat		
	20%	25%	30%
1200	27	33	40
1300	29	36	43
1400	31	39	47
1500	33	42	50
1600	36	44	53
1700	38	47	57
1800	40	50	60
1900	42	53	63
2000	44	56	67
2100	47	58	70
2200	49	61	73
2300	51	64	77
2400	53	67	80
2500	56	69	83
2600	58	72	87
2700	60	75	90
2800	62	78	93
2900	64	81	97
3000	67	83	100

Example:

If you are trying to limit your caloric intake for the day to 2000 and you are trying to limit your fat intake to 25% of these calories, then you can see that you can consume 56 g of fat for the day.

The calculations for the three food items listed previously are as follows:

Extra-lean ham
Serving size—1 oz
Calories—30
Fat—1 g
Protein—5 g
Calories from fat—1 × 9 = 9
Percentage of calories from fat—9/30 = 30%

2% Milk
Serving size—1 cup
Calories—121
Protein—8 g
Fat—5 g
Carbohydrates—12 g
Calories from fat—5 × 9 = 45
Percentage of calories from fat—45/121 = 37%

Ground beef—extra lean—16% fat
Serving size—3 oz
Calories—225
Protein—24 g
Fat—13 g
Carbohydrates—0 g
Calories from fat— 13 × 9 = 117
Percentage of calories from fat—117/225 = 52%

NOTE: These figures are much higher than the figures listed on the label referring to fat by weight. The following box will help you to evaluate foods according to the percentage of their calories coming from fat.

The Percentage of Fat Calories for Common Foods

>90%	Bacon, butter, cooking oils, margarine, mayonnaise, salad oils, sour cream, tartar sauce, vegetable shortening
80%-89%	Avocadoes, bologna, frankfurters, olives
60%-79%	Beef, ham, cheese, enchiladas, nuts, peanut butter, pork, potato chips, salami, veal
40%-59%	Beef (lean), brownies, bread stuffing, chicken (fried), cookies, corn chips, croissants, doughnuts (cake), fish (fried), french-fried potatoes, ice cream, milk (whole), popcorn (with oil), potato salad, scallops (breaded)
20%-39%	Bran muffins, cakes, dinner rolls, cereal (granola), ground beef (extra-lean), ham (lean), lamb (lean—roasted), pancakes (made from mix), tuna (oil packed), waffles (made from mix), yogurt (low fat)
<20%	Bagels, baked potatoes, breakfast cereal (except granola), chicken (broiled or baked), crackers (low fat), fish (broiled or baked), fruits, legumes, lentils, muffins (English), pasta, popcorn (air popped), tortillas, tuna (water packed), vegetables

Case Study

JOHN and JOE

John and Joe are both trying to lose weight by reducing their percentage of body fat. They often go out to eat lunch together. John has learned the importance of reducing the amount of fat he eats and has become knowledgeable about the foods which are high in fat. Joe, on the other hand, has not learned the importance of reducing fat but still thinks he is eating well. A typical lunch for John and Joe is as follows:

John—Chicken Sandwich	Joe—Chicken Club Sandwich
Whole-wheat bread—2 slices	Whole-wheat bread—2 slices
Chicken—white meat, no skin, 3 oz	Chicken—white meat, no skin, 3 oz
Mustard—1 tbsp.	Mayonnaise—1 tbsp
Lettuce—2 slices	Lettuce—2 slices
Tomato—2 slices	Tomato—2 slices
Cantaloupe—¼ small	Cantaloupe—¼ small
Strawberries—½ c	Strawberries—½ c
	Bacon—3 small strips
	Cheese—1½ oz

Notice that Joe makes just three small changes in the way he orders his sandwich as compared to John. He substitutes mayonnaise for mustard and adds three small strips of bacon and 1½ oz of cheddar cheese.

Nutritional Analysis

	John	Joe
Calories	334	757
Protein	34 g	49 g
Carbohydrates	36 g	48 g
Fat	6 g	41 g

The nutritional analysis shows that for John, this is a good lunch providing 334 cal with only 6 g of fat, which means that John is getting less than 20% of his calories from fat. Joe on the other hand, simply cannot believe it when he finds out that by making these three insignificant changes, he has increased the calories from 334 to 757 and the fat grams from 6 to 41. The percentage of calories from fat for Joe is 49.

If Joe was to add 2 oz of poato chips to this meal, it would add an additional 284 cal and an additional 19 g of fat. What started out as a healthy meal with 334 cal and 6 g of fat has now increased to 1041 cal with 60 g of fat.

Table 7-7 compares foods which are relatively high in fat to those that have a low-fat content. You can use this information to make some changes in the foods you select. These changes could result in a significant reduction in the amount of fat that you eat.

PROTEIN

The most important of the energy nutrients is **protein.** It is appropriate that this word is derived from the Greek word "protos," which means *in first place* or *of prime importance*. If you mention the word *protein* to average people, they usually associate the word with animal products and relate it to meat, fish, poultry, milk, or eggs. However, remember that there are both plant and animal proteins.

Proteins are large complex molecules consisting of anywhere from 24 to as many as 300 **amino acids** joined together in a particular sequence. A great variety of proteins exist because different amino acids combine in unique sequences to form individual proteins. For ex-

ample, some proteins are flexible and elastic—such as the protein of hair, whereas others are firm and rigid—such as the protein of fingernails.

There are 22 different amino acids that are found in foods, and all but 9 of these are also made by the body. The nine that cannot be made by the body are called *essential amino acids*; they must be obtained regularly and in sufficient quantities from the foods that we eat. The nine essential amino acids are as follows:

Histidine	Methionine	Tryptophan
Isoleucine	Phenylalanine	Valine
Leucine	Threonine	Lysine

Food	Amount	Fat Grams	Food	Amount	Fat Grams
		Table 7-7 Comparison of Foods Relatively High in Fat to Those That Have a Low Fat Content			
Whole milk	8 oz	8	Skim milk	8 oz	0
Croissant	1 medium	12	Bagel	1 medium	2
Hash browns	1 cup	18	Baked potato	1 medium	0
Granola cereal	1 oz	5	Shredded wheat cereal	1 oz	0
Danish—fruit filled	1 medium	13	English muffin with jelly	1 medium	1
Peanuts-roasted	¼ cup	10	Raisins	¼ cup	0
Cream cheese	1 oz	10	Cottage cheese 1%	1 oz	1
Corn chips	1 oz	9	Pretzels	1 oz	0
T-bone steak	8 oz	56	Chicken breast	8 oz	8
Fried shrimp	3 oz	10	Broiled shrimp	3 oz	1
Bologna	3 oz	24	Extra-lean ham	3 oz	1
Chicken salad	3 oz	22	Chicken breast	3 oz	4
Ritz crackers	3 oz	18	Ry-Krisp crackers	3 oz	0
Baked potato—sour cream	1 medium	8	Baked potato—picante sauce	1 medium	0
Cheesecake	1 slice	18	Angelfood cake	1 slice	0
Mayonnaise	1 tbsp	11	Mustard	1 tbsp	0
Potato salad	1 cup	21	Boiled potatoes	1 cup	0
Cream of mushroom soup	1 cup	14	Black bean soup	1 cup	2
Glazed donut	1 medium	12	Ginger snap cookies	2	1
Bacon	1 oz	14	Canadian bacon	1 oz	2
Lamp chop—broiled	3 oz	25	Leg of lamb—lean	3 oz	6

Functions of protein in the body

Proteins perform a variety of important functions in the body. They are crucial to the minute-by-minute functioning of our bodies.

- Growth and repair of body tissues
  Muscles, hair, skin, bones, teeth, tendons, ligaments, and so on, are made from protein.
- Regulation of body functions
  Enzymes: These are specific proteins that speed up nearly every chemical reaction in the body. There are over 1000 enzymes in the human body. Lactase is an example; it is the enzyme necessary to break down the lactose found in milk.
  Hormones: These are specific proteins that are internal chemical messengers. Insulin is an example. When your blood glucose level is too high, your body produces insulin. This signals the cells to remove insulin from the bloodstream.
  Antibodies: These are blood proteins that attack foreign proteins found in the body, such as bacteria and viruses.
- Transport of nutrients
  Hemoglobin is a protein that transports oxygen. Fats also need protein to be transported in the bloodstream.
- Maintenance of the salt and fluid balance
  Proteins push potassium in and force sodium

out of nerve cells to maintain the salt balance. This is also important in maintaining the fluid balance.

- Blood clotting
  Fibrin is a protein and plays an important part in blood clotting.
- Source of energy
  This is not what protein is designed for; it occurs only if your total caloric intake is inadequate.
- Source of glucose
  This will occur only in the absence of sufficient carbohydrates.

Protein requirements

As indicated previously, both the quantity and the quality of your protein intake are important.

Protein: Primary food substance formed from amino acids and used by the body to build, repair, regulate, and replace cells.

Amino acids: The constituents of protein—an adequate amount of each is necessary for the body to make protein.

Table 7-8	**Comparison of Protein and Fat Content for Complete Protein Sources**			
Food	Serving Size	Protein (grams)	Fat (grams)	Calories
Meat (lean)	1 oz	7	3	55
Fish	1 oz	7	3	55
Poultry (lean)	1 oz	7	1-3	40-55
Milk (low fat)	8 oz	8	1	80
Milk (whole)	8 oz	8	8	150
Cheese	1 oz	6-8	6-9	100-120
Yogurt	8 oz	8	8	140
Egg	1 large	7	6	80

Quantity of protein

There is an RDA for protein. It is based on your body weight and is calculated as follows:

1. Calculate your body weight in kilograms
   Body weight (lb)/2.2 = Body weight (kg)
2. Multiply your body weight in kilograms by 0.8. This will give you your protein requirement in grams.
   Example:
   Body weight = 154 lb
   Step 1: 154/2.2 = 70 g
   Step 2: Protein requirement = 70 × 0.8 = 56 g

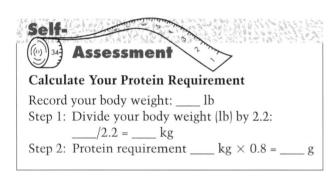

Calculate Your Protein Requirement

Record your body weight: _____ lb
Step 1: Divide your body weight (lb) by 2.2:
   _____ /2.2 = _____ kg
Step 2: Protein requirement _____ kg × 0.8 = _____ g

This protein requirement should be considered the minimum amount needed by an *inactive* person. If you exercise regularly for 45 minutes or more and you want to be sure that you are getting a sufficient amount of protein, you probably should multiply your body weight (kg) by 1.2 rather than 0.8.

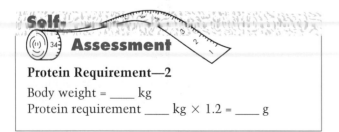

Protein Requirement—2

Body weight = _____ kg
Protein requirement _____ kg × 1.2 = _____ g

Quality of protein

Complete protein   Any food containing all nine of the essential amino acids is classified as a **complete protein.** All animal products are complete proteins; these include meat, fish, poultry, eggs, and dairy products. The amount of protein available from the complete protein sources is given in Table 7-8.

Incomplete protein   All other proteins are called **incomplete proteins.** They contain insufficient amounts of one or more of the essential amino acids. The incomplete protein sources can basically be divided into four groups—grain products, green leafy vegetables, seeds and nuts, and legumes. Information concerning the amount of protein available in each of these groups is presented in Table 7-9 for select foods.

Selecting incomplete proteins   In selecting incomplete proteins, it is important to consider which amino acids are missing with each of the groups of foods. These are presented below. (The *X*'s indicate that the designated amino acid is missing from that particular food group.)

Food group	Lysine	Methionine	Threonine	Tryptophan
Grain products	X	—	X	—
Green leafy vegetables	—	X	—	—
Nuts and seeds	X	—	—	—
Legumes	—	X	—	X

Different incomplete proteins can be combined to complement one another and provide all the amino acids that are needed by the body. It is important to consume foods from two of these groups so that the same essential amino acid is not lacking in each group. The following combinations will give you all the essential amino acids:

- A grain product with a green leafy vegetable— *Example:* Potato with broccoli

Table 7-9	Protein and Fat Content from Incomplete Protein Sources			
Food	**Serving Size**	**Protein (grams)**	**Fat (grams)**	**Calories**
Grain products (includes starchy vegetables)				
Bran cereal	½ cup	3-5	0-2	90
Bread	1 slice	2-3	0-2	60-80
Oatmeal (cooked)	1 cup	5	2	130
Rice (cooked)	1 cup	4-5	2	150-200
Potato (baked)	1 medium	5	0	220
Green leafy vegetables (raw)				
Broccoli	1 cup	5	0	45
Brussels sprouts	1 cup	6	0	55
Most other green vegetables	1 cup	2-5	0	50
Seeds and nuts				
Sesame seeds	¼ cup	10	21	221
Sunflower seeds	¼ cup	7	19	208
Walnuts	1 cup	30	71	759
Cashews	1 cup	21	63	787
Peanut butter	1 tbsp	5	8	95
Dry-roasted peanuts	1 cup	39	71	840
Legumes				
Peas-green	½ cup	4	0	70
Beans-navy	1 cup	16	1	259
Beans-lima	1 cup	15	1	217
Beans-pinto	1 cup	14	1	235
Beans-garbanzo	1 cup	15	4	269

- A grain product with a legume—*Example:* Rice and beans
- A green leafy vegetable with nuts or seeds—*Example:* Brussel sprouts and cashews
- A legume with nuts or seeds—*Example:* Garbanzo beans with dry roasted peanuts

Note that two of the four combinations involve nuts and seeds. These are not good choices if you are trying to limit your fat intake.

Regardless of the source of the protein, for protein in food to be used in the body, it must be broken down by digestion into amino acids, absorbed into the blood, and transported to the cells of the body where they are used to build different proteins. The formation of proteins is summarized in Figure 7-9.

Note what happens if the body does not get a sufficient amount of all the necessary amino acids at the same time. It cannot use any of them unless it has all of them, and because it has no place to store them—like it does for carbohydrates and fat—the only other option your body has is to convert them to fat and store them as fat. This explains why many vegetarians, even though they do not usually have a weight problem, tend to accumulate excess fat. The reason is that because of what they eat and do not eat, they have difficulty getting a sufficient amount of all the essential amino acids.

Protein intake

Until recently, it was not difficult for the average American to take in an adequate amount of protein. In fact, many consumed almost double the amount of protein that they needed. However, in recent years we have seen a significant reduction in the amount of fat consumed. Because many of the foods that are high in fat are also high in protein, this has also reduced the total amount of protein that many people get. Those who limit their intake of meat and milk are frequently lacking in protein.

A listing of foods that are high in protein and relatively low in fat appears in Table 7-10. If you need to increase your protein intake these will be good choices for you. Also included in this table is a listing of foods that are high in protein and also fat. When possible, you should limit your intake of foods from this list.

Complete protein: Any food containing all nine of the essential amino acids—includes meat, fish, poultry, eggs, and dairy products.

Incomplete protein: Any food containing protein that does not contain all nine of the essential amino acids—includes grain products, green leafy vegetables, nuts and seeds, and legumes.

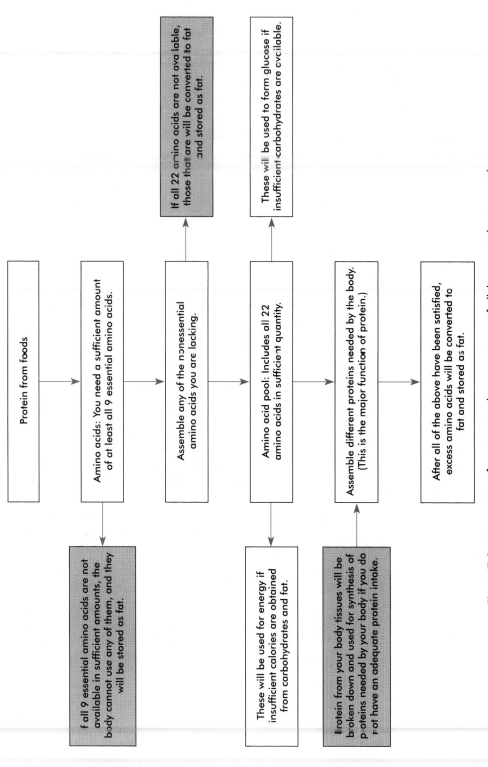

Figure 7-9   Importance of getting an adequate amount of all the essential amino acids.

Table 7-10				**Protein and Fat Contents of Select Foods**			
Food	Amount	Fat	Protein	Food	Amount	Fat	Protein
Whole milk	8 oz	8	7	Skim milk	8 oz	0	7
Salami	3 oz	30	18	Turkey	3 oz	3	24
Bacon	2 oz	28	18	Canadian bacon	2 oz	4	16
Shrimp/fried	3 oz	10	21	Shrimp-broiled	3 oz	1	21
Avocado	1 medium	30	4	Pinto beans	½ cup	0	7
Yogurt	8 oz	8	8	Yogurt	nonfat	0	9
Bologna	3 oz	24	9	Corned beef-lean	3 oz	3	21
Granola cereal	2 oz	10	6	Oatmeal	2 oz	0	10
Peanut butter	2 tbsp	16	10	Vegetarian chili	2 oz	0	10
Tuna salad	1 cup	19	33	Tuna-water packed	3 oz	1	30
Croissant	1 medium	12	5	Bagel	1 medium	2	7
French fries	20	16	4	Baked potato	1 medium	0	5
Creamy coleslaw	4 oz	15	1	Black beans	½ cup	0	8
Creamy chicken mushroom soup	1 cup	7	3	Split pea soup with ham	1 cup	4	10
Cheddar cheese	1 oz	9	7	Low-fat cottage cheese	1 oz	1	14

VITAMINS

Vitamins are organic compounds needed in small quantities by the body to perform specific functions important to growth and development and the work of nerves and muscles. Although vitamins do not provide energy, they play an important role in releasing energy from the foods that we eat.

Vitamins cannot be manufactured within the body and therefore must be supplied from the foods that we eat. The best method of ensuring an adequate supply of vitamins is to have a well-balanced diet from a variety of foods.

There are presently 13 vitamins that are known to be required by the body and must be consumed. They can be classified into two groups—fat-soluble vitamins and water-soluble vitamins. The most important difference between the two groups is that the fat-soluble vitamins can be stored in fat in the body, so it is not necessary to eat them each day. There is some danger in consuming extremely large amounts of these vitamins. Water-soluble vitamins cannot be stored in large amounts in the body and must therefore be consumed on a daily basis. Each of the vitamins is identified in Table 7-11. Information is provided for each of them relative to their RDA, food sources, and basic functions in the body.

MINERALS

Minerals are inorganic substances needed by the body in small amounts. They serve a variety of functions within the body, such as maintaining the water and acid-base balance. In addition, they assist in blood clotting, absorption of nutrients, oxygen transportation, and nerve transmission.

Minerals are classified into two categories—macrominerals and microminerals—depending on the amount needed by the body. You need 100 mg or more of macrominerals. These include calcium, phosphorus, sulfur, sodium, potassium, chlorine, and magnesium. Microminerals are needed in extremely small amounts. These include iron, copper, zinc, fluorine, iodine, chromium, selenium, and manganese. Specific information relating to the most important minerals is contained in Table 7-12.

WATER

Water is the most important nutrient needed by the body. If you are deprived of food, you can live for several weeks but without water, you can live for only a few days. It has been described as an indispensable nutrient on which all forms of life depend. Water is second only to oxygen in its importance for sustaining life.

Vitamins: Organic compounds needed in small quantities by the body to perform specific functions.

Minerals: Inorganic substances needed by the body for specific functions.

Table 7-11	**Nutrient Needs of the Body: Vitamins**			
	Adult RDA			
Vitamin	**Men**	**Women**	**Food Sources**	**Functions**
Fat-soluble vitamins				
A	1000 µg	8000 µg	Most dark green leafy vegetables—carrots, pumpkins, sweet potatoes, peaches, apricots, cantaloupe, eggs, milk, fish, butter, and margarine	Promotes good vision; helps keep skin and mucous membrane linings healthy; resistance to certain infectious diseases
D	5 µg	5 µg	Fortified milk, fish-liver oils; some may be produced in the body in response to sunlight; small amounts also contained in butter, liver, egg yolk, salmon, and sardines	Promotes strong bones and teeth and regulates calcium and phosphorus absorption
E	10 µg	8 µg	Plant sources include nuts, vegetable oils, green leafy vegetables, and whole grains	Assists body to use vitamin K; important for formation of red blood cells
K	No specific RDA (70-140 micrograms may be adequate)		Cauliflower, cabbage, spinach, broccoli, and cereals	Assists in formation of blood clots
Water-soluble vitamins				
B_1 (Thiamine)	1.4 mg	1 mg	Bran and whole-wheat bread, dried beans, pork, fish, liver, and lean meats	Assists in energy release from carbohydrates; necessary for efficient functioning of heart and nervous system
B_2 (Riboflavin)	1.6 mg	1.2 mg	Cheese, milk, green vegetables, ice cream, enriched bread, and cereals	Assists in the release of energy from food; assists in respiration
B_3 (Niacin)	18 mg	13 mg	Meat, poultry, fish, peanuts, whole grain, or enriched cereals and breads	Needed for carbohydrate metabolism and fat synthesis; promotes normal appetite
B_6 (Pyridoxine)	2.2 mg	2 mg	Meat, poultry, fish, sweet potatoes, vegetables, and whole grains	Aids in absorption of protein; helps convert complex carbohydrates to simple carbohydrates; assists in production of red blood cells
B_{12}	3 mg	3 mg	Animal foods only, such as meat, fish, eggs, cheese, and chicken	Necessary for development of red blood cells; maintenance of normal functioning of nervous system
Folacin (folic acid)	400 µg	400 µg	Whole-wheat products, green vegetables, organ meats, fish, poultry, and eggs	Acts together with vitamin B_{12} to produce hemoglobin
Pantothenic acid	No specific RDA (safe range may be 4-7 mg)		Whole grains, dried beans, eggs, nuts, lean meats, and spinach	Assists in release of energy from foods; assists in hormone synthesis
Biotin	No specific RDA (safe range may be 100-200 mg)		Yeast, liver, egg yolks, and milk	Assists in metabolism of amino acids and carbohydrates; important in formation of fatty acids
C (ascorbic acid)	60 mg	60 mg	All citrus fruits and juices, cabbage, broccoli, green and red peppers, sweet potatoes, and spinach	Tooth and bone formation; promotes iron absorption; necessary for the healing of wounds

| Table 7-12 | **Nutrient Needs of the Body: Minerals** |

Vitamin	Adult RDA		Food Sources	Functions
	Men	Women		
Calcium	800 mg	800 mg	Milk and milk products, dark green vegetables, and shellfish	Builds bones and teeth and maintains bone density and strength; helps muscles contract and relax normally; delays fatigue
Chromium	No specific RDA (safe range may be 0.05-0.20 mg)		Liver, meat, cheese, whole-grain cereals, and yeast	Important for glucose metabolism
Phosphorus	800 mg	800 mg	Fish, poultry, meat, dairy products, soft drinks, and nuts	Necessary for normal muscle metabolism, skeletal growth, and tooth development; controls acid-base balance
Sodium	No specific RDA (safe range may be 2000-3000 mg)		Table salt, and most packaged goods where it is used as a preservative	Helps regulate the water balance; assists in maintaining blood pressure
Potassium	No specific RDA (safe range may be 1500-6000 mg)		Bananas, orange juice, most fruits, potatoes, peanuts	Promotes regular heart beat; controls water balance; contributes to control of blood pressure
Iron	10 mg	18 mg	Liver, kidney, red meat, poultry, egg yolk, whole-grain products, dark green vegetables	Formation of hemoglobin, contributes to energy release during metabolism
Copper	No specific RDA (safe range may be 2-3 mg)		Liver, kidney, shellfish, meats, nuts, whole-grain cereals	Aids in formation of red blood cells, assists in production of certain enzymes
Magnesium	350 mg	300 mg	Meat, whole-grain cereal, nuts, peas, beans, milk, green leafy vegetables	Bone growth; assists in nerve and muscle functioning; regulation of normal heart rhythm
Zinc	15 mg	15 mg	Seafood, beef, liver, eggs, whole wheat bread, oysters	Maintains normal taste and smell; important in healing
Fluorine (fluoride)	No specific RDA (safe range may be 1.5-4 mg)		Water, fish	Increases resistance of teeth to disease; may help prevent osteoporosis
Manganese	No specific RDA (safe range may be 2.5-5 mg)		Nuts, whole-grain cereals, peas, beans, coffee, tea, egg yolk	Normal bone growth; activation of enzymes used in carbohydrates and protein metabolism
Iodine	15 mg	15 mg	Iodized salt, seafood, vegetable oil	Necessary for normal functioning of thyroid gland; essential for normal cell function

Importance of water

Water is the most abundant nutrient in the human body, accounting for approximately 60% of your total body weight. Your body uses water for a variety of functions, including the following:

- Water is important for food digestion and metabolism, acting as a medium for various enzymatic and chemical reactions.

- Water is an important fluid in your blood that carries various nutrients and oxygen to the cells and transports waste products.

- Water helps regulate the body temperature by dissipating heat through the skin.

- Water is necessary for efficient movement at each joint, because it contributes to lubrication.

- Water keeps the lungs and respiratory passages moist to facilitate the efficient intake of oxygen and excretion of carbon dioxide.

- The efficient removal of waste products from the body depends on an adequate supply of water, because these waste products must be dissolved in water.

- Water is a natural diuretic. Without an adequate intake of water, your body will tend to retain more water than it should.

It can clearly be seen that if you do not drink sufficient water to maintain a normal fluid balance, your body will not be able to function efficiently. It is essential that your body maintain its crucial water balance. When the fluid balance is low, dehydration occurs. Severe dehydration can cause death.

How much water should you drink?

Not all the water in the body comes from water that we drink. Many of the foods and other fluids we drink contain large amounts of water. Milk, for example, is made up mainly of water, and most fruits and vegetables have a high percentage of water. Some water is also created in your body as the end product of carbohydrate, fat, and protein metabolism.

On a typical day, your body will normally give up the equivalent of 10 to 12 cups of water in one form or another. The water contained in your food will normally provide the equivalent of only 2 to 4 cups per day. This means that you probably need to drink between six and eight glasses of water per day just to maintain your fluid balance. If you exercise a lot or live in a hot climate or you are trying to lose weight, then you probably need to drink even more.

Water intake and weight loss

Adequate water intake is essential if any weight-loss program is to be effective. There are several reasons for this:

- Water suppresses the appetite. If you drink one or two glasses of water before a meal, you will probably not eat as much as you would have eaten if you had not drunk the water.
- An adequate intake of water is essential if the body is to metabolize fat efficiently. The reason for this is that your kidneys will not function efficiently without sufficient water, and the liver will be forced to perform some of their functions. One of the primary functions of the liver is to metabolize fat, and if it is forced to perform additional functions, it will not be as efficient as it should be at metabolizing fat.
- With an insufficient intake of water, your body will actually retain more water than it normally would. When your body gets very little water, it treats this as a threat to survival and tries to hold on to all the water that it has. This often shows up in the form of swelling in the feet, legs, and hands. The best way to alleviate this problem and to make sure that an adequate fluid balance exists is to drink lots of water.

Does it make a difference which beverage you drink?

Obviously you can obtain water by consuming such beverages as fruit juice, soft drinks, beer, wine, coffee, tea, and milk. However, there is a difference in the way your body treats pure water and other beverages that contain water.

Apart from the fact that most of these other beverages contain a significant number of calories, many of them contain substances that are not healthful. Following are some examples:

- Beer and wine contain alcohol, which is a toxic substance. In addition, for every ounce of alcohol consumed you need an additional 8 oz of water to metabolize it. This often seriously distorts your fluid balance.
- Many of these beverages contain caffeine. Caffeine itself is a diuretic, which also has several negative effects on the body.
- Fruit juices and soft drinks contain lots of sugar. Sugar requires extra water for metabolism.
- Most of the soft drinks are high in sodium.
- Many of the diet beverages contain chemicals such as preservatives and colorings. These often irritate the stomach lining, and the liver and kidneys require extra water to dispose of them.
- Many of the alternatives to water contain significant amounts of phosphoric acid. This may inhibit the ability of your body to absorb calcium.

In Summary

Drinking pure water eliminates all these problems. It contains no extra calories to slow down digestion or add unwanted fat, and it contains no irritants or chemicals to aggravate sensitive linings of the digestive tract.

THE FOUR FOOD GROUP PLAN

A well-balanced diet from a variety of foods is essential if all nutrients required by the body are to be obtained. The four food group plan was developed to categorize foods that are similar in origin and nutrient content. A number of servings is recommended from each group to meet the basic daily nutritional requirements. Basic information on the four food group plan is presented in Table 7-13. In principle, the four food group plan is very simple to use. However, depending on the choices you make within each group, you may finish with a caloric intake that is high in fat, cholesterol, sugar, or salt, and you may eat too many calories.

Table 7-13	**Four Food Group Plan**		
Food Group	**Servings Per Day**	**Sample Foods and Serving Size**	**Major Nutrient Contributions**
Milk and milk products	2*	1 cup (8 oz) milk, 1 cup yogurt, 1½ cups cottage cheese, 2 cups ice cream, 1-2 oz cheese, 1 cup milk pudding	Calcium Protein Riboflavin Zinc Vitamin B_{12}
Fruits and vegetables	4†	½ cup fruit, vegetable, or juice, 1 medium apple, orange, banana, or peach	Vitamin A Vitamin C Folacin
Grains (bread and cereal products)	4‡	1 slice bread, ½ cup cooked cereal, or 1 oz ready-to-eat cereal (1 cup); ½ hamburger bun, hot dog bun, or English muffin; ½ cup cooked rice, grits, macaroni, or spaghetti; 2 tbsp flour; 6 saltines; 1 6-inch tortilla	Niacin Iron Thiamine Fiber Zinc
Meat and meat substitutes	2	2 to 3 oz cooked meat, fish, or chicken; ¼ cup tuna; 2 eggs; 4 tbsp peanut butter; 1 cup cooked legumes; ½ cup nuts	Protein Iron Riboflavin Niacin Zinc Vitamin B_{12} Thiamine

*Children, teenagers, pregnant women, and nursing mothers need three to four servings or more.
†One selection should be rich in vitamin C, and one should be rich in vitamin A.
‡Enriched or whole-grain products are the best.

THE NEW AMERICAN EATING GUIDE

Because of these problems, the Center for Science in the Public Interest has prepared a modified version of the four food group plan that provides additional information so that you can make wise choices concerning the foods you select within each group.

With this plan, foods within each of the four groups are divided into three categories. Those you can eat any time are the ones that are low in fat, sugar, and salt. The grain foods in this category are those which are mostly unrefined and therefore are high in fiber and some of the trace minerals.

The second category comprises those foods you should eat in moderation. They may contain moderate amounts of fat and may be high in salt, sugar, sodium, or cholesterol. A coding system is used to indicate why each food is listed in this category.

The third category of foods comprises those you should eat only now and then or possibly not eat at all. They are foods that are usually high in fat—particularly saturated fat—or sugar, salt, or cholesterol. It is suggested that if these foods are eaten, they are to be eaten less frequently and in small amounts.

This plan is referred to as the *New American Eating Guide*. Basic information relative to each of the classifications within each of the four groups is summarized in Table 7-14.

THE FOOD PYRAMID

In 1992 the U.S. Department of Agriculture released new standards for a recommended diet in the form of a food pyramid. With this system, foods are divided into six categories; the recommended number of servings for each of these is given in Figure 7-10. This plan suggests that we need to eat less fat and sugar and eat more fruits, vegetables, and grains.

THE FOOD EXCHANGE SYSTEM

The best system for planning meals and the only one that allows you to analyze your meals is the food exchange system. With this system, foods are classified into six categories, or lists. Some lists contain subgroups. Each food on any given list contains approximately the same number of calories as any other food on the list and approximately the same amount of each of the energy nutrients. With some of the lists the portion size must be adjusted to obtain the desired results. A listing of the exchange groups and their caloric value together with other nutritional information is presented in Table 7-15 (p. 164).

A listing of the individual foods that make up each of the six exchanges is presented in Appendix A. In addition, Laboratory Experience 7-2 is designed so that you can use the exchange lists to determine the adequacy of your diet.

Table 7-14   New American Eating Guide (Modified Four Group Plan)

Anytime	In Moderation	Now and Then
1. Milk products (three to four servings per day for children, two for adults)		
Buttermilk (from skim milk)	Cocoa with skim milk[e]	Cheesecake[d,e]
Low-fat cottage cheese	Cottage cheese, regular[a]	Cheese fondue[d,g]
Low-fat milk (1%)	Frozen yogurt[e]	Cheese souffle[d,g,h]
Low fat yogurt	Ice milk[e]	Eggnog[d,e,h]
Nonfat dry milk	Low-fat milk (2%)[a]	Hard cheeses: blue, brick,
Skim-milk cheeses	Low-fat yogurt, sweetened[e]	Camembert, cheddar, muenster,
Skim milk	Mozzarella, part-skim[d,g]	Swiss[d,g]
Skim-milk and banana shake		Ice cream[d,e]
		Processed cheeses[d,f]
		Whole milk[d]
		Whole-milk yogurt[d]
2. Fruits and vegetables (four or more servings per day)		
All fruits and vegetables except those at right	Avocado[c]	Coconut[d]
Applesauce (unsweetened)	Cole slaw[c]	Pickles[f]
Unsweetened fruit juices	Cranberry sauce[e]	
Unsalted vegetable juices	Dried fruit	
Potatoes, white or sweet	French fries[a or b]	
	Fried eggplant[b]	
	Fruits canned in syrup[e]	
	Gazpacho[b,g]	
	Glazed carrots[e,g]	
	Guacamole[c]	
	Potatoes au gratin[a,g]	
	Salted vegetable juices[b]	
	Sweetened fruit juices[e]	
	Vegetables canned with salt[f]	
3. Beans, grains, and nuts (four or more servings per day)		
Bread and rolls (whole grain)	Cornbread[i]	Croissant[d,i]
Bulgur	Flour tortilla[i]	Doughnut[c or d;e,i]
Dried beans and peas	Granola cereals[a or b]	Presweetened cereals[e,i]
Lentils	Hominy grits[i]	Sticky buns[a or b;e,i]
Oatmeal	Macaroni and cheese[a,g,i]	Stuffing (with butter)[d,g,i]
Pasta, whole-wheat	Matzoh[i]	
Rice, brown	Nuts[c]	
Sprouts	Pasta, refined[i]	
Whole-grain hot and cold cereals	Peanut butter[c]	
Whole-wheat matzoh	Pizza[f,i]	
	Refined unsweetened cereals[i]	
	Refried beans[a or b]	
	Seeds[c]	
	Soybeans[b]	
	Tofu[b]	
	Waffles or pancakes with syrup[e,g,i]	
	White bread and rolls[i]	
	White rice[i]	

Modified from the Center for Science in the Public Interest, Washington, DC, 1982.
[a]Moderate fat, saturated.
[b]Moderate fat, unsaturated.
[c]High fat, unsaturated.
[d]High fat, saturated.
[e]High in added sugar.
[f]High in salt or sodium.
[g]May be high in salt or sodium.
[h]High in cholesterol.
[i]Refined grains.

Analysis using the exchange lists By consulting the exchange lists (see Appendix A) you can determine how many exchanges you must count for each of the food items. The daily meal plan can now be analyzed quickly by adding the number of exchanges and using the information contained in Table 7-15. A summary of this information follows.

Analysis using the nutritional information tables

A more comprehensive analysis may be obtained by using the information contained in a table of nutritional information for foods (see Appendix B). This is a tedious and time-consuming task. Fortunately, many computer software packages have been developed that

	Food	Amount	Exchanges
Breakfast	Orange juice	1 cup	2 fruit
	Bran cereal	1 cup	2 starch
	Skim milk	1 cup	1 milk
	Banana	1 large	2 fruit
	Blueberries	¾ cup	1 fruit
	English muffin	1 large	2 starch
	Margarine	1 tsp	1 fat
Lunch	Chicken breast	3 oz	3 meat
	Whole-wheat bread	2 slices	2 starch
	Mayonnaise (diet)	1 tbsp	1 fat
	Tomato	3 slices	1 vegetable
	Strawberries	1¼ cup	1 fruit
	Shredded wheat	½ cup	1 starch
	Skim milk	1 cup	1 milk
Dinner	Mixed green salad	2 cups	2 vegetable
	French dressing	2 tbsp	2 fat
	Carrots (cooked)	½ cup	1 vegetable
	Green beans (cooked)	½ cup	1 vegetable
	Tenderloin steak (lean)	3 oz	3 meat
	Potato (baked)	1 small	2 starch
	Margarine (diet)	1 tbsp	1 fat
	Whole-wheat bread	2 slices	2 starch
	Margarine (diet)	2 tbsp	1 fat

Exchange	Total	Total Carbohydrate (Grams)	Total Fat (Grams)	Total Protein (Grams)
Starch	11	165	—	33
Meat	6	—	18	42
Vegetable	5	25	—	10
Fruit	6	90	—	—
Milk	2	24	—	16
Fat	6	—	30	—
TOTALS		304	48	101

Total calories can be estimated as follows:

	Grams	×	Cal/G	=	Calories
Carbohydrates	304	×	4	=	1216
Fats	48	×	9	=	432
Proteins	101	×	4	=	404
TOTAL CALORIES					2052

The percentage of the total calories from each of the three nutrients is as follows:

Carbohydrates	=	1216/2052	=	59%
Fats	=	432/2052	=	21%
Proteins	=	404/2052	=	20%

Sample Computer Program Output for Nutritional Analysis

Prucal

Planning your diet to meet PRUDENT guidelines

Diet Analysis for:	Freddie Fitness
Age:	21
Height:	5 ft 11 inches
Recommended Weight:	158 lb
Sex:	Male
Frame:	Medium
Activity:	Moderate

This program estimates your individual energy needs (kcal) based on your sex, the desirable weight for your height and frame size, and your activity level.

The goals are set as follows:

Kcal 2686

Calorie distribution

Protein	13%
Total Carbohydrates.....................	57%
Total Sugars	20%
Fat	30%
Saturated Fat............................	10%
Polyunsaturated Fat.................	10%

Dietary Fiber	15 g/1000 kcal
Cholesterol......................................	300 mg/day
Sodium	2000 mg/day

Vitamin and mineral goals are set to meet the RDAs based on sex and age. The potassium goal is set at the midpoint of Estimated Safe and Adequate Daily Intake.

Freddie Fitness   Day One   8/17/95

Comparison of Nutrient Intake and Goals by Percentage

Nutrients	Percent of goal
Kcal	77
Protein	118
Total Sugars	85
Dietary Fiber	101
Fat	76
Saturated Fat	50
Polyunsat Fat	70
Cholesterol	62
Sodium	121
Potassium	127
Vitamin A	275
Vitamin C	475
Thiamin	133
Riboflavin	161
Vitamin B6	152
Calcium	127
Iron	210
Zinc	96

Goals indicated by an *O* are maximum goals and should not be exceeded.

Goals indicated by an *X* are minimum goals and should be met or exceeded.

Goal indicated by an *M* is the midpoint of the Safe and Adequate Range.

The graph lines for total sugars, fats, saturated fats, and polyunsaturated fat should not be longer than the kcals line.

Your diet provides 2071 calories distributed as follows:

Protein....................................	20%	Fat..	25%
Total Carbohydrate	55%	Saturated Fat.....................	7%
Total Sugars........................	22%	Polyunsaturated Fat	9%

Your actual intake per day of the following nutrients is:

Protein.............. 104 g	Cholesterol....... 188 mg	Riboflavin....... 2.7 mg
Total sugars...... 115 g	Sodium .... 2428 mg	Vitamin B6..... 3.3 mg
Dietary fiber....... 41 g	Potassium....... 4793 mg	Calcium....... 1022 mg
Fat...................... 68 g	Vitamin A...... 13794 IU	Iron .... 20.8 mg
Saturated fat... 14.9 g	Vitamin C......... 285 mg	Zinc .... 14.5 mg
Polyunsat fat... 20.9 g	Thiamin............. 2.0 mg	

Modified from Colorado State University, Department of Food Science and Human Nutrition, Fort Collins, Colorado.

---

will perform most of this busy work for you and will provide you with a large amount of valuable information. Following is a summary for the previously analyzed meal plan using the PRUCAL computer software package. With this program, goals are established based on the specific information for each person relative to age, height, gender, activity level, and frame size. These results show that the foods consumed provided 2071 cal with 20% from protein, 55% from carbohydrate, and 25% from fat. The actual intakes for each of the 17 important nutrients is given and compared with the RDA values to determine whether the dietary goals are being met.

Several other similar programs are available to assist you in analyzing your caloric intake. The results from these programs can then be used to assist you in making changes in what you eat and how much you eat, so that you can achieve your objectives.

EATING OUT

Eating out has become an important part of the American lifestyle. This is possibly because of the growing number of families in which both the husband and wife work and because of the increase in the number of people living alone who find it easier to eat out rather than cook for themselves. An increase in the number of fast-food outlets available makes it much easier for a person to eat quickly.

However, consumers have become much more concerned about the nutritional content of food, and many restaurants and fast-food chains have been forced to alter their menus to cater to the needs of the consumers. Despite these changes, it is still very difficult to eat well when dining out. Consider, for example, the following typical steakhouse meal:

> Tossed salad with French dressing
> Rib-eye steak (8 oz)
> Baked potato with butter and sour cream
> Coffee with sugar and cream

An analysis shows that this one meal provides over 1600 cal, with 63% of these calories coming from fat and only 24% from carbohydrates. It is no wonder that the typical American diet is so high in fat.

Eating at fast-food restaurants can be just as bad or worse, depending on the selection of foods. Consider the following selections:

> Bacon cheeseburger
> French fries
> Apple turnover
> Chocolate milkshake

This meal contains approximately 1700 cal, with slightly less than 50% of these calories coming from fat. Additional information relating to the nutritional content for fast foods is included in Appendix C.

Chapter Summary

The following summary will help you to identify some of the important concepts covered in this chapter:

- Most Americans are confused about nutrition, and many of them have poor eating habits.
- There are approximately 40 essential nutrients that the body needs. The secret to eating well is to learn how to get adequate amounts of all of these without gaining weight or getting fat.
- Fat is a concentrated source of energy, containing more than twice as many calories as protein and carbohydrates.
- The average American needs to learn how to increase his or her intake of carbohydrates while significantly reducing his or her intake of simple refined sugar.
- Fat, sugar, and alcohol contain "empty" calories and basically contribute very few if any of the essential nutrients.
- Complete proteins from animal products contain all nine of the essential amino acids. All other sources of protein are considered incomplete. Incomplete proteins; however, can be combined to complement one another.
- Because many of the foods that are high in fat are also high in protein, many people now get a less than adequate amount of protein when reducing their fat intake.
- Water is the most important essential nutrient needed by the body. We need to drink at least eight glasses of water each day.
- Various eating plans have been devised to enable you to obtain a well-balanced diet from a variety of foods. The food exchange lists are probably the best available.

References

1. Althoff SA, Svobada M, Girdano DA: *Choices in health and fitness for life,* ed 2, Scottsdale, Ariz, 1992, Gorsuch Scarisbrick.
2. American Diabetes Association, Inc., American Dietetic Association: *Exchange lists,* Chicago, 1995, The Association.
3. Brown JE: *Nutrition now,* Minneapolis, 1995, West Publishing.
4. Center for Science in Public Interest: *How sweet is it?* Washington, DC, 1985, The Center.
5. Church CF, Church HN: *Food values of portions commonly used,* ed 10, Philadelphia, 1985, JB Lippincott.
6. Cotteman SK: *Y's way to weight management,* Champaign, Ill, 1985, Human Kinetics.
7. Crow VCR: *Nutrient needs at a glance,* College Station, Tex, 1985, The Texas Agriculture Extension Service, Texas A & M University System.
8. DuPuy NA, Mermel VL: *Focus on nutrition,* St Louis, 1995, Mosby.
9. Guthrie HA, Picciano M: *Human nutrition,* St Louis, 1995, Mosby-Year Book.
10. Hurley JS: *Nutrition and health,* Guilford, Conn, 1992, The Dushkin Publishing Group.
11. Katch FI, McArdle WD: *Nutrition, weight control and exercise,* ed 4, Philadelphia, 1993, Lea & Febiger.
12. Lecos C: *Water: the number one nutrient,* In *FDA consumer,* 1984, US Government Printing Office.
13. McLaren M: *Weight loss and nutrition,* San Diego, 1986, Health Media of America.
14. Nutritive value of foods, *Home garden bulletin* No. 72, 1981 Washington, DC, United States Department of Agriculture.
15. Prentice WE: *Fitness for college and life,* ed 4, St Louis, 1994, Mosby.
16. PRUCAL: *Prudent diet analysis user's guide,* Fort Collins, Colo, 1986.
17. *Recommended dietary allowances,* ed 9, Washington, DC, 1980.
18. Rosato FD: *Fitness and wellness—the physical connection,* ed 3, St Paul, Minn, 1994, West.
19. Texas Agriculture and Extension Service: *Hidden sugar in foods,* College Station, Tex, 1985, The Service.
20. Vitamins: fact and fancy, University of California, Berkeley, Calif, *Wellness Letter* 2:1, October 1985.
21. Wardlaw GM, Insel PA: *Perspectives in nutrition,* ed 3, 1996, Mosby-Year Book.
22. Wardlaw GM, Insel PA, Seyler MF: *Contemporary nutrition: issues and insights,* ed 2, 1994, Mosby.
23. Williams MH: *Nutrition for fitness and sport,* ed 4, Dubuque, Ia, 1995, Brown and Benchmark.
24. Young EA et al: Fast foods 1986: nutrient analyses, *Dietetic Currents* 13:6, 1986.

Estimating Your Daily Fiber Intake

Name _____   Section _____   Date _____

Following is a listing of many of the foods containing fiber. This list shows the amount of fiber for the designated serving size.

Try to recall the foods that you ate yesterday, and check these off in column 1 on this list.

Next to each item checked off, estimate the grams of fiber you obtained from each item. This will be based on how much of the food you ate in relation to the serving size. Write this value in column 2.

Total up the estimated grams of fiber for the day.

Fiber content of foods

Column 1	Column 2	Food	Serving Size	Fiber—Grams
		Fruits		
_____	_____	Apple with skin	1 medium	3.5
_____	_____	Banana	1 medium	2.4
_____	_____	Cherries	10	1.2
_____	_____	Cantaloupe	¼ melon	1.0
_____	_____	Peach with skin	1	1.9
_____	_____	Pear with skin	½	3.1
_____	_____	Prunes	3	3.0
_____	_____	Raisins	¼ cup	3.1
_____	_____	Raspberries	½ cup	3.1
_____	_____	Strawberries	1 cup	3.0
_____	_____	Orange	1 medium	2.6
		Vegetables—cooked		
_____	_____	Asparagus	½ cup	1.0
_____	_____	Beans—green	½ cup	1.6
_____	_____	Broccoli	½ cup	2.2
_____	_____	Brussels sprouts	½ cup	2.3
_____	_____	Cabbage	½ cup	2.0
_____	_____	Potato with skin	1 medium	2.5
_____	_____	Spinach	½ cup	2.5
_____	_____	Sweet potato	½ medium	1.7
_____	_____	Zucchini	½ cup	1.8
		Vegetables—raw		
_____	_____	Lettuce	1 cup	1.0
_____	_____	Tomato	½ cup	1.1
_____	_____	Celery	½ cup	1.1
_____	_____	Cucumber	½ cup	0.4
_____	_____	Mushrooms	½ cup	0.9
		Legumes		
_____	_____	Baked beans	½ cup	8.8
_____	_____	Peas—dried, cooked	½ cup	4.7
_____	_____	Kidney beans—cooked	½ cup	7.3
_____	_____	Lima beans—cooked	½ cup	4.5

Continued

Fiber content of foods—cont'd

Column 1	Column 2	Food	Serving Size	Fiber—Grams
_____	_____	Lentils—cooked	½ cup	3.7
_____	_____	Navy beans—cooked	½ cup	6.0
		Nuts and seeds		
_____	_____	Almonds	10 nuts	1.1
_____	_____	Peanuts	10 nuts	1.4
_____	_____	Popcorn—air popped	1 cup	1.0
		Bread and pasta		
_____	_____	Whole-wheat bread	1 slice	1.4
_____	_____	Other breads	1 slice	1.0
_____	_____	Bran muffin	1 medium	2.5
_____	_____	Bagel	1 medium	0.6
_____	_____	Rice—cooked	½ cup	1.0
_____	_____	Pasta—cooked	½ cup	1.1
		Breakfast cereals		
_____	_____	All Bran with extra fiber (Kellogg's)	1 oz	14.0
_____	_____	Fiber One (General Mills)	1 oz	12.0
_____	_____	All Bran (Kellogg's)	1 oz	10.0
_____	_____	100% Bran with oat bran (Nabisco)	1 oz	8.0
_____	_____	Uncle Sams (U.S. Mills)	1 oz	8.0
_____	_____	40% Bran type	1 oz	4.0
_____	_____	Raisin bran type	1 oz	4.0
_____	_____	Shredded wheat	1 oz	2.6
_____	_____	Oatmeal—regular, quick, or instant	1 oz	1.6

Record your total fiber intake for the day, in the space provided below:

Name: _____

Date: _____

Total fiber intake: _____ g

If your total fiber intake is less than 25 g, look carefully at the foods containing fiber and select some additional foods you can eat to increase your intake to at least 25 g each day.

Laboratory Experience 7-2

Estimation and Analysis of Daily Caloric Intake

_____   _____   _____
Name   Section   Date

The purpose of this Laboratory Experience is to analyze your caloric intake to determine the number of calories and the percentage of these calories that come from fat, carbohydrates, and protein.

INSTRUCTIONS

1. You must record everything that you eat and drink for 2 days—a weekday and a weekend day. Try to select typical days that will reflect your true eating habits. Simply fill out the first two columns for each day on each of the prepared sheets that are provided.
2. Consult the food exchange lists (see Appendix A) to estimate how many of the exchanges each food item contains. (An example is given on p. 167 to show you how this is done.)
3. Consult Table 7-15 to determine the number of grams of fat, carbohydrate, and protein in each food. (If the food item does not appear on the exchange list, you may obtain this information from the food label, or you may need to consult Appendix B or a more complete table showing the nutritional content of foods.)
4. Total the values for the day so that you know exactly how many grams of carbohydrates, fat, and protein that you consumed.
5. Perform the calculations as shown on the summary sheet. (See p. 167 and 168 for an example showing how to do this.)

Continued

ANALYZING CALORIC INTAKE USING THE FOOD EXCHANGE LISTS Name _____

DAY 1

Food or beverage	Approximate amount	Number of exchanges											Carbohydrate* (g)	Protein* (g)	Fat* (g)
		Milk (skim)	Milk (low fat)	Milk (whole)	Fat	Vegetable	Starch/grains	Meat (lean)	Meat (medium fat)	Meat (high fat)	Fat	Sugar			

TOTALS ___ ___ ___

*Information can be determined from exchange list information or can be obtained directly from food label.

ANALYZING CALORIC INTAKE USING THE FOOD EXCHANGE LISTS Name _____

DAY 2

Food or beverage	Approximate amount	Number of exchanges											Carbohydrate* (g)	Protein* (g)	Fat* (g)
		Milk (skim)	Milk (low fat)	Milk (whole)	Fat	Vegetable	Starch/grains	Meat (lean)	Meat (medium fat)	Meat (high fat)	Fat	Sugar			

TOTALS ___ ___ ___

*Information can be determined from exchange list information or can be obtained directly from food label.

Summary Sheet—Estimation of Calories Consumed

DAY 1

	Total Grams	**× Cal/g**	**= Calories**
Carbohydrates	____	× 4 =	____
Protein	____	× 4 =	____
Fat	____	× 9 =	____
TOTAL CALORIES			____

% Carbohydrates $= \dfrac{\text{Calories from carbohydrates}}{\text{Total calories}}$

$= $ ____

$= $ ____ %

% Protein $\quad\dfrac{\text{Calories from protein}}{\text{Total calories}}$

$= $ ____

$= $ ____ %

% Fat $\quad= \dfrac{\text{Calories from fat}}{\text{Total calories}}$

$= $ ____

$= $ ____ %

DAY 2

	Total Grams	**× Cal/g**	**= Calories**
Carbohydrates	____	× 4 =	____
Protein	____	× 4 =	____
Fat	____	× 9 =	____
TOTAL CALORIES			____

% Carbohydrates $= \dfrac{\text{Calories from carbohydrates}}{\text{Total calories}}$

$= $ ____

$= $ ____ %

% Protein $\quad\dfrac{\text{Calories from protein}}{\text{Total calories}}$

$= $ ____

$= $ ____ %

% Fat $\quad= \dfrac{\text{Calories from fat}}{\text{Total calories}}$

$= $ ____

$= $ ____ %

Interpretation of Results

You can now compare your total calories for each day to your RDA value (see Table 7-2). Remember the RDA value for calories is for those trying to maintain their present weight. If you are trying to lose weight you will need to subtract either 500 or 1000 calories from this value depending on how much weight you are trying to lose. Record your scores in the spaces provided below.

Name: _____

Date: _____

Recommended daily caloric intake: _____ calories

Caloric intake Day 1: _____ calories

Caloric intake Day 2: _____ calories

Record the percentages of calories from carbohydrates, fats, and protein in the spaces provided below.

Percentage of Calories	Day 1	Day 2	Recommended Percentage
Carbohydrates	_____	_____	>58%
Fats	_____	_____	<30%
Protein	_____	_____	>12%

You can also determine whether your total protein intake is adequate. Record the total number of grams of protein consumed each day in the space provided below and also record your calculated RDA values for protein (see p. 154).

Name: _____

Date: _____

Total protein intake:

   Day 1: _____ g

   Day 2: _____ g

RDA value for protein:

   RDA value is 0.8 g for each kg of body weight:

    $= $ _____ g

If you exercise regularly for at least 30 minutes three times a week, you should probably multiply by 1.2 rather than 0.8

    $= $ _____ g

If your protein intake is more than or less than the appropriate value, you should suggest some additions, deletions, or substitutions you can make to your food intake.

Chapter Eight **Exercise and Body Composition**

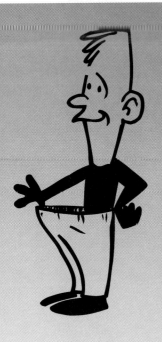

CHAPTER OBJECTIVES
Check off each objective you achieve.

- ❏ Define the terms *obese* and *overweight*, and know how to determine each of them.
- ❏ Evaluate your body composition, and determine your ideal weight.
- ❏ Discuss the disadvantages associated with excess body fat.
- ❏ Determine your daily caloric expenditure, and be able to plan a weight-loss or weight-management program based on these results.
- ❏ Explain the importance of exercise in a weight loss program, and determine how much exercise is necessary and at what intensity you must exercise if you are to be successful at losing body fat.
- ❏ Implement a successful exercise program for weight loss or weight management.

One of the major health problems in the United States today relates to controlling body weight and/or body fat. A 1995 survey showed that only 18% of the American adult population considered their weight to be within an acceptable range, 68% indicated that they would like to weigh less, and 14% indicated that they would like to weigh more. This same survey showed that 75% of the men were over their recommended weight range compared with 60% of the women.[17]

Despite the health craze of the '80s and the fact that more people are now aware of the importance of good nutrition and regular exercise and the negative effects of obesity on health, there has been a 30% increase in the prevalence of overweight in the United States during the last 20 years.[10]

The results from a national survey showed conclusively that the number of Americans who are seriously overweight, after holding steady for 20 years at 25%, suddenly jumped to 33% in 1991. This represents an increase of more than 30%; there are now 58 million Americans over the age of 25 who are 20% or more above their ideal weight.[10] The results from this survey are compared with three previous studies in Figure 8-1. In addition, it would appear that the situation for the next generation is even worse. The percentage of teenagers that are overweight, which had held steady at 15%, has increased dramatically to 21%.[2]

Fitness Flash

The *Healthy People 2000* goal was to reduce the percentage of overweight Americans from 25% to 20% by the year 2000. It is now obvious that this goal will not be met.

Facts and Figures

The economic costs of illness associated with overweight were estimated to be in excess of $39 billion per year.

Even though there is more leisure time available, many individuals are actually less active now than they were in previous years. This is partly because of the introduction of the home computer and video games and the expansion of cable television, which now features special channels for sports, music, and first-run movies. If the time now spent on these activities was previously spent on some form of active recreation, then there is a significant decrease in daily caloric expenditure.

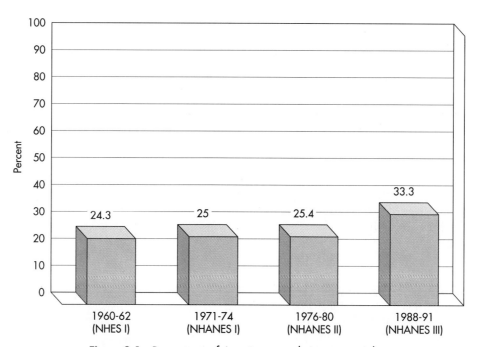

Figure 8-1 Percentage of American population overweight.

The start of obesity or overweight problems for many people is associated with a decrease in physical activity. Professional or college athletes during training usually have very little trouble maintaining their weight, even though they eat all the food that they want. Yet many athletes do not maintain their activity level or decrease their food intake when they retire and therefore experience a problem controlling their weight. This is a problem also encountered by many individuals when they finish college and go to work. If their job is sedentary or inactive, these people tend to be less active but usually continue to eat as much as ever. The result, of course, is that their weight increases very rapidly.

In Summary

If more people are to be successful in controlling their weight, they need to learn behavior modification skills where they incorporate a good exercise program and a good nutritional program into their lifestyle.

DEFINITION OF TERMS

It is important to differentiate clearly between the terms **overweight** and **obese.**

Overweight

An overweight person is one who weighs more than his or her **desirable weight.** A person's desirable weight has been defined as one at which he or she looks good, feels good, and can function efficiently. Originally, simple tables based on a person's height, age, and gender were used to determine desirable weight. In 1963 the Metropolitan Life Insurance Company introduced a new standard table based on different principles. The company recognized the undesirability of a continued increase in weight during adulthood past the termination of growth and realized at least in theory that people vary according to body build. Weight ranges were then presented for three classes of frame size—small, medium, and large. However, determination of the category in which each individual was to be classified was apparently left to the subjective judgment of the examiner; no criteria were presented for classification purposes.

The present method recommended for determination of frame size involves the measurement of elbow breadth (Figure 8-2). To measure your elbow breadth, flex your forearm so that there is approximately a 90° angle at the elbow joint. Use a pair of calipers to measure the exact distance between the most prominent projection on either side of your elbow.

The range of values presented in Table 8-1 can be used to determine your frame size. The values pre-

sented are for medium frame size for men and women. Note that they vary according to your height. If your score is within this range, you would be considered to be a medium frame size. If your score is greater than the score for your height and gender, you would be considered to have a large frame; if your score is lower, you would be considered to have a small frame size.

The most recent tables available for determination of desirable weight are Tables 8-2 (men) and 8-3 (women).

Even though these height/weight tables are used extensively, they have some serious limitations.

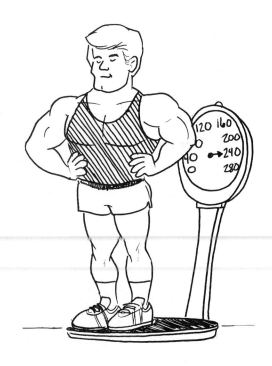

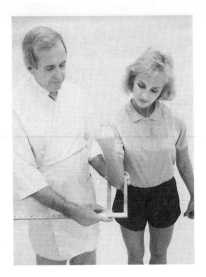

Figure 8-2   Measurement of elbow breadth for determination of frame size.

Table 8-1	**Determination of Frame Size**		
Height (women)	Elbow Breadth	Height (men)	Elbow Breadth
<4'11"	2¼"-2½"	<5'3"	2½"-2⅞"
4'11"-5'2"	2¼"-2½"	5'3"-5'6"	2⅝"-2⅞"
5'3"-5'6"	2⅜"-2⅝"	5'7"-5'10"	2¾"-3"
5'7"-5'10"	2½"-2¾"	5'11"-6'6"	2¾"-3⅛"
>5'10"	2½"-2¾"	>6'2"	2⅞"-3¼"

Table 8-2	**Metropolitan Life Insurance Height/Weight Tables for Men***		
Height	Small Frame	Medium Frame	Large Frame
5'2"	128-134	131-141	138-150
5'3"	130-136	133-143	140-153
5'4"	132-138	135-145	142-156
5'5"	134-140	137-148	144-160
5'6"	136-142	139-151	146-164
5'7"	138-145	142-154	149-168
5'8"	140-148	145-157	152-172
5'9"	142-151	148-160	155-176
5'10"	144-154	151-163	158-180
5'11	146-157	154-166	161-184
6'0"	149-160	157-170	164-188
6'1"	152-164	160-174	168-192
6'2"	155-168	164-178	172-197
6'3"	158-172	167-182	176-202
6'4"	162-176	171-187	181-207

Data from Metropolitan Life Insurance Co.
*Weight is in pounds, with clothing weighing 5 lb; height is with shoes with 1-inch heels.

- The method used for determination of frame size appears to be inadequate.

- The desirable range of weight for a particular height is very large. For example, the recommended weight for a 6-foot man ranges from 149 to 188 lb. Even for a particular frame size the range is very large—164 to 188 lb for this 6-foot man.

- These tables make no allowances for differences in the development of musculature among individuals. Most highly trained athletes, particularly football players, would be considerably overweight by these standards. However, if these athletes are examined more closely, this excess weight is seen to be caused by muscular development and their percentage of body fat is usually quite low. It is not uncommon to find professional football players who weigh 250 lb or more with 12% body fat or less. It is not how heavy a person is that is important, but how much fat he or she has.

Despite these disadvantages, these tables are still used frequently. The most frequently used standard to determine whether you are classified as overweight is 10%. If you weigh 10% or more above your desirable weight, you are considered to be overweight. The procedures that are used to determine this are included in Laboratory Experience 8-1.

Overweight: An excessive accumulation of body weight

Obese: An excessive accumulation of body fat.

Desirable weight: The weight at which a person looks good, feels good, and functions efficiently.

Table 8-3	Metropolitan Life Insurance Height/Weight Tables for Women*		
Height	**Small Frame**	**Medium Frame**	**Large Frame**
4'10"	102-111	109-121	118-131
4'11"	103-113	111-123	120-134
5'0"	104-115	113-126	122-137
5'1"	106-118	115-129	125-140
5'2"	108-121	118-132	128-143
5'3"	111-124	121-135	131-147
5'4"	114-127	124-138	134-151
5'5"	117-130	127-141	137-155
5'6"	120-133	130-144	140-159
5'7"	123-136	133-147	143-163
5'8"	126-139	136-150	146-167
5'9"	129-142	139-153	149-170
5'10"	132-145	142-156	152-173
5'11	135-148	145-159	155-176
6'0"	138-151	148-162	158-179

From Metropolitan Life Insurance Co.
*Weight is in pounds, with clothing weighing 3 lb; height is with shoes with 1-inch heels.

BODY MASS INDEX

The body mass index is another method that is widely used to evaluate your weight. It is based solely on your height and weight, so it has the same limitations as the height/weight tables. The procedures to follow to determine your body mass index are given in Laboratory Experience 8-2. Although this procedure does not take into account crucial factors such as percent body fat, frame size, and overall build, it does indicate to you if your weight falls within an "acceptable" range.

Obese

An obese person is one who has an excessive accumulation of body fat. This raises the question of how much fat you need to have to be considered obese. Unfortunately, there is no clear-cut answer. Instead, fatness should be considered to exist on a continuum, just like your level of aerobic fitness. Based on norms that are available, arbitrary standards are established to evaluate your scores. These norms for both men and women are included in Laboratory Experience 8-3.

Scores for **percent of body fat** have continued to rise in recent years. In 1968 the average percentage of body fat for college-age students was 12% for men and 20% for women. By 1980 these figures had increased to 15% for men and 22% for women, and by 1990 these scores were 18% for men and 23% for women. The terms "desirable" and "normal" should not be confused. Men wishing to attain a desirable amount of body fat for optimal health and fitness should probably strive for 12% or less; women should strive to be between 14% and 18%.

BODY COMPOSITION

The term **body composition** refers to the percentage of your body weight that is composed of fat in relation to that composed of fat-free tissue. Your fat-free weight is also referred to as your **lean body weight.** It has been established that the real threat to good health is not total weight but excess body fat.

Determination of percentage of body fat

It is important to be able to determine your body composition so that you can ascertain how much fat you have and what proportion of your body weight can be

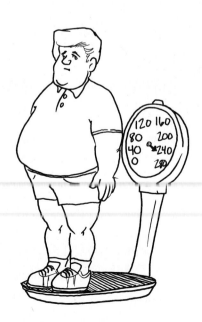

attributed to this. By knowing this, you will be able to determine more exactly how much you should weigh. Certainly, this procedure is much better than simply consulting the standard height/weight charts that have previously been discussed.

Your percentage of body fat may be determined by a variety of techniques. Perhaps the best method is to use the underwater weighing technique to determine body density and then use this figure to calculate your percentage of body fat and lean body weight. However, this technique is not practical for use with large groups of people and requires expensive equipment.

Several other approaches have been developed that attempt to estimate a person's percentage of body fat. The most common and possibly the most accurate method involves the use of skinfold measurements, provided the person who is taking the measurements is experienced and takes each measurement accurately.

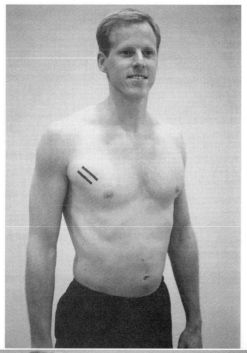

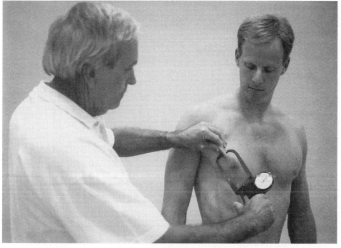

Figure 8-3 Measurement of chest skinfold thickness.

Taking skinfold measurements

Taking skinfold measurements requires practice to obtain consistent results. The following are suggestions for measuring skinfold thickness:

- Firmly grasp the fold of the skin between the left thumb and forefinger, and pull the fold away from the body.
- Place the contact surfaces of the calipers approximately ½ inch from the tips of the fingers.
- The caliper should be held perpendicular to the skinfold by the right hand, with the skinfold dial up so that it can be read.
- Wait for approximately 2 seconds until the needle becomes relatively stable.
- Read the measurement to the nearest 0.5 mm.
- Three measurements should be taken at each site, with at least two of these measurements equal. If not, additional measurements must be made until consistency is obtained.
- All measurements should be made on the right side of the body.
- Marking each anatomical site with a black felt pen will enhance consistency.
- Measurements should not be taken when the skin is moist or through leotards or tights.
- Measurements should not be taken immediately after exercise or when the subject is overheated because the shift in body fluid to the skin may increase the skinfold size.
- Practice is necessary to be able to grasp the same size of skinfold consistently at the same location each time.

Skinfold sites

Following are locations for skinfold measurements:

1. *Chest.* Take a diagonal fold on the front of the chest. For men this should be midway between the right nipple and the front border of the armpit. For women this should be two thirds of the way from the right nipple to the front border of the armpit (Figure 8-3).

Percent body fat: The percentage of total body weight that is attributable to fat.

Body composition: The percentage of your body weight that is composed of fat in relation to that classified as fat free.

Lean body weight: The total amount of body weight that is not attributed to body fat.

Skinfold measurement: The measurement of fat at a particular site using skinfold calipers.

2. *Subscapular.* Take a diagonal fold immediately below the interior angle of the scapula. The natural fold to be measured is located away from the midline of the body downward (Figure 8-4).

3. *Triceps.* Take a vertical fold at the back of the right arm, running parallel to the length of the arm, midway between the shoulder and the elbow joints. The arm should be hanging naturally at the side in a relaxed position (Figure 8-5).

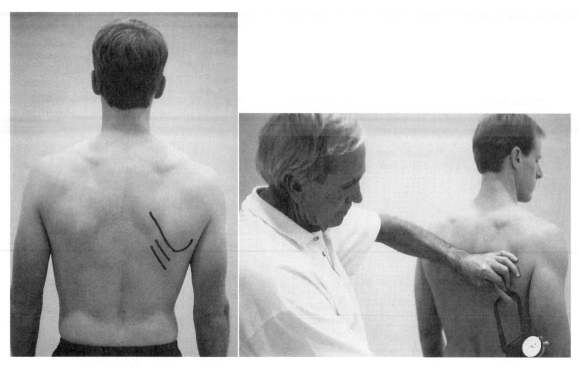

Figure 8-4   Measurement of subscapular skinfold thickness.

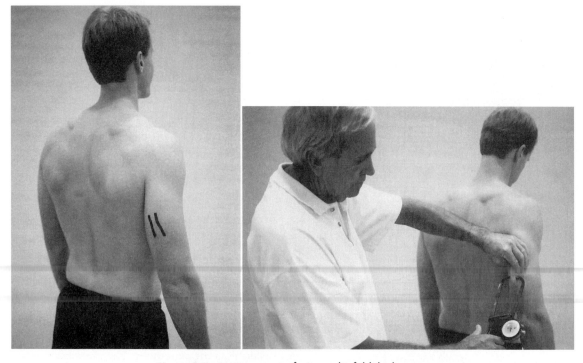

Figure 8-5   Measurement of triceps skinfold thickness.

4. *Thigh.* Take a vertical fold on the front of the right thigh midway between the hip and knee joints. NOTE: It is often easier to take this measurement if the subject is seated with the knee slightly flexed, with weight not supported on that leg (Figure 8-6).

5. *Abdominal.* Take a vertical fold approximately 1 inch to the right of the umbilicus (Figure 8-7).

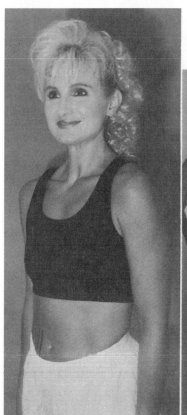
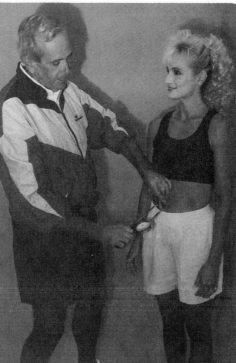

Figure 8-6 Measurement of thigh skinfold thickness.

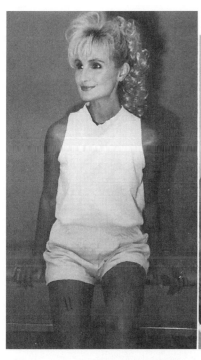
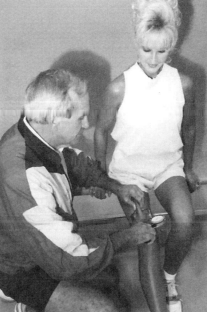

Figure 8-7 Measurement of abdominal skinfold thickness.

6. *Suprailiac.* Take a vertical fold at the front of the hips immediately above the crest of the ilium (Figure 8-8).
7. *Midaxillary.* Take a vertical fold at the side of the body on the midaxillary line, level with the lower part of the sternum (Figure 8-9).

PREDICTION OF PERCENT BODY FAT

There are many different regression equations available that use various combinations of these measurements.[6,7] The most recent trend has been to use generalized equations that have been developed using large heterogenous samples and that include age as a variable. You can determine your percentage of body fat by completing Laboratory Experience 8-3.

DETERMINATION OF DESIRABLE WEIGHT

It is now possible to determine your desirable weight using your body weight and your existing percentage of body fat. This is probably the most accurate method available to determine what you should weigh.

The example that is on p. 186 can be used for a person weighing 180 lb with 21% body fat who wants to reduce his or her percentage of body fat to 12%.

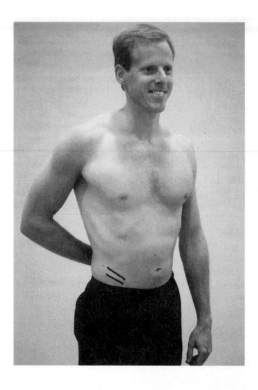

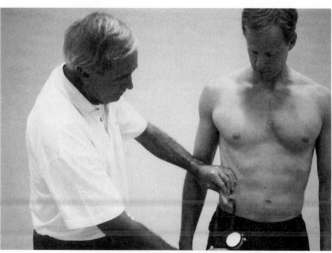

Figure 8-8   Measurement of suprailiac skinfold thickness.

DISADVANTAGES OF EXCESS WEIGHT OR FAT

Many disadvantages are associated with an excess accumulation of weight or fat, including the following:

■ There is an increased incidence of cardiovascular disease. Results from the Framingham study showed that obesity is independently related to an increased risk of coronary artery disease. The excess weight places additional stress on the heart, which then must work harder to perform the same amount of work. In addition, obesity is associated with other cardiovascular risk factors. For example, hypertension is found twice as frequently in those considered to be obese, and atherosclerosis is three times more prevalent in those who are overweight than in those whose weight is normal.

■ Mortality at a younger age is higher in those who are obese or overweight, resulting in a decrease in life expectancy.

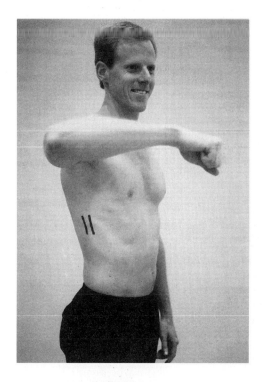

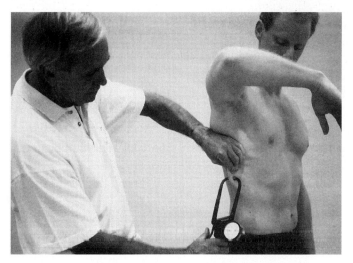

Figure 8-9 Measurement of midaxillary skinfold thickness.

Determination of Desirable Weight

Step 1. Determine your body weight and percentage of body fat.
Body weight = 180 lb
Body fat = 21%

Step 2. Calculate the weight attributable to fat.
Fat weight = 180 × 0.21
          = 37.8 lb

Step 3. Determine the existing lean body weight.
Lean body weight = Body weight − fat weight
                 = 180 − 37.8
                 = 142.2 lb

Step 4. Arbitrarily determine the desired percentage of body fat.
Ideal percentage of body fat selected is 12%

Step 5. Calculate the desired body weight for 12% body fat.
Desired weight = Lean body weight/1 − desired % body fat
               = 142.2/1 − 0.12
               = 142.2/0.88
               = 162 lb (to the nearest pound)

This 180-lb person should weigh 162 lb if he or she is to decrease his or her percentage of body fat from 21% to 12%. This would be a realistic goal for this person. For those who have a very high percentage of body fat, a goal more realistic than 12% for men or 18% for women should be selected initially. For these people, a more realistic goal might be to reach the "average" percentage of body fat. These figures are 18% for men and 23% for women. You can determine your desirable weight by completing Laboratory Experience 8-4.

- An excess accumulation of fat, particularly in the legs, can impede the return of blood to the heart and can contribute to an increase in the incidence of varicose veins.

- Overweight and obese persons experience more problems with muscles and joints because the extra weight places additional stress on their joints. This is particularly evident in areas such as the knees, hips, and lower back. The incidence of low back pain is much higher in those who are obese.

- Obesity is associated with increased incidence of diabetes. The incidence of diabetes is three times higher in obese subjects compared with nonobese subjects.

- Blood cholesterol levels are much higher in obese subjects compared with subjects who are at their desirable weight.

- Obesity is associated with an increased incidence of other health problems, such as cirrhosis of the liver and various respiratory problems.

- It has been shown that those who are obese or overweight have more accidents, surgical complications, and complications during pregnancy. In addition, their exercise tolerance is reduced considerably.

- People who are overweight or obese are also at a social and economic disadvantage. Because of their reduced life expectancy, they must pay higher insurance premiums. They are also often discriminated against when applying for a job.

ENERGY BALANCE

Regardless of whether a person tries to control weight by diet or by exercise, the balance between food intake and energy expenditure is very important.

Neutral energy balance

A **neutral energy balance** exists when the **caloric intake** is equal to the **caloric expenditure.** Under these conditions the body weight should remain constant and should neither increase nor decrease by any appreciable amount.

Positive energy balance

A **positive energy balance** exists when the caloric intake is greater than the caloric expenditure. The excess food is stored in the form of fat, and the body weight will increase.

Negative energy balance

With a **negative energy balance,** the number of calories used will be greater than the number of calories consumed. Stored fat will be used for energy, and the body fat and body weight should be reduced.

Case Study

JOE

Body weight: 180 lbs
Caloric balance: +100 cal/day
Weight gain: +10 lb/yr for last 2 years

Exercise program: Joe now weighs more than he has ever weighed in his life, so he decides to get very serious about losing weight. He decides on an exercise program where he walks 2 miles 3 days each week. However, he does not change his eating habits.

Results: After exercising for 3 months, Joe is very disappointed because he has not lost any weight.

Reason for not losing weight: Each time Joe walks 2 miles, he burns an additional 240 calories. As he does this 3 times each week, he will accumulate an additional 720 extra calories as a result of his exercise program. However, this barely balances out the "extra" calories that he is getting each day, and this is why he does not lose any weight.

Exercise
$$-240 \times 3 = -720 \text{ cal}$$
Caloric intake
$$100 \times 7 = +700$$

If Joe was to increase his exercise from 30 minutes to 45 minutes and exercise 5 days each week instead of just 3, this would be sufficient for him to lose approximately 1/3 lb of fat each week. This may sound like very little for the amount of exercise. However, if Joe exercises all 52 weeks, this is the equivalent of 17 lb in a year, and this is without modifying his eating habits. This emphasizes the importance of consistency each week in relation to exercise.

I see a large number of people just like Joe who are unsuccessful because they do not know how to plan their exercise program to achieve their desired results. You can see that there is a logical explanation as to why Joe did not lose any weight despite the fact that he exercised very regularly for 3 months.

THE IMPORTANCE OF AEROBIC EXERCISE IN WEIGHT MANAGEMENT

There are several reasons why regular aerobic exercise is important if you are to successfully manage your weight.

Exercise burns body fat

You have probably heard that it takes 10 hours of tennis or 30 miles of walking to burn the 3500 calories that you must use to lose 1 lb of fat. This certainly sounds intimidating, particularly if you have lots of weight to lose. However, you do not have to burn all these calories at once.

Playing tennis 1 hour a day 5 days each week will account for 1 lb of fat every 2 weeks or 26 lb of fat in 1 year if you find time for this much exercise each week.

To burn fat efficiently, it is important not to exercise at too high an intensity level. You should probably not exercise above 80% of your maximum heart rate if you want to burn fat most effectively. The reason for this is that carbohydrates—glycogen—can provide energy more efficiently than does fat. When you force your body to work at a high intensity, it will use mainly carbohydrates and very little fat. Your maximum heart rate can be estimated by subtracting your age from 220.

Example:

A 40-year-old person would have a maximum heart rate of approximately 180 beats per minute and should therefore keep his or her heart rate below 144 beats per minute if he or she is trying to burn fat while exercising.

Maximum heart rate	= 220 − age
	= 220 − 40
	= 180
Fat burning limit	= 180 × 0.80
	= 140

In Summary

Exercise goal for fat loss: exercise longer, not harder

Exercise speeds up your metabolism

When you decrease your caloric intake or lose weight, your metabolism will usually slow down. This is counterproductive to losing weight, and you will usually find that your rate of weight loss slows down considerably or else you reach the point where you see no further weight loss. At this point in time, most of us become very discouraged, and we may be tempted to quit our weight loss program.

By including exercise in your program or, if you are already exercising, by increasing the amount of exercise that you are doing, you can often counteract this problem. Exercise not only burns calories while you are exercising, but it has a significant effect on your metabolism for several hours after a good aerobic workout.

the caloric intake is less than the caloric expenditure).

A difference of only 200 calories per day between caloric intake and caloric expenditure might seem like an insignificant amount. It is equivalent to 12 french fries, less than 1½ cans of beer or soda, 2 oz of hamburger meat, 1 cup of potato chips, or six strips of bacon. However, in 6 months this small deficit can have a significant effect on your weight.

Example:

Initial body weight	= 180 lb
Caloric intake	= 3200 cal/day
Caloric expenditure	= 3000 cal/day
Deficit	= 200 cal/day
Cal/week	= 200 × 7
	= 1400 cal/wk
Cal/6 months	= 1400 × 26
	= 36,400
Equivalent lbs fat	= 36,400/3500*
	= 10.4 lb fat

*There are 3500 calories in 1 lb fat.

This person has several options to control and/or reduce his or her weight:

■ Caloric intake can be reduced by 300 calories per day, while caloric expenditure remains the same. This would create a negative energy balance of 100 calories per day, which would result in a weight loss of approximately 5 lb in 6 months, bringing the weight down to approximately 175 lb.

■ Caloric intake could remain the same, and a 4-mile walk could be substituted for 1 hour normally spent sleeping 4 days per week. On the days of the walk, an additional 410 calories would be burned. This would account for a weight loss of approximately 6 lb in 6 months and a final weight of approximately 174 lb. Remember that this is actually a weight shift of 16 lb because if this person does not make any changes, he or she will weigh 190 lb at the end of 6 months. Remember also that this weight change is achieved without reducing caloric intake.

■ Caloric intake can be reduced by 200 calories per day while the moderate exercise program of walking 4 miles 4 days each week is incorporated. This program would result in a daily reduction of caloric intake and an increase in caloric expenditure 4 days per week. The net result will be a weight loss of almost 12 lb, bringing the weight down to 168 lb in 6 months.

This example emphasizes the importance of regular exercise in weight control. People must be concerned with the long-term effects of a small daily caloric deficit.

WEIGHT LOSS AND EXERCISE

The maximal rate at which weight should be lost is approximately 1 lb per week. To achieve this, you will need a daily caloric deficit of 500 calories per day. Weekly weight-loss goals should be set, and if these are not met, then a further adjustment should be made in either caloric intake or caloric expenditure. The following example helps to illustrate the "long-range" concept of weight control.

Example:

Present body weight	= 180 lb
Desired body weight	= 170 lb
Rate of weight loss	= 1 lb/wk

The plan can be summarized as follows:

Week	Date	Target Body Weight
1	Jan 7	179
2	Jan 14	178
3	Jan 21	177
4	Jan 28	176
5	Feb 3	175
6	Feb 10	174
7	Feb 17	173
8	Feb 24	172
9	Mar 3	171
10	Mar 10	170

It will take this person 11 weeks to reach the desired goal. If this person were to start on January 1, by March 10 he or she will have achieved the goal if he or she has the determination to adhere regularly to the program.

Most people have no problem achieving the goals for the first few weeks, and frequently they lose more than they "have to" during this time. This often tempts them to get off their diet or skip their exercise, and before they know it they are right back where they started. It takes determination, hard work, and discipline to complete a program such as the one illustrated. However, the end results are very rewarding.

How much exercise do you need for weight loss?

If your objective is simply to improve your level of aerobic fitness so that your body functions more efficiently, you need to exercise only 3 to 4 times each week for 20 to 30 minutes at the right level of intensity. However, if your objective is to lose weight and/or body fat, you really need to make a commitment to exercise for 45 minutes 5 times each week.

Exercise can increase your lean body weight

Maintaining your lean body weight while losing fat is essential for long-term weight control. If you maintain your lean body tissue while reducing your body fat, you will burn more calories performing your everyday activities because muscle is more metabolically active than fat.

Exercise not only preserves your existing muscle mass, but it is likely to increase the amount that you have. This will also have a positive influence on your metabolism.

Summary of Research Study

Group 1	Group 2
Caloric intake:	Caloric intake:
1000 cal/day	1000 cal/day
Exercise: 3 days per week	Exercise: No exercise
Weight loss: 19 lb	Weight loss: 18 lb
Fat loss: 23 lb	Fat loss: 11 lb
Lean body weight: +4 lb	Lean body weight: −7 lb

The results from this study clearly show that dieting alone results in a decrease in lean body weight, whereas dieting plus exercise results in an increase in lean body weight. Despite the fact that both groups lost approximately the same amount of weight, there was a big difference in the type of weight lost.

The increase in lean body weight is one reason why several participants in weight management programs that include exercise do not see large changes in their body weight. At the same time that they are losing fat, they are gaining lean body weight. This is particularly true for those who greatly increase the amount of exercise that they participate in, particularly, if the exercise includes weight-bearing activity and/or weight training. Even though you do not see large changes when you weigh yourself, you should notice a difference in the way your clothes fit you.

Fitness Flash

Extra Benefits From Aerobic Exercise
Exercise is an appetite suppressant.
Exercise increases your chances of maintaining weight loss.
Exercise reduces anxiety and depression.
Exercise improves self-esteem and discipline.

STARTING A SUCCESSFUL EXERCISE PROGRAM AND STICKING WITH IT

Research shows that over 60% of adults who start an exercise program drop out within the first month. Some of these dropouts try again, but most of them soon quit again. This high dropout rate is unfortunate. There are many who drop out simply because they are misinformed. They think that exercise takes too much time and effort and that it is boring and very inconvenient. This is not necessarily true.

It is important to realize that exercise will take time and effort and will involve discipline and determination. However, it does not mean that it cannot be enjoyable, and you will probably discover that you do not have to work as hard as you thought you would. The old "no pain, no gain" philosophy has been replaced with "gain without pain." Initiating a successful weight management/exercise program and sticking with it involves several steps. These are as follows:

1. You need to make a commitment to exercise

The first step in beginning an exercise program is to make a commitment that exercise is important to you. Over 95% of freshmen entering college indicate that exercise is important to them, yet less than 35% exercise at least three times each week. If exercise is important to you, you will do something about it and find a way to make sure that you exercise regularly.

Consistency is very important. The most successful participants in our weight management programs are those who find a way to ensure that they get their 5 days of exercise every week, whereas those who are not as successful come up with excuses as to why they are unable to exercise as frequently as they need to. I see many clients who are frequently out of town on business. Some of them use this as an excuse not to exercise. These people are rarely successful at controlling their weight.

2. Schedule exercise into your everyday routine

To achieve your specific objectives, you must participate on a regular basis. Those who wait until they "find" time to exercise do not exercise very frequently. If you believe strongly enough in exercise, you will make time available on a regular basis and exercise will become a habit. There is no reason that you cannot schedule exercise each day just like you schedule other activities. At the beginning of each week, look at your schedule for the week. Look carefully at what major commitments you have for the week. You should then tentatively decide which 5 days would be most convenient for you to exercise, and you should mark these days in your schedule book. Each night before you go to bed, look at your schedule for the next day. If it is a day that you had planned to exercise but you now have a very busy schedule, you may have to get up an hour earlier than you normally would if you are to "find" time to exercise.

3. Be patient and start slowly

It is important to start out slowly, to be patient, and not to expect too much too soon. The first few weeks are very important. During this time a large number of people become disheartened and give up. It should be emphasized that you cannot start out at too low a level. It has probably taken you a long time to get out of shape and gain those extra pounds of fat. It will take you more than a few weeks to get back in shape and to lose the extra weight that you have. You need patience and determination.

Moderation is the key to starting an exercise program. Too much too soon may lead to excessive muscle soreness and will increase the chance of musculoskeletal injuries.

4. Determine personal goals

You can waste much time and effort if you do not establish specific goals for your program. These goals should be based on your individual needs. Your goals need to be realistic, and you need to allow a reasonable amount of time to achieve them so that you can experience some degree of success. Losing 20 lb in a month or running 10 miles in an hour are unrealistic goals for most people. A realistic goal for you might be to average five exercise sessions for 15 consecutive weeks and accumulate from 12 to 16 miles per week by walking at an intensity sufficient to maintain your heart rate in the desired target zone. Another realistic goal might be to average 20 miles per week walking and to reduce your caloric intake so that in 12 weeks you will lose 15 pounds. You need to determine goals that are important to you, that are realistic, and that will require discipline, determination, and effort.

5. Be willing to work

In any field of endeavor, the people who are the most successful are those who work hard at it. The familiar phrase "I know I should but . . ." is not part of a winner's vocabulary. It has been stated that "man is the architect of his own destiny." You must believe that this is true when it comes to controlling your body weight. Regular exercise is very important if this is to occur.

Many people who do not exercise use the excuse that they just do not have enough energy. You should not let the grind of your daily routine keep you from exercising. Regular exercise will actually increase your energy level and enable you to be more productive in your everyday tasks. You should feel refreshed after a good workout. If you are completely exhausted and have no energy left, in all likelihood you are doing too much or you are working at a higher intensity than what you should be.

6. Monitor your progress

It is important to monitor your progress on a regular basis. You can do this be keeping a record of your workouts. This enables you to chart your progress and can be used to establish the success of your program. Keep track of such things as the number of exercise sessions each week, the total miles accumulated, the calories burned, and changes in body weight. Many different computer programs are available that can be used on home computers for this purpose. A sample printout from an exercise logging program is included in Chapter 12 so that you can see samples of the type of information that these programs provide for you.

MISCONCEPTIONS ABOUT WEIGHT CONTROL

Until recently the role of exercise in weight control programs has been minimized. The reason for this appears to be that many persons lack sufficient knowledge about the relationship between exercise and weight control. Many of the basic misconceptions that exist are discussed briefly.

Misconception 1: Exercise burns relatively few calories and therefore makes an insignificant contribution to changing the energy balance

Everyone has heard from time to time that it takes several hours of golf or tennis or some other activity to lose 1 lb of fat. The actual figures for several of these activities for a 170-lb person are summarized in Table 8-8.

These figures, although correct, are very misleading. As shown in the previous sections, a difference of only 200 calories per day will make a difference in body weight of 10 lb in 6 months. The activity does not have to be performed continuously, nor does the heart rate

Table 8-8	**Caloric Expenditure and Weight Control for Certain Activities for a 170-lb Man**	
Activity	**Cal/hr**	**Hours to Lose 1 lb of Fat**
Walking (3 mph)	285	12.28
Basketball	612	5.72
Volleyball	306	11.44
Golf	367	9.54
Tennis	459	7.63

have to reach the target zone as it does for cardiovascular endurance. The following example will help you to again emphasize the role that exercise can play in weight control:

Example:

A person who weighs 170 lb decides to substitute 1 hour of tennis for 1 hour of watching television (tennis requires 0.045 cal/min/lb, and sitting watching television uses 0.008 cal/min/lb.)

Calories burned playing tennis for 1 hour	$= 170 \times 0.045 \times 60$ $= 459$
Calories that would have been spent watching television	$= 170 \times 0.008 \times 60$ $= 81$
Extra calories burned	$= 459 - 81$ $= 378$

If this person were to play tennis four times per week for 6 months, this would account for 39,312 extra calories being burned. This is the equivalent of just over 11 lb of fat. A reduction in body weight of 11 lb in 6 months might seem like an insignificant value; however, it must be remembered that this is obtained without reducing the caloric intake.

Misconception 2: An increase in physical activity will automatically result in an increase in the amount of food eaten

This statement is definitely false for the average person who exercises up to 1 hour per day. Laboratory tests using rats have shown that when the amount of exercise performed is moderate, from 20 minutes to 1 hour, the food intake does not increase—in fact, it actually decreases. These results are presented in Figure 8-10. Not only was there a decrease in the daily caloric intake, but there was also a decrease in body weight. With long periods of sustained activity, the food intake did increase; however, the

weight remained constant at this optimal level, since the extra activity balanced out the extra caloric intake.

Mayer also was able to obtain similar results working with adults. This study was conducted in India, where it was possible to adequately control many relevant factors. The results of this study are presented in Figure 8-11. These results indicate that light and medium work result in a decrease in caloric intake and a decrease in body weight and that heavy and very heavy work result in an increase in caloric intake but that the body weight remains constant.

Misconception 3: Exercise can be used to reduce fat from a specific area of the body

Many people believe that they can perform localized exercises and that this, combined with the correct diet, will significantly reduce fat in a particular area of the body. Research, however, does not document this theory. Instead, it shows that fat los will occur in proportion to the amount of fat in the body and that those areas with the greatest amount of fat will lose more than will the areas where there is less fat.

There are seven areas in the body where the majority of the fat accumulates. These have been identified and described previously. In women the two most troublesome areas are usually the triceps and the thighs; in men the highest concentration of fat usually occurs in the abdominal area.

Exercise is an important part of weight reduction because, if it is performed regularly, it will use a substantial number of calories and help to prevent loss of

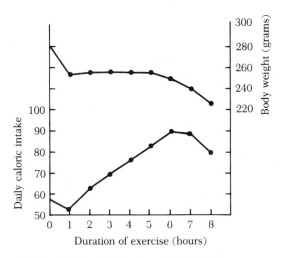

Figure 8-10 Relationship between food intake, energy expenditure, and body weight. (Modified from Mayer J: *Overweight: causes, cost and control,* Englewood Cliffs, NJ, 1968, Prentice Hall.)

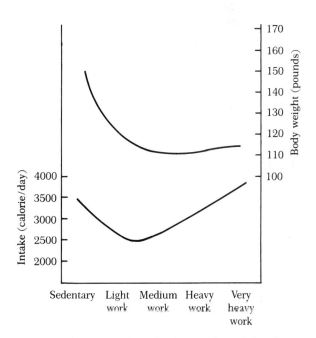

Figure 8-11 Body weight and caloric intake as related to physical activity in humans. (Modified from Mayer J: *Overweight: causes, cost and control,* Englewood Cliffs, NJ, 1968, Prentice Hall.)

lean body weight. However, regardless of the amount or kind of exercise for any specific body part, it will not reduce the fat in that particular area. It should be noted that it may increase muscular development in the specific area and may result in a shift or change in body fluids. These factors may considerably enhance the appearance but will not significantly reduce the amount of fat in that particular area.

Misconception 4: Saunas and steam baths are effective for losing weight

You do lose weight through sweating when you take a sauna or steam bath. However, this is only a temporary weight loss; the fluid will quickly be replaced, and your weight will return to its original level. No permanent weight loss results from saunas and steam baths. They are, however, useful for relaxation.

Misconception 5: Passive exercise machines can be used to reduce body weight

Many people think that they can get a machine that will exercise for them and reduce body fat. An example of this type of device is the electrically powered Exercycle. You turn it on, and all you have to do is sit on it and let it do all the work. Many health clubs and spas have similar devices, such as vibrators, rollers, and whirlpools. None of these assist in the reduction of body fat or in the shifting of fat deposits from one area to another.

Chapter Summary

The following summary will help you to identify some of the important concepts covered in this chapter:

- Obesity is one of the major health problems in America—many people have a hard time achieving and maintaining a desirable body weight and an optimal level of body fat.
- The term *overweight* refers to excess weight, whereas *obese* refers to excess fat.
- To accurately determine your desirable weight, you need to know your percentage of body fat.
- Regular exercise can positively affect your caloric balance if you exercise for 45 minutes, 5 days each week.
- Exercising at the right intensity is important if you are going to burn fat.
- Exercise of up to an hour per day will not usually result in an increase in the amount of food that you eat.
- Exercises for a specific area of your body are not effective for reducing fat in that particular area. Continuous aerobic exercise at a low intensity must be used to lose fat.

References

1. Colditz GA: Economic costs of obesity, *Am J Clin Nutr* 55:503S-507S, 1992.
2. Dewitt PE: Fat times,*Time,* pp 56-66, Jan 16, 1995.
3. Golding LA, Myers CR, Sinning WE: *The Y's way to physical fitness,* ed 2, Chicago, 1982, National Board of YMCA.
4. Hoeger WWK: *Principles and laboratories for physical fitness and wellness,* ed 3, Englewood, Colo, 1994, Morton.
5. Jackson AS, Pollock ML: Practical assessment of body composition, *The Physician and Sportsmedicine* 13(5):76, 1985.
6. Jackson AS, Pollock ML: Prediction accuracy of body density, lean body weight and total body volume equations, *Med Sci Sports Exerc* 9(4):197, 1977.
7. Jackson AS, Pollock ML, Ward A: Generalized equations for predicting body density of women, *Med Sci Sports Exerc* 12(2):175-182, 1980.
8. Jackson AS, Ross RM: *Understanding exercise for health and fitness,* Houston, Tex, 1986, Mac J-R Publishing CSI Software.
9. Katch FI, McArdle WD: *Nutrition, weight control and exercise,* ed 4, Philadelphia, 1993, Lea & Febiger.
10. Kuczmarski RJ et al: Increasing prevalence of overweight among US adults. The national health and nutrition evaluation survey 1960-1991, *JAMA* 20:272:3, 1994.
11. McArdle WD, Katch FI, Katch VL: *Exercise physiology, energy, nutrition and human performance,* ed 3, Philadelphia, 1991, Lea & Febiger.
12. Nieman DC: *Fitness and sports medicine—an introduction,* Palo Alto, Calif, 1990, Bull Publishing.
13. Paffenberger RS Jr et al: The association of changes in physical activity level and other lifestyle characteristics with mortality among men, *N Engl J Med* 328:536-45,1993.
14. Pi-Sunyer FX: Health implications of obesity, *Am J Clin Nutr* 53:1595S-1603S, 1991.
15. Prentice WE: *Fitness for college and life,* ed 4, St Louis, 1994, Mosby.
16. Sinning W: Use and misuse of anthropometric estimates of body composition, *Journal of Health, Physical Education and Recreation* 51:43, 1980.
17. *The Prevention Index 1995 Summary Report,* Emmaus, Penn, 1995, Rodale Press.

Laboratory Experience 8-1

Determination of Percentage Overweight

_____   _____   _____
Name   Section   Date

Complete the following steps to determine what percentage you are overweight or underweight. (Refer to the example at the end of this section if you need help.)

1. Record your actual weight to the nearest pound.
   Weight _____ lb

2. Determine your frame size from your elbow breadth.
   Elbow breadth _____ inches
   Frame size (see Table 7-1) _____

3. Consult Table 8-2 *(men)* or 8-3 *(women)* to determine the range for your desired weight.
   From _____ to _____ lb

4. Determine the midpoint of this range. This figure will be referred to as your desired weight.
   Desired weight _____ lb

5. Determine the difference between your desired weight and your actual weight.
   Difference = Actual weight − desired weight
   $$= \underline{\hspace{1cm}} - \underline{\hspace{1cm}}$$
   $$= \underline{\hspace{1cm}} \text{ lb}$$

6. Divide this difference by your desired weight to determine the percentage you are overweight or underweight.
   Percentage overweight or underweight = _____ / _____
   $$= \underline{\hspace{1cm}} \text{ (indicate + or −)}$$

Interpretation of Score

If you are more than 10% above your desirable weight, you would be classified as overweight.

EXAMPLE:
Name: Joe Jock
Height: 70 inches
Weight: 180 lb
Frame Size: Medium
   Desired weight range
   (From Table 7-2)   = 151-163 lb
   Midpoint   = 157 lb
   Difference   = Actual weight − desired weight
                          = 180 − 157
                          = +23 lb
   Percentage overweight = 23/157
                          = 0.15
                          = 15%

Laboratory Experience 8-2

Evaluation of Weight Using the Body Mass Index

_____   _____   _____
Name   Section   Date

Your body mass index is calculated as follows (an example is given below if you need help):

1. Record your name, height, and weight in the spaces provided below:
   Name _____
   Height _____ inches
   Weight _____ lb

2. Convert your height to meters by dividing by 39.4 (1 meter = 39.4 inches).
   Height (meters) = Height/39.4 (inches)
            = _____ /39.4
            = _____ meters (correct this to two decimal places)

3. Convert your weight to kilograms by dividing your weight in pounds by 2.2.
   Weight (kg) = Weight (lb)/2.2
            = _____/2.2
            = _____ kg

4. Calculate your body mass index (BMI)
   BMI = Weight (kg)/Height (meters)^2
            = _____ / (_____ × _____)
            = _____ / _____
            = _____

Interpretation of Score

You can interpret your score as follows:

<20	Below normal weight
20-25	Normal weight
25-30	Overweight
>30	Extremely overweight

EXAMPLE:
   Name: Joe Jock
   Height: 70 inches
   Weight: 180 lb

1. Height (meters) = 70/39.4
                  = 1.78
2. Weight (kg)   = 180/2.2
                  = 81.82 kg
3. BMI   = 81.82/(1.78)^2
                  = 81.82/3.17
                  = 25.81

Laboratory Experience 8-3

Determination of Percentage of Body Fat

Name _____   Section _____   Date _____

Record your skinfold measurements in the spaces provided below:

MEASUREMENT   SCORE (MM)

Chest   _____

Subscapular   _____

Triceps   _____

Thigh   _____

Abdominal   _____

Suprailiac   _____

Midaxillary   _____

You can calculate your percentage of body fat using one of the following formulas or you can use the nomogram from Figure 8-12. To use this nomogram, you must use the three specific measurements as indicated for men and for women. Take the total of these three measurements, draw a straight line from this value to your age, and read off the percentage from the appropriate place.

Prediction Equations—Body Density

WOMEN:

Body density = 1.0994921 − 0.0009929 (sum of three skinfolds) + 0.0000023 (sum of three skinfolds)^2 − 0.0001392 (age)

Measurements: triceps, suprailiac, thigh

MEN:

Body density = 1.1093800 − 0.0008267 (sum of three skinfolds) + 0.0000016 (sum of three skinfolds)^2 − 0.0002574 (age)

Measurements: chest, abdominal, thigh

Percent body fat = [(4.95/body density) − 4.5] × 100

Record your percentage of body fat in the space provided below:

Name _____

Date _____

Percentage of body fat: _____ lb

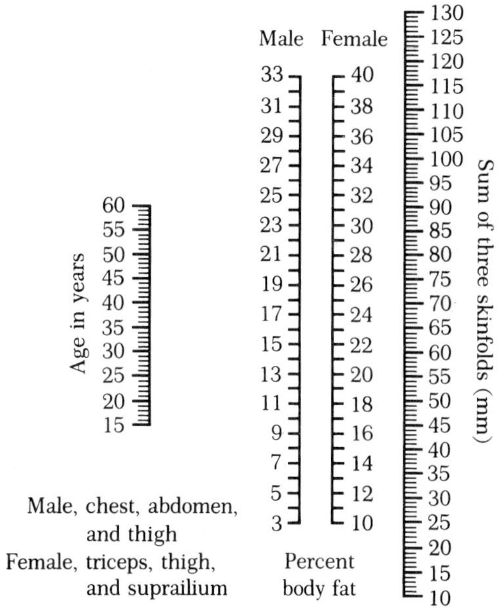

Figure 8-12 Nomogram for determination of percentage of body fat using age and three designated skinfold measurements.

Interpretation of Scores

The norms for percentage of body fat and for each of the skinfold measurements are presented in Table 8-9 *(men)* and Table 8-10 *(women)*. Circle each of your scores on the appropriate chart. You will be able to evaluate your total percentage of body fat, and you will also be able to see how this fat is distributed.

Ideal percentages are 12% or less for men and 18% to 14% for women. If you achieve these values, all your scores should be in the "good" or "excellent" categories and you should be happy with your distribution of fat.

Tablo 8-9 — Norms for Percent Body Fat and for Skinfold Measurements (Men)

Category	Percent Body Fat	Chest	Subscapular	Triceps	Thigh	Abdominal	Suprailiac	Mid-axillary
Excellent	6	2	3	2	4	6	2	5
	7	3	4	3	5	7	3	6
	8	4	5	4	6	8	4	7
	9	5	6	5	7	9	5	8
	10	6	7	6	8	10	6	
		7	8		9	11	7	
		8						
Good	11	9	9	7	10	12	8	9
	12	10	10	8	11	13	9	10
	13	11	11	9	12	14	10	11
	14	12	12	10	13	15	11	12
	15		13			16	12	13
								14
Average	16	13	14	11	14	17	13	15
	17	14	15	12	15	18	14	16
	18	15	16	13	16	19	15	17
	19	16	17	14	17	20	16	18
	20	17	18	15	18	21	17	19
	21	18	19		19	22	18	20
		19			20	23	19	21
						24	20	
						25		
						26		
Fair	22	20	20	16	21	27	21	22
	23	21	21	17	22	28	22	23
	24	22	22	18	23	29	23	24
	25	23	23	19	24	30	24	25
		24				31	25	26
						32	26	
						33		
						34		
Poor	26	25	25	20	25	35	27	27
	27	26	26	21	26	36	28	28
	28	27	27	22	27	37	29	29
	29	28	28	23	28	38	30	30
	30	29	29	24	29	39	31	31
	31	30	30	25	30	40	32	32
	32	31	31		31			
		32	32		32			

Table 8-10 — Norms for Percent Body Fat and for Skinfold Measurements (Women)

Category	Percent Body Fat	Chest	Subscapular	Triceps	Thigh	Abdominal	Suprailiac	Mid-axillary
Excellent	11	3	3	5	12	6	3	5
	12	4	4	6	13	7	4	6
	13	5	5	7	14	8	5	7
	14	6	6	8	15	9	6	8
	15	7	7	9	16	10	7	
				10		11		
						12		
Good	16	8	8	11	17	13	8	9
	17	9	9	12	18	14	9	10
	18	10	10	13	19	15	10	11
	19	11	11	14	20	16	11	12
	20	12			21	17	12	13
					22	18		
Average	21	13	12	15	23	19	13	14
	22	14	13	16	24	20	14	15
	23	15	14	17	25	21	15	16
	24	16	15	18	26	22	16	17
	25	17	16	19	27	23	17	18
	26	18	17	20	28	24	18	19
		19			29	25	19	
					30	26		
					31			
Fair	27	20	18	21	32	27	20	20
	28	21	19	22	33	28	21	21
	29	22	20	23	34	29	22	22
	30	23	21	24	35	30	23	23
	31		22	25	36	31	24	24
					37	32		
Poor	31	24	22	25	38	33	25	25
	32	25	23	26	39	34	26	26
	33	26	24	27	40	35	27	27
	34	27	25	28	41	36	28	28
	35	28	26	29	42	37	29	29
	36	29	27	30	43	38	30	30
	37	30	28	31	44	39	31	31
	38	31	29			40	32	32

Laboratory Experience 8-4

Determination of Desirable Weight

Name _____   Section _____   Date _____

NOTE: Refer to the example given on p. 186.

Name _____
Date _____

Step 1. Determine your body weight and percentage of body fat.
      Body weight = _____ lb
      Body fat   = _____ %

Step 2. Calculate the weight attributable to fat.
      Fat weight = Body weight $\times$ percentage of body fat
                = _____ $\times$ _____
                = _____ lb

Step 3. Determine the existing lean body weight.
      Lean body weight = Body weight $-$ fat weight
                    = _____ $-$ _____
                    = _____ lb

Step 4. Arbitrarily determine the desired percentage of body fat.
      Ideal percentage of body fat selected is _____ %

Step 5. Calculate the desired body weight for this percentage of body fat.
      Desired weight = Lean body weight/1 $-$ desired % body fat
               = _____ /1 $-$ _____
               = _____ / _____
               = _____ lb (to the nearest pound)

Laboratory Experience 8-5

Determination of Daily Caloric Expenditure

Name _____   Section _____   Date _____

Refer to the example given on p. 190 for additional instructions and help. You need to record your activities for 2 days a weekday and a weekend day. Try to select "typical" days. Start each day at midnight and make sure that the total time for each day adds up to 1440 minutes—the number of minutes in 1 day. Record these activities on Tables 8-11 and 8-12.

After each daily caloric expenditure form has been completed, you need to group some of the activities together and transfer them to the daily caloric expenditure summary forms (Tables 8-13 and 8-14). The example presented previously on p. 190 may help you in calculating your values.

Table 8-11   Daily Caloric Expenditure Form

Name _____   Date _____

Starting Time	Finishing Time	Type of Activity or Task	Number of Minutes

TOTAL   1440 minutes

Table 8-12	**Daily Caloric Expenditure Form**		

Name _____ Date _____

Starting Time	Finishing Time	Type of Activity or Task	Number of Minutes

TOTAL 1440 minutes

Table 8-13   Daily Caloric Expenditure Summary Form

Name _____

Date _____   Body weight _____ lb

Activity	Cal/min/lb	×	Total Time (min)	×	Body Weight (lb)	=	Calories Used
Sleeping and lying quietly	0.008	×	_____	×	_____	=	_____
Sitting (total all your activity you performed while sitting)	0.011	×	_____	×	_____	=	_____
Standing with little or no movement	0.013	×	_____	×	_____	=	_____
Standing with light activity	0.015		_____		_____	=	_____
Walking							
Slow (2 mph)	0.020	×	_____	×	_____	=	_____
Fast (3 mph)	0.030	×	_____	×	_____	=	_____
Other (specify all other activity)							
_____	_____	×	_____	×	_____	=	_____
_____	_____	×	_____	×	_____	=	_____
_____	_____	×	_____	×	_____	=	_____
_____	_____	×	_____	×	_____	=	_____
_____	_____	×	_____	×	_____	=	_____
_____	_____	×	_____	×	_____	=	_____

TOTAL TIME [1440]   TOTAL CALORIES USED [   ]

Table 8-14   Daily Caloric Expenditure Summary Form

Name _____

Date _____   Body weight _____ lb

Activity	Cal/min/lb	×	Total Time (min)	×	Body Weight (lb)	=	Calories Used
Sleeping and lying quietly	0.008	×	_____	×	_____	=	_____
Sitting (total all your activity you performed while sitting)	0.011	×	_____	×	_____	=	_____
Standing with little or no movement	0.013	×	_____	×	_____	=	_____
Standing with light activity	0.015		_____		_____	=	_____
Walking							
Slow (2 mph)	0.020	×	_____	×	_____	=	_____
Fast (3 mph)	0.030	×	_____	×	_____	=	_____
Other (specify all other activity)							
_____	_____	×	_____	×	_____	=	_____
_____	_____	×	_____	×	_____	=	_____
_____	_____	×	_____	×	_____	=	_____
_____	_____	×	_____	×	_____	=	_____
_____	_____	×	_____	×	_____	=	_____
_____	_____	×	_____	×	_____	=	_____

TOTAL TIME [1440]   TOTAL CALORIES USED [   ]

Chapter Nine Weight Management

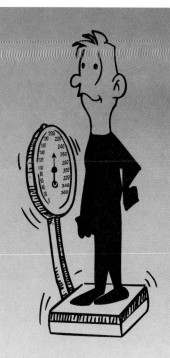

CHAPTER OBJECTIVES
Check off each objective you achieve.

❑ Explain why very few people who use "dieting" as a means to lose weight are successful at losing the weight and keeping it off.

❑ List the problems associated with very low-calorie diets.

❑ Identify specific objectives you would like to achieve, and know how to achieve these objectives.

❑ Identify five positive outcomes associated with eating regularly throughout the day.

❑ Explain why people who skip breakfast are more likely to accumulate body fat than those who eat a nutritious breakfast.

❑ Explain why an adequate amount of both carbohydrates and proteins are an essential part of a good breakfast.

❑ Evaluate the consistency of your eating and exercise habits, and know what changes you need to make.

❑ List the 11 guidelines that are essential to any successful weight-management program.

Losing weight has become an obsession for a large percentage of the American population. Following is a listing of some statements that have appeared in different books, magazines, and journals during the last several years. Whether they are 100% accurate is not important. They reflect the situation that exists in this country.

- Almost 90% of Americans think that they weigh too much.
- Sixty-five million Americans are presently on some type of diet.
- Twenty million Americans are spending an estimated $1 billion annually on liquid diets and programs.
- Americans spend almost $5 billion each year in an attempt to lose weight.
- Each year, Americans spend over $200 million on over-the-counter drugs that contain caffeine and amphetamine-related compounds.
- The sale of low-calorie frozen foods has increased 15% each year for the past several years.
- Of American women, 16% consider themselves to be perpetual dieters.
- From age 25, the average American woman gains almost 1½ lb of fat each year.

It is obvious that despite this obsession, the majority of Americans have not been successful at losing the excess weight or fat and keeping it off.

WHY DIETS FAIL

It has become clear in recent years that dieting is not the answer for weight management. There are several reasons for this.

Most diets restrict your caloric intake so that your metabolism slows down

For many years now most people have been told that if they want to lose weight, they must limit the amount of food that they eat and select foods that are low in calories. However, most experts now agree that drastically reducing your caloric intake can significantly slow down your metabolism, which is counterproductive to losing weight.

It is theorized that our bodies have a built-in mechanism—sometimes referred to as the set point—that drives our bodies to maintain a certain amount of body fat. When your caloric intake is restricted, your body will attempt to compensate by "slowing down" to conserve the amount of body fat that you have. One study showed that when caloric intake was severely restricted, the resting metabolic rate was reduced by almost 45%.

If you are female and eating less than 1200 calories per day, or male and eating less than 1500 calories per day, it is likely that such a low caloric intake will have a negative effect on your resting metabolic rate, thus making continuous weight loss difficult, if not impossible. Most college students can eat a much larger number of calories than this and still be successful at losing weight.

Dieting usually results in depression, which is counterproductive to losing weight

For many people, dieting becomes an antisocial event. People give up friends, meals, and in many cases eating out because they are afraid that they might eat something that they are not supposed to eat. This usually results in depression and anxiety, which frequently sets the stage for overeating as people turn to food for comfort. Those who diet will be constantly losing weight and gaining it right back again.

Most diets do not encourage permanent lifestyle changes

Good eating habits require a lifetime commitment; otherwise, they will result in temporary changes. As your weight goes up and down, this creates definite health problems and may have a negative effect on your metabolism.

There are many weight-loss programs available that involve preplanned "packaged" foods. These programs may initially result in significant weight loss because the meals are carefully planned and the portion sizes relatively small. However, it does not make sense to eat packaged food for the rest of your life, and frequently when people who have been on these programs start to make their own choices and buy food from the grocery store, they begin to regain the lost weight. In many of these programs an attempt is made to "educate" clients while they are in the program about what constitutes good eating. However, it does not make sense to tell people this is how you are supposed to eat and then have them eat preplanned packaged foods. One of the major reasons why they do this is that they make most of their money from the sale of their packaged food.

With low-calorie diets, weight lost is usually lean body weight

Several studies show that in weight-loss programs where the caloric intake is severely restricted, a large percentage of the weight lost is lean body weight. Many of those who participate in such programs do not have a weight problem, but they have large amounts of excess fat. I frequently evaluate many women who weigh less than 130 lb and who have over 30% body fat, and I see a significant number of men who weigh less than 180 lb who have 25% body fat or more. You do not necessarily have to weigh a lot to be obese. In many of these cases the problem is caused by not eating sufficient calories each day.

CRITERIA ASSOCIATED WITH A GOOD WEIGHT-LOSS PROGRAM

With society's current obsession for thinness, together with concerns about the effects of obesity on health, the number of weight-loss programs and associated services has increased tremendously during recent years.

Fitness Flash

There has been a continued growth in the diet industry—now estimated to have revenues in excess of $50 billion per year.

Many of these programs are very expensive, and it is often very difficult to evaluate them and decide which program might be best for you. The following criteria might be helpful to you in evaluating your options.

A successful weight-management program should:

- Encourage you to adopt permanent lifestyle habits that you can live with for the rest of your life
- Teach you how to select and prepare the foods that you eat and how to control the portion sizes
- Teach you how to set reasonable goals, and show you how to achieve these goals
- Not restrict your caloric intake to the extent that you are constantly hungry or craving certain foods
- Not result in your being consistently lacking in energy throughout the day
- Advocate regular aerobic exercise, and teach you how to design a program based on your specific needs
- Promote a realistic weight loss of ½ lb to 1 lb per week
- Promote eating a variety of foods
- Teach you to identify and modify the behavior patterns that may be contributing to your weight problem
- Encourage you to take personal responsibility for the everyday decisions that you make relative to your exercise and eating habits

ADOPTING A HEALTHY LIFESTYLE

To be successful, you need to adopt a healthy lifestyle—one you can live with for the rest of your life. Permanent weight loss will rarely occur if your motivation comes from wanting to look good in a new swimsuit for the summer or from wanting to lose 10 pounds so that you can wear a specific dress and look good at a wedding or class reunion. In cases such as these, maintaining weight is always going to be a problem because as soon as a specific goal is achieved, you will likely return to your old habits and the lost weight will quickly be regained. This is the same problem that most people encounter with most commercial weight-loss programs.

Case Study

TOM

Tom was a 40-year-old attorney who enrolled in one of our Looking Good Weight Management/ Exercise Programs in September 1989. He weighed 200 lb and had been constantly fighting his weight for years. By dieting he would lose 10 lb and then put the 10 lb right back on again. He decided that he wanted to take charge of his eating and exercise habits so that he could permanently lose the 25 to 30 extra pounds that he did not need. He learned quickly the changes he needed to make in his eating habits, but at the same time he was careful to make sure that he was adopting changes that he could live with for the rest of his life. He quickly noticed that he had more energy each day and was not constantly hungry. At the same time he learned exactly how much exercise he needed to do to regularly lose 1 lb each week. Because he learned what to do and because he believed that he could be responsible in controlling his habits, he was successful. He lost the 25 lb in 6 months and at the same time reduced his percentage of body fat from 21% to 13%.

GETTING STARTED AND BEING SUCCESSFUL

For you to develop new lifestyle habits relative to exercise and nutrition, you need to learn how to make the right choices each day. These choices relate to when you eat, what you eat, how much you eat, and whether you exercise. You must realize that the choices you make each day relative to each of these will determine how successful you will be at achieving your goals. The following suggestions may be helpful to you in getting started.

Step 1. Have a positive mental attitude and believe in your ability to succeed

It is extremely important that you believe in yourself. It does not make sense for you not to be able to control your exercise and eating habits. If you believe in yourself, you will be much more likely to try harder and stick with your program. You will handle success and failure much better and should experience less stress.

The material in this chapter shows you what you need to do if you are to be successful, but you must believe that this is important and that by implementing these changes each day in your lifestyle you can be successful.

In Summary

Your belief in yourself and your determination will determine how successful you will be.

Step 2. Learn how to set realistic objectives

You need to learn how to set realistic objectives, making sure that you allow yourself a reasonable amount of time to achieve these objectives. Much time and effort can be wasted unless objectives are established and unless these objectives are organized into specific tangible goals with priorities. These objectives should be based on your individual needs. Do not expect too much too soon.

Many weight-reduction programs concentrate simply on how much weight you need to lose. The material in the previous chapter showed you that losing fat is more important than losing weight. However, because it is much easier to monitor changes in weight, losing weight is usually the most important objective for most participants in a weight-management program. A number of important objectives are identified below.

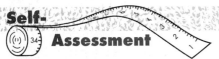

Self-Assessment

Possible Overall Objectives for a Good Weight-Management Program

Check off each of the following objectives that apply to you.
I would like to:

- Reduce my body weight
- Have less body fat
- Have more energy throughout the day
- Look and feel better
- Increase my level of aerobic fitness
- Lower my cholesterol level
- Learn how to eat well
- Reduce my chances of cardiovascular disease
- Develop consistent exercise habits
- Reduce my level of stress

If one of your objectives is to lose weight, it is very important that you plan to lose this weight slowly and gradually. This is the most effective way to keep it off. Research shows that 95% of all the people who lose weight quickly on low-calorie diets gain most or all of it back—usually within the first year. Also, when you lose weight rapidly, the majority of the weight loss is caused by a change in your fluid balance or, if you are on a very low-caloric diet, a large percentage of the weight lost will be lean body weight. Most people who weigh more than they would like to are trying to reduce their weight by losing *fat*. With most quick weight-loss programs, this does not occur.

Most experts now agree that the maximum rate for weight loss should be ½ lb to 1 lb each week. Consistently losing more weight than this each week is very difficult for the majority of those trying to lose weight and is very hard to achieve even for those who are extremely overweight or obese to begin with. It is also important to realize that weight will usually come off faster at first and that you will find it more difficult to lose the closer you get to your goal weight. This is usually because as you weigh less, you use fewer calories performing the same everyday tasks and because as you lose weight, your metabolism will slow down.

Step 3. Implement a plan to achieve your objectives

Not only do you need to know where you are going, but you must have a plan as to how to get there. It is important to establish a step-by-step approach that is systematic and carefully designed. It is helpful if it is in writing so that you can constantly evaluate this plan, update it if necessary, and modify it if it does not work for you. It is important to remember that you must be patient rather than wanting everything at once.

This plan must include specific objectives each week that you will attempt to achieve that will contribute to your overall success. As these objectives regularly become part of your new lifestyle, you can add new objectives. You need to work *constantly* at achieving each of these objectives rather than working with concentrated spurts of energy.

To establish specific objectives, you need first to carefully evaluate your existing eating habits to determine which habits need to be changed and you will then need to develop specific strategies for changing these behaviors. You can evaluate your existing habits by completing Laboratory Experiences 9-1 and 9-2.

At this time, having evaluated your existing habits, you should now attempt to establish some specific objectives relative to your exercise and eating habits. The questions included at the end of Laboratory Experience 9-2 should provide clues to you as to some of the changes you need to make. Use Table 9-1 to list your objectives. Each day that you are successful at achiev-

| Table 9-1 | **Weekly Objectives Relative To Exercise And Eating Habits** |

Name: _____   WEEK COMMENCING: _____

List your specific objectives for the week. Place a check next to each objective each day that you successfully achieve it.
√ = successful at achieving the objective
x = failed to achieve the objective

Specific Objective	Date:	Sun	Mon	Tue	Wed	Thu	Fri	Sat
1. _____								
_____		___	___	___	___	___	___	___
2. _____								
_____		___	___	___	___	___	___	___
3. _____								
_____		___	___	___	___	___	___	___
4. _____								
_____		___	___	___	___	___	___	___
5. _____								
_____		___	___	___	___	___	___	___
6. _____								
_____		___	___	___	___	___	___	___
7. _____								
_____		___	___	___	___	___	___	___
8. _____								
_____		___	___	___	___	___	___	___

ing each objective on your list, place a check mark in the appropriate place. At the end of each day and the end of each week, you can then evaluate how consistent you have been. If your weekly goals have been carefully determined and you meet these consistently, you will be moving in a positive direction toward your overall objectives.

Later in this chapter you will find a weekly self-evaluation scoresheet. This includes 11 guidelines that I have found are very important in any weight-management/exercise program. A simple scoring system is included so that you can evaluate yourself each week and determine more precisely the consistency of your eating and exercise habits.

Step 4. Work hard at achieving each of your objectives

In any endeavor, those who are the most successful are those who work the hardest. You must be willing to work hard each day at achieving each of your objectives. If you want something bad enough, you will find a way to achieve it. Motivation must come from within.

Step 5. Stick with your program

More than 60% of those who start a weight-management/exercise program drop out within the first month. It is important that you learn to be patient. It will take you time to get to where you want to be, and it certainly will involve lots of hard work and discipline. However, the benefits will far outweigh the effort spent. If you implement the steps outlined in this chapter, you will be much more likely to stick with your program.

One way to increase your motivation is to monitor your progress. For some people, changes will show up almost immediately in terms of weight loss. However, simply measuring your body weight may be very misleading, particularly if you are exercising more. If you have not exercised regularly for some time and you initiate a good exercise program, you are likely to develop muscle tone at the same time that you start to lose fat. This may result in very little if any change in your body weight at first, but you should soon begin to notice that your clothes start to fit more loosely. This is a positive sign.

You must also realize that for women during the menstrual cycle, there will be changes in body weight because of excess fluid retention. Also, the amount of carbohydrates and sodium that you eat each day can cause daily fluctuations in your fluid balance that are reflected in your body weight.

The thing to remember is that if you continue to make better choices relative to your eating habits and if you exercise regularly to the extent advocated for weight loss in the previous chapter, your body fat should gradually decrease and these changes will eventually show up on the scales. You should also notice many other positive changes as a result of your new lifestyle. You should have more energy so that you do not become tired so easily, and you should not be constantly hungry throughout the day and be craving certain foods.

Let's Get Started

If you are to be successful at permanently changing your behavior, you need to:

1. **Become more knowledgeable concerning exercise and nutrition.** How successful you will be will basically depend on several choices you make each day. These choices determine your everyday habits. They relate to when you eat, what you eat, and how much you eat. In addition, each day you must decide whether to exercise or not. If you do decide to exercise, then you must make additional choices as to how long to exercise, how hard to exercise, and which activities to include in your program. By becoming more knowledgeable, you will be able to make better decisions concerning these issues.

2. **Assess your existing eating and exercise habits.** As you study the consistency of your eating and exercise habits, you should be able to determine why you have not been successful in the past. For example, you may find that snacking gets out of control while watching television or reading, or you may find that you eat out at fast food restaurants far too frequently. Forms are included in Laboratory Experience 9-2 with instructions to help you evaluate your present eating habits.

3. **Identify those habits that need to be changed.** Decide which habits you can live with and which habits you feel need to be changed. Plan your strategy as to how you are going to change these habits.

4. **Implement planned changes.** Plan changes gradually, making sure you only adopt changes you can live with for the rest of your life.

5. **Monitor your consistency.** Use the weekly self-evaluation scoresheets to monitor the consistency of changes you make in your eating and exercise habits.

DIETARY GOALS AND GUIDELINES

Three separate publications have been released in recent years in an attempt to encourage good eating habits. These are listed below:

- *Dietary Guidelines for Americans*—Published by the U.S. Department of Agriculture and the U.S. Department of Health and Human Services, 1985
- *Dietary Goals for the United States*—Published by the Senate Select Committee on Nutrition and Human Needs, U.S. Government Printing Office, Washington, D.C., 1985
- *The Surgeon General's Report on Nutrition and Health*—Published by the U.S. Department of Health and Human Services, Washington, D.C., 1989

These publications provide general guidelines relative to what we should and should not be eating. However, they provide very little new information. For example, we have known for some time that if you are to be successful, you need to do the following:

- Avoid too much fat, saturated fat, and cholesterol.
- Eat more fruits, vegetables, and grain products.
- Limit your intake of sodium and salt.
- Reduce your consumption of simple refined sugar.
- Limit your intake of alcohol.

However, there are two basic problems associated with these guidelines. The average person does not know how much is too much, and he or she does not really know how to implement these recommendations. For example, how do you know how many servings of fruits, vegetables, and grain products you need to eat, and what constitutes a serving? It is also obvious that these guidelines do not focus on the issue of when to eat. When you eat your meals is probably just as important as what you eat.

THE IMPORTANCE OF EATING REGULARLY

Each day you decide how often you are going to eat and when you will eat. The decisions you make as to what time of the day you eat and how you space your meals throughout the day can significantly affect how much you will weigh and how much fat you will accumulate.

A large number of people who are overweight or obese suffer from the same problem. It is often referred to as *nighttime eating syndrome*. It is defined as an eating pattern where the majority of the calories for the day are eaten in either one or two meals, with a large number of these calories often eaten late in the day.

Case Study

MARY

Mary is a regular exerciser who walks 3 or 4 miles at least 4 days each week. She either skips breakfast each day, or else breakfast consists of coffee and a bran muffin. If she eats lunch, it usually consists of half of a bagel, a small green salad, or a piece of fruit. She usually eats nothing during the afternoon, despite the fact that she feels tired and is usually lacking in energy.

By early evening she is famished and feels that she can reward herself by eating or drinking just about anything. Snacking often gets out of control, and she frequently consumes several alcoholic drinks that she feels she deserves, since she has eaten so little during the day. She then eats a large evening meal that is usually high in fat, and she will often continue snacking until late into the evening.

Because she eats so many of her calories late in the day, when she wakes up in the morning she does not feel like eating anything for breakfast and she will repeat the same cycle over and over.

Mary does not have a weight problem, but despite the fact that she has been exercising consistently for several years, she has been unable to reduce the excess fat that she would like to get rid of.

When we eat more frequently, we are more likely to make better choices

In today's world, particularly with all the fast foods readily available, we can get a large number of calories in a small volume of food that can be eaten very quickly. For example, a cheeseburger, french fries, and a chocolate milkshake—which can be eaten in less than 10 minutes—supplies over 1500 calories. A meal such as this is high in fat and sodium and contains very little if any fiber.

Because a meal such as this contains so many calories, many of us tend to eat less frequently throughout the day. In fact, a recent national survey showed that only 39% of Americans eat the traditional three meals each day. What many of us need to do is adopt a more natural eating pattern, where we eat smaller meals more frequently. By doing this, we are more likely to eat more fruits, vegetables, and grain products and fewer animal products, which are usually high in fat.

In Summary

When you eat only one or two meals each day, snacking often gets out of control and you frequently make poor choices about what you eat.

Eating more frequently reduces the amount of insulin produced by the body

When you eat several small meals throughout the day instead of one or two larger meals, your body will actually produce less insulin. A recent study showed that when two groups followed the exact same diet, those who consumed their calories over several small meals during the day produced significantly less insulin than those who ate the traditional three meals. Insulin production was 28% lower in those who ate several small meals spaced regularly throughout the day. For those who eat only one or two meals each day, the amount of insulin produced is likely to be even higher. The reason is that insulin is responsible for fat storage and production of fat in the body. The less frequently you eat, the longer the meal is likely to be and the amount of food eaten will usually be greater than what your body can use at that time. When this happens, your body will produce more insulin than normal in an attempt to store the excess calories as fat.

This is nothing new. We have known for some time that those who eat less frequently tend to accumulate more fat. During the last 10 years, over 80% of the people I have tested for body composition who have had a serious fat problem have had poor eating habits relative to when they eat and/or how frequently they eat. Skipping meals is not the answer for those who are trying to reduce their percentage of body fat.

Insulin production affects your appetite

You are much more likely to control your appetite if you eat more frequently, particularly if the meals and snacks are planned in advance. The reason for this again relates to the amount of insulin produced by the body.

Increased levels of insulin production in the body quickly result in a decrease in your blood glucose level. When your blood glucose falls to a low level, you will usually feel tired and hungry and will want to eat again.

Those who eat frequently do a better job maintaining a constant blood glucose level, and by eating before they get too hungry, they will not become famished and want to eat anything or everything in sight. They will usually be less likely to crave sweets or fats. Maintaining a constant blood glucose level within normal limits also allows you to concentrate better, particularly during the late afternoon hours. You should therefore be more productive as a result of this.

Long lapses of time between meals can distort your appetite. You may find that you actually consume more calories in the one or two meals that you eat than you would have had you eaten three or four planned meals.

Skipping meals may also affect your metabolism

Your metabolic rate determines the rate at which your body burns calories. If your metabolism slows down, you will burn calories at a slower rate and a greater amount of the calories consumed will be stored as fat. Increasing the number of meals that you eat each day—particularly if they are high in protein, complex carbohydrates, and fiber—has been shown to increase certain hormones in your body that increase your metabolism. Conversely, we have known for some time that skipping meals is likely to result in a reduction in your metabolic rate.

Eating more frequently can increase your energy level

Skipping meals can significantly reduce your energy level. Including nutritious snacks between meals can increase your energy level. This is extremely important if you exercise late in the day. If you do a good job of scheduling your meals and snacks throughout the day, you should have more energy and not feel as tired at the end of the day.

BREAKFAST: THE MOST IMPORTANT MEAL OF THE DAY

Each day millions of Americans rush out the door without eating breakfast, thinking that by not eating they are saving calories and that this will contribute to weight loss. This is just not so. In fact, a large number of people who are overweight or obese seldom eat breakfast.

Common sense should tell us that breakfast is important. It does not make sense to start the day with just a cup of coffee, a glass of juice, or a slice of toast. You need more food than this for breakfast to get a sufficient amount of the various nutrients that you need and to start the day filled with energy so that you can perform at an optimal level throughout the day. The results from a recent national survey showed that the majority of those surveyed felt that they were less productive when they skipped breakfast and more productive when they ate a healthy breakfast. They stated that a good breakfast "gave them more energy" and "helped to get them going in the morning."

It is now well established that breakfast is the most important meal of the day. Despite this, a recent national survey[14a] showed that less than 50% of the population reported eating breakfast each day. People who did not eat breakfast were asked why; the following are the three most common responses:

- "I am on a diet and I want to save calories."
- "I just do not have the time."
- "I am not hungry in the morning."

If you eat a nutritious breakfast each morning, you will usually have more energy as a result of this and will therefore feel better throughout the day. You will also usually be more successful at controlling your weight and percentage of body fat. There are several reasons for this.

Eating breakfast can positively affect your metabolism

One reason that breakfast is important is that it can positively influence your metabolism. When you wake up in the morning, your body is in a slow fasting state, with your metabolic rate very low. If you do not eat breakfast, your body will not only remain at a low level but will slow down even further. Studies have shown that those who do not eat breakfast have metabolic rates below normal. One reason for this is that each meal that we eat increases the rate at which we burn calories. This is referred to as the thermic effect of food. If you eat just one large meal each day, you will actually burn fewer calories than does someone who eats the same amount of food spread over three meals. In addition, because you will not be getting the carbohydrates and protein that you need, you will often feel tired and weak and be lacking in energy. You will be "dragging" for most of the day. This will mean that you will be less active throughout the day, which will also negatively influence your metabolism.

> **In Summary**
>
> Those who skip breakfast to "save" calories frequently find that they are not successful at losing weight or fat.

Many breakfast foods are low in fat

Those who skip breakfast and eat only one or two meals each day are much more likely to consume a higher percentage of their calories from fat. The reason for this is that there are so many foods that are available for breakfast that contain very little fat, whereas many of the foods that traditionally are eaten later in the day contain large amounts of fat. Cereal, skim milk, and fruit are traditional breakfast foods that contain practically no fat. Of course, if you eat bacon, eggs, and hash browns for breakfast, your fat intake will be extremely high.

WHAT YOU EAT FOR BREAKFAST IS IMPORTANT

Making healthy choices is important when deciding what to eat for breakfast. It is important that your breakfast each day contains an adequate amount of complex carbohydrates and protein and is very low in fat and simple sugar.

Importance of complex carbohydrates

Each day carbohydrates are needed to supply energy. Your body can store a limited amount of carbohydrates in the form of glycogen in the muscles and in the liver, usually approximately 1600 calories worth. If you do not eat breakfast, your carbohydrate stores will become depleted and this will greatly reduce the amount of energy that you will have throughout the day. This is particularly true if you also skip lunch. One of the most frequent comments that I get from the participants in our weight-management classes who start eating breakfast is that "I can't believe how much more energy I now have throughout the day since I have started eating breakfast."

Remember that you need an adequate intake of carbohydrates to metabolize fat efficiently. When you skip breakfast or another meal, your body will metabolize fat less efficiently; those who skip breakfast are much more likely to accumulate more fat compared with those who eat a nutritious breakfast each day.

Importance of protein

Protein performs a variety of functions in your body, yet your body does not store protein for use in the body like it stores fats and carbohydrates. It is important to eat foods containing an adequate amount of protein at regular intervals throughout the day.

When you skip a meal, your body will continue to function normally, but because you get no protein coming in, you will force your body to use its own protein to perform the important functions that require protein. Your body will usually use protein from your muscle tissue because it is most readily available. This will often then result in an imbalance between the amount of fat and muscle in your body. This also explains why very–low-calorie diets often result in loss of a significant amount of lean body weight. With a very low caloric intake, it is almost impossible to get the necessary amount of protein that your body needs and your body will use part of its own protein to perform the functions that are necessary in your body. An 8 oz glass of milk—preferably skim milk or 1% milk—and a bowl of cereal provide approximately 12 to 15 grams of protein. This would appear to be an adequate amount of protein for the average person to consume for breakfast. If you eat just a piece of fruit, a glass of juice, or a slice of toast with coffee for breakfast, you will be depriving your body of the essential protein that it needs.

Making healthful choices

Making healthful choices is important when deciding what to eat for breakfast. A good breakfast should contain an adequate amount of complex carbohydrates and protein and be very low in fat. Because many of the traditional breakfast foods are very low in fat, your total fat intake for breakfast should be well below the maximum daily recommendation of 30% if you make wise choices.

Four different breakfast plans are included where the total calories are close to 300 and where the percentage of calories from fat is 20% or less.

Typical low-fat breakfast—cereal, milk, and fruit

Item	Serving size	Calories
Skim milk	1 cup	90
Cereal		
All bran	⅓ cup	45
Bran flakes	½ cup	70
Apple	1 medium	110

Nutritional information—Calories 315

		% of calories
Protein	15 g	19
Carbohydrates	69 g	76
Fat	2 g	6

Egg, muffin, and milk

Item	Serving size	Calories
English muffin	1	140
Jelly	1 tbsp	60
Poached egg	1	80
Skim milk	½ glass	40

Nutritional information—Calories 320

		% of calories
Protein	15 g	19
Carbohydrates	49 g	61
Fat	7 g	20

Grapefruit, pancakes, and milk

Item	Serving size	Calories
Grapefruit	½ medium	30
Pancakes	2	140
Syrup	1 tbsp	50
Skim milk	1 cup	80

Nutritional information—Calories 300

		% of calories
Protein	19 g	15
Carbohydrates	51 g	75
Fat	2 g	6

Bagel, fruit, and milk

Item	Serving size	Calories
Bagel	1 medium	170
Cream cheese	2 tsp	30
Banana	½ medium	55
Skim milk	½ cup	40

Nutritional information—Calories 295

		% of calories
Protein	11 g	15
Carbohydrates	52 g	70
Fat	5 g	15

Because of the importance of protein, each of the four breakfast plans includes milk. Milk is a very nutrient-dense food that has little fat.

If you have lactose intolerance or simply dislike milk, it is difficult to get the necessary protein for breakfast without getting a lot of fat with it. If you can substitute nonfat or low-fat yogurt, you will get a comparable amount of protein. Another alternative is to eat an omelet made with one egg and two additional egg whites or one made with egg substitutes. If these alternatives to milk are not possible, then you may want to take a protein supplement and mix it with juice and fruit.

Milk—nutritional information
Serving size 1 glass (8 oz)

	Fat grams	Calories
Skim milk	0.4	86
1% milk	2.6	102
2% milk	4.7	121
Whole milk	8.2	150

MAKING POOR CHOICES AT BREAKFAST

It is easy to select low-fat, nutritious breakfast items, but if you are not careful, you may find that you are getting as many as half your calories for the day in one meal, with 50% or more calories coming from fat.

It may surprise you that this meal contains over 1200 calories with 70 grams of fat. It is impossible to be successful with a weight-management program if you are eating this many calories for breakfast with such a high percentage of calories coming from fat.

Typical high-fat breakfast

Item	Serving size	Calories
Orange juice	8 oz	106
Bacon	3 slices	120
Eggs—fried	2	160
Hash-brown potatoes	1 cup	340
Toast	2 slices	140
Jelly	2 tbsp	120
Butter	2 tbsp	210
Coffee	1 cup	0
Cream—Half & Half	2 tbsp	40

Nutritional information—Calories 1236

		% of calories
Protein	28 g	9
Carbohydrates	124 g	40
Fat	70	51

WEIGHT CYCLING: THE YO-YO SYNDROME

With diets, particularly very–low-calorie diets, weight that is lost is usually not maintained and a large percentage of the weight lost is usually lean body weight. The following example (Figure 9-1) shows what frequently happens when you gain weight slowly and try to lose it quickly. This will usually have a very detrimental effect on your distribution of body fat.

Notice that by means of a crash diet, Mary was quickly able to lose the 20 lb she had gained; however, she now has 31% body fat instead of the 25% that she had originally, despite the fact that she weighs the same now as she did when she was 23.

The bad news doesn't end there because when you lose lean body weight, your metabolism will slow down. It has been estimated that for each pound of lean body weight that you lose, you will require 50 fewer calories just to maintain your weight. As Mary lost 10 lb of lean body weight, simply to now just maintain her weight of 115 lb, she would have to reduce her caloric intake by approximately 500 calories. Yo-yo dieting is not the answer and is probably the quickest way to mess up your metabolism.

ACCUMULATION OF BODY FAT

Many weight-reduction programs simply concentrate on how much weight you need to lose. In most cases your ideal or goal weight is determined by consulting the standard height/weight tables. These tables work fine with some people, but because they do not differentiate between muscle and fat, they have some serious drawbacks. The following case study will illustrate this point:

Case Study

JERRY and ROBERT

Variable	Jerry	Robert
Age (years)	43	52
Height (inches)	71	70
Weight (lb)	170	173
Percent body fat	27	13

Notice that even though these two men were almost identical relative to height and weight, Jerry had more than twice as much body fat as Robert. The standard height/weight charts showed that for each of them, their body weight was within the normal range. However, the body composition analysis showed that Jerry was obese and Robert was very lean.

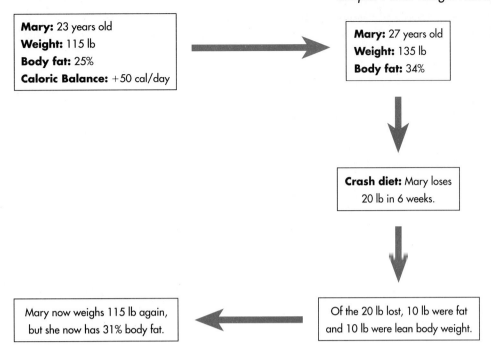

Mary: 23 years old
Weight: 115 lb
Body fat: 25%
Caloric Balance: +50 cal/day

Mary: 27 years old
Weight: 135 lb
Body fat: 34%

Crash diet: Mary loses 20 lb in 6 weeks.

Of the 20 lb lost, 10 lb were fat and 10 lb were lean body weight.

Mary now weighs 115 lb again, but she now has 31% body fat.

Figure 9-1   The effect of yo-yo dieting on body composition.

Fat accumulation—possible causes

For many years it was thought that fat accumulation was directly related to the amount of food eaten and that those who ate more than they should accumulated large amounts of body fat. The situation is much more complex than this; it would appear as if there are a number of possible reasons as to why some people accumulate more body fat than others. These are summarized in the self assessment below.

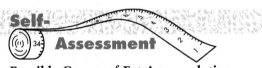

Self-Assessment

Possible Causes of Fat Accumulation

Please check those that apply to you:
- High fat intake
- Skipping meals
- Low protein intake
- High intake of simple sugar
- Excessive alcohol intake
- Very high caloric intake
- Very low caloric intake
- Lack of regular exercise
- Yo-yo dieting
- Low fiber intake

Information pertaining to each of the possible causes for fat accumulation identified in the self assessment above has been included at appropriate places throughout the book. You should now have sufficient knowledge so that you can make the changes that are necessary for you to be successful.

PUTTING IT ALL TOGETHER: THE 11 GUIDELINES

The importance of the choices that you make each day relative to when you eat, what you eat, how much you eat, and whether to exercise have been discussed previously. The consistency with which you make wise choices concerning each of these will basically determine how successful you will be in your weight-management/exercise program.

This weight-management/exercise program is based on 11 specific guidelines that you can use each day to evaluate the consistency of your eating and exercise habits. These guidelines are identified in this chapter, and the importance of each of them is briefly described. Detailed information relative to each of these guidelines has been presented at various places throughout this text.

1. Eat a nutritious breakfast within an hour of waking up

You have probably been told time and time again that "breakfast is the most important meal of the day." This is certainly true if you are trying to lose weight and reduce your body fat. By eating a nutritious breakfast each day, you can positively influence your metabolism, you will have more energy throughout the day, and you will be much more likely to control your snacking throughout the day. A good breakfast must provide an adequate amount of protein and carbohydrates. It is important to eat as soon as you can when you get up in the morning because your metabolism is low and the food will help to increase your metabolism.

2. Eat at least three planned meals spaced regularly throughout the day

When you eat frequently throughout the day, your metabolism will increase and you will burn more calories than you would have if you had eaten only one or two meals during the day. Skipping meals contributes to an increase in the amount of stored fat in your body. If you plan your meals, you will also be much more likely to make better choices about what to eat and will probably find it easier to control how much you eat. Long lapses of time between meals can distort your hunger, and you will often find that when you do eat you will eat more calories in one or two meals than you would if you had eaten three or four planned meals.

3. Eat your evening meal as early as possible

When you eat your evening meal is very important, particularly if it is your biggest meal of the day—which is the case for most people. Eating a large amount of food late in the day is likely to result in more of these calories being stored as fat in your body. The reason for this is that we are usually much less active during the evening hours. There are very few ways you can use many of these calories.

4. Drink water frequently throughout the day

This is one concept that just about every weight-loss program agrees on. This is necessary if you are to maintain a normal fluid balance in your body and if your body is to metabolize fat efficiently. By drinking water frequently throughout the day, you will also find it easier to control the amount of calories that you consume. Remember that water is the only fluid that you can drink that contains no calories.

5. If you drink alcoholic beverages, limit your intake

The secret to eating well is to get all the nutrients that you need each day without getting excess calories and without gaining excess weight or fat. Alcohol provides a considerable number of calories with little or no nutritional value. These calories are often referred to as "empty calories." For this reason even moderate drinkers need to drink less if they are overweight or have excess fat. Excessive consumption of alcohol is frequently associated with nutritional deficiencies and may contribute to several serious diseases. In addition to creating a loss of appetite and poor food intake, drinking too much alcohol also results in an impairment of the absorption of nutrients.

6. Limit your between-meal snacks to low-calorie, nonfat, or low-fat foods

Snacking can be good for you if you plan your snacks and make sensible choices as to what you eat. On the other hand, snacking can be bad if it is not planned and if you eat impulsively because the foods that you will usually choose will be very low in nutritional value or very high in fat or sugar. You need to learn which foods you can eat regularly and which foods you need to eat sparingly.

7. Limit your intake of simple refined sugars

Similar to alcohol, simple sugars provide calories but few other nutrients. Also, in most cases the more simple sugars you eat, the more you crave. For these reasons it is important that your intake of simple sugars be kept to a minimum. Many of the new low-fat or nonfat foods that are available contain a considerable amount of simple sugar.

8. Limit your intake of sodium and salt

Excessive sodium or salt may be hazardous to your health and is likely to create an imbalance in your fluid balance and contribute to an increase in your blood pressure. Since most Americans consume much more sodium than is needed, you should learn how to use less table salt and you need to read food labels carefully so that you can limit your intake of those foods that contain large amounts of sodium.

9. Limit the amount of fat that you eat each day

If you are to be successful at reducing your body weight and percentage of body fat, you must learn how to limit your fat intake. Not only does fat provide more than twice as many calories as protein or carbohydrates, but we now know that people who eat more fat accumulate more fat in specific areas of their body. With all the new low-fat and nonfat products now available, it is much easier to reduce the amount of fat that you eat each day.

10. Increase your intake of dietary fiber

Fiber is one of the most neglected nutrients, with the average American consuming less than half the recommended amount of fiber each day. You need to eat lots of fruits, vegetables, and grain products to increase your intake of fiber. If you select a breakfast cereal with lots of fiber, this will help to increase your intake. There are different types of fiber that perform different functions in your body, so you need to make sure that you get your fiber from different sources.

11. Exercise regularly

Regular aerobic exercise is important in any weight-management program. If you exercise at the right intensity, you will burn fat, which is probably what you are most concerned with. In addition, exercise has a positive effect on your metabolism. After aerobic exercise, your metabolism stays elevated for some time. Also, exercise can be used to increase your muscle mass. Muscle is more metabolically active than is fat. So by reducing your amount of fat and increasing your lean body tissue, your body will actually burn more calories each day while you are performing your everyday tasks. More fat and less muscle tissue are lost in weight-loss programs that incorporate exercise. The amount of exercise necessary for weight management is discussed in Chapter 8.

THE WEIGHT-MANAGEMENT/EXERCISE PROGRAM

Implementing the guidelines

If you are to be successful, you need to be constantly striving to implement these guidelines into your daily routine. The problem, however, is that most people simply do not know how to do this, or else they lack the motivation that is necessary to establish consistent eating and exercise habits.

A simple scoresheet has been devised using these guidelines so that you can evaluate your eating and exercise habits each day and you can then determine how consistent you are. At the same time as you evaluate yourself, you will learn how to make changes relative to each of these guidelines so that you can be successful. This self-evaluation form is presented in Table 9-2.

How to use the self-evaluation form

Following are the instructions for using the self-evaluation scoresheet:

- Rate yourself each day on each of these guidelines using the specific scoring system identified on the form.
- For each guideline there is a maximum number of points that you may earn and a maximum number of points that you may record. For example, with the first guideline there are 9 possible points you can earn. However, you can record only a maximum of 7 points.
- At the end of each day, add up all 11 scores for the day and record your total points for the day in the appropriate place. There is a maximum of 100 points each day.
- At the end of each week, add up your 7 daily totals and record this total in the appropriate place.

- Determine your average points per day for the week by dividing the total points for the week by 7. Record this value in the appropriate place.

In Summary

Your average points per day for the week on the self-evaluation scoresheet is the score that will indicate how consistent you have been for the week.

What does it take to be successful?

If you are trying to lose weight or body fat, we have found that to be successful at losing gradually, you need to meet each of the following three criteria each week.

- Eat a nutritious breakfast every day. (You will need to score 7 points for guideline 1 each day.)
- Make a commitment to exercise continuously for at least 45 minutes for a minimum of 5 days each week in any type of weight-bearing activity such as walking, jogging, basketball, racquetball, aerobics, or stair-climbing. If you have not been exercising regularly when you start this program, it may take you 2 or 3 weeks to gradually increase the length of each exercise session until you can participate continuously for 45 minutes. Start out at a very low level until 45 minutes of continuous work feels comfortable, and then gradually increase the intensity. (You will need to score 45 points for guideline 11, 5 days each week.)
- Average 70 or more points per day for each week. This total is based on 5 days of exercise. If you exercise 6 days, then you will need to average 75 points, and if you exercise all 7 days, then this total needs to be 80 or more points.

Does the program work?

It has taken over 4 years to develop the scoring system for the weekly self-evaluation scoresheet and to determine the criteria that you need to meet to be successful. Over 80% of the clients enrolled in our weight-management/exercise programs who meet the above three criteria each week and who have weight or body fat to lose are successful at gradually losing this weight or fat. Some lose only ½ to 1 lb of weight per week, whereas others lose up to 2 lb. Some lose very little weight initially but significantly reduce their percentage of body fat. The case study on p. 222 is one of hundreds of successful participants in this weight-management program. It shows how successful you can be if you decide to take charge of your eating and exercise habits.

| Table 9-2 | **Weight-Management/Exercise Program–Weekly Scoresheet** |

Rate yourself on the following 11 guidelines each day and record your score for each of them. At the end of each day, add up all 11 scores to determine your daily total.

Name:	Day: Date:	Mon	Tues	Wed	Thu	Fri	Sat	Sun
1. Eat a nutritious breakfast within an hour of when you wake up. 　3 points—if your breakfast includes a full glass of either skim milk, 1% milk, low-fat yogurt or ½ cup low-fat cottage cheese 　2 points—if your breakfast includes cereal or whole grain toast 　2 points—if your breakfast includes fruit or fruit juice 　2 points—if you eat breakfast and it does not include bacon, eggs, or hash browns	MAXIMUM 7 points	☐	☐	☐	☐	☐	☐	☐
2. Eat at least 3 planned meals spaced regularly throughout the day. 　0 points—if you eat less than 3 meals a day	MAXIMUM 3 points	☐	☐	☐	☐	☐	☐	☐
3. Eat your evening meal as early as possible. 　4 points—if you eat before 6 PM 　2 points—if you eat before 7 PM 　0 points—if you eat after 7 PM	MAXIMUM 4 points	☐	☐	☐	☐	☐	☐	☐
4. Drink water frequently throughout the day (1 glass = 8 oz.) 　4 points—if you drink 8 or more glasses 　3 points—if you drink 6 or 7 glasses 　2 points—if you drink 4 or 5 glasses 　1 point—if you drink 2 or 3 glasses 　0 points—if you drink less than 2 glasses	MAXIMUM 4 points	☐	☐	☐	☐	☐	☐	☐
5. Limit your alcoholic beverages each day. 　5 points—if you have 0 drinks 　3 points—if you have 1 or 2 drinks 　0 points—if you have 3 drinks 　−2 points—for each drink above 3 (maximum −10 points)	MAXIMUM 5 points MINIMUM −10 points	☐	☐	☐	☐	☐	☐	☐
6. Limit your between-meal snacks to fruit, vegetables, nonfat yogurt, pretzels, or air-popped popcorn (no butter or salt). 　3 points—if you do not snack or limit your snacks to the above foods 　1 point—if you have one snack other than the above (<150 cal)	MAXIMUM 3 points	☐	☐	☐	☐	☐	☐	☐

Table 9-2	**Weight-Management/Exercise Program-Weekly—cont'd**

Rate yourself on the following 11 guidelines each day and record your score for each of them. At the end of each day, add up all 11 scores to determine your daily total.

	Day: Date:	Mon	Tue	Wed	Thu	Fri	Sat	Sun

Name: _____

7. Limit your intake of simple sugars from sources other than fruit.
   - 2 points—if you do not eat jelly, jam, honey, or candy and you do not drink soda (you may drink <3 diet sodas).
   - 2 points—if you do not eat baked foods such as cookies, doughnuts, twinkies, cakes, pies, or desserts (you may record 1 point if these foods contain <100 cal).

   MAXIMUM 4 points ☐ ☐ ☐ ☐ ☐ ☐ ☐

8. Limit your intake of sodium and salt.
   - 2 points—if you do not add salt to your food or cook with salt.
   - 1 point—if you consistently select foods low in sodium

   MAXIMUM 3 points ☐ ☐ ☐ ☐ ☐ ☐ ☐

9. Limit the amount of fat that you eat each day.
   - 2 points—if you eat no butter or margarine
   - 2 points—if all your dairy products are low fat
   - 3 points—if you eat no cheese
   - 3 points—if your meat intake consists only of fish, turkey, chicken without skin, or 4 oz or less of lean red meat
   - 2 points—if you eat no food cooked in oil, no fried food, and no products with tropical oils

   MAXIMUM 12 points ☐ ☐ ☐ ☐ ☐ ☐ ☐

10. Increase your intake of dietary fiber.
    - 1 point—for each serving of fruit and vegetables (maximum–5 pts)
    - 1 point—for each serving from grain products and legumes (maximum–5 pts)
    - 1 point—for each 4 g of fiber from breakfast cereals (maximum–3 pts)

    MAXIMUM 10 points ☐ ☐ ☐ ☐ ☐ ☐ ☐

11. Exercise regularly.
    - 1 point—for each minute of organized continuous aerobic exercise where you are on your feet and supporting your body weight and moving
    - ½ point—for each minute of organized continuous exercise that does not meet the above criteria

    MAXIMUM 45 points ☐ ☐ ☐ ☐ ☐ ☐ ☐

    TOTAL POINTS PER DAY — MAXIMUM 100 points ☐ ☐ ☐ ☐ ☐ ☐ ☐

TOTAL POINTS FOR THE WEEK (add total points for all 7 days) _____

AVERAGE POINTS/DAY (divide the total points for the week by 7) _____

Case Study

LYLIAN

Lylian was a nonexerciser who enrolled in our weight-management/exercise program in September 1990. She had extremely poor eating habits, was overweight, and had an excessive amount of fat. She decided that it was time to make a commitment and to take charge of her eating and exercise habits.

During the 10 weeks she was in this program, there was not one morning that she did not eat breakfast and there was not one week that she did not exercise at least 5 times for 45 minutes. Her average points per day for each of the 10 weeks ranged from 72 to 96. Her average for the 10 weeks was 81. Before the program started, she was averaging less than 40 points per day. These scores reflect major changes in her eating and exercise habits.

She was very consistent during the program, and because of this she was very successful. Following is a comparison between her initial and final test results.

Measurement	September 1990	December 1990
Body weight (lbs)	170	148
Percent body fat	41	30
Body fat measurements		
Subscapular	28	19
Triceps	32	24
Thigh	46	33
Abdominal	48	33
Suprailiac	41	24
Midaxillary	40	24
Cholesterol (mg/dl)	186	139
Aerobic fitness (ml/kgbw/min)	19	28

Not everyone is alike, and it may be necessary to "fine-tune" this program so that you determine the amount of exercise you need to do each week to balance out the eating habits that you have established. Do not be discouraged if you do not see a change in your body weight initially. The reason for this has been explained previously. A number of clients who go through our weight-management/exercise program see only minimal changes in their body weight; however, when their body fat is measured again at the end of the program, they are surprised by the amount of fat that they have lost.

If you initially have extremely poor eating habits and have not been exercising regularly for some time, do not expect to immediately achieve all three criteria that you need to meet to be successful. It is unlikely that you will be able to make all the necessary changes at once. Work on them one at a time. As specific objectives regularly become part of your lifestyle, you can concentrate on becoming more consistent with each of the other objectives. You should see an increase each week in the average number of points for the week.

Evaluating your exercise and eating habits

Use the self-evaluation scoresheet (Table 9-2) to evaluate a "typical" day for you. By doing this, you will see which of these guidelines are already part of your lifestyle and you should be able to identify changes that you can make immediately. In Laboratory Experience 9-3, you will evaluate yourself for an entire week. This will give you a much better idea of the consistency of your eating and exercise habits.

Make 10 copies of Table 9-2 so that you can use these for 10 consecutive weeks. We have found that most people will take more than a week or so to change some of their habits. By working each week at getting more consistent with each of these and recording your score each week, you will be more motivated to stick with your program. You will be able to see progress in your weekly scores if you are more consistent.

Chapter Summary

The following summary will help you to identify some of the important concepts covered in this chapter:

- Despite the fact that weight loss has become an obsession in America, very few people have been successful at losing excess weight and keeping it off.
- Most diets fail because they restrict your food intake and do not encourage permanent lifestyle changes.
- For permanent weight loss, you should lose weight slowly by making changes in your lifestyle that you can live with for the rest of your life.
- Initially in a weight-loss program, you can lose fat but you may not lose any weight.
- You need to eat at regular intervals throughout the day. Skipping meals is counterproductive to losing body fat.
- Eating a nutritious breakfast is essential if you are to be successful at controlling the amount of body fat that you have.
- The day-to-day consistency of your exercise and eating habits will determine how successful you will be.

References

1. Alford BB et al: The effects of variations in carbohydrate, protein and fat content of the diet upon weight loss, blood values, and nutrient intake of adult obese women, *J Am Diet Assoc* 90(4):534-540, 1990.
2. Boyle MA, Zyla G: *Personal nutrition*, ed 2, St Paul, Minn, 1992, West Publishing.
3. Burgess NS: Effect of a very low calorie diet on body composition and resting metabolic rate in obese men and women, *J Am Diet Assoc* 91(4):430-434, 1992.
4. Christian JL, Greger JL: *Nutrition for living*, ed 4, Redwood City, Calif, 1994, Benjamin-Cummings.
5. Coats C, Smith P: *Alive and well in the fast food lane*, Orlando, Fla, 1987, Carolyn Coats Bestsellers.
6. Cottrell RR: *Wellness—weight control*, Guilford, Conn, 1991, Dushkin.
7. *Dietary Guidelines for Americans*, US Department of Agriculture and Department of Health and Human Services, Washington, DC, 1985.
8. *Dietary Guidelines for the United States*, Senate Select Committee on Nutrition and Human Needs, US Government Printing Office, Washington, DC, 1985.
9. DuPuy NA, Mermel VL: *Focus on nutrition*, St Louis, 1995, Mosby.
10. Lewis CJ et al: Nutrient intakes and body weights of persons consuming high and moderate levels of added sugars, *J Am Diet Assoc* 92(6):705-713, 1992.
11. Miller WC et al: Dietary fat, sugar and fiber predict body fat content, *J Am Diet Assoc* 94(6):612-615, 1994.
12. Nash JD: Weight control programs—what's the best choice? *Healthline* 7:1-4, Jan 1988.
13. Pritikin: Is snacking good for you? *Vantage Point* 1:6, April 1991.
14. Schelkun PH: The risk of riding the weight-loss roller coaster, *The Physician and Sportmedicine* 19(6):149-156, 1991.
14a. Schoeborn CA, Cohen BH: Trends in smoking, alcohol consumption, and other health practices among US adults, 1977-1983, *Advance data* Jun 30, 1986, p 118.
15. Shapiro L: Feeding frenzy, *Newsweek*, May 27, 1991, pp 46-53.
16. Walker P: Theories of weight management, *Idea Today*, April 1994, p. 49-53.
17. *The Surgeon General's Report on Nutrition and Health*, US Department of Health and Human Services, Washington, DC, 1989.
18. Wardlaw GM, Insel PM, Seyler MF: *Contemporary nutrition*, ed 2, St Louis, 1994, Mosby.

Laboratory Experience 9-1

Do Your Daily Habits Encourage Weight Management?

Name _____ Section _____ Date _____

To determine whether your daily habits encourage weight management and to help you to identify changes that you need to make, simply circle the appropriate number in response to each question.

How Often Do You:	RARELY	SOMETIMES	OFTEN
1. Eat fried foods rather than foods that are baked, broiled, or boiled?	3	2	1
2. Eat a nutritious breakfast?	1	2	3
3. Choose low-fat or nonfat foods?	1	2	3
4. Plan ahead of time the foods that you eat?	1	2	3
5. Skip meals?	3	2	1
6. Overeat and wish that you had not eaten so much?	3	2	1
7. Eat at fast-food restaurants because you do not have time to sit down and relax and enjoy a quiet, leisurely meal?	3	2	1
8. Get up in time so that you can eat breakfast at home?	1	2	3
9. Crave for a dessert after eating an adequate meal?	3	2	1
10. Buy troublesome foods such as chips, ice cream, cookies, etc.?	3	2	1
11. Eat in one main place when eating at home?	1	2	3
12. Engage in other activities, such as reading or watching television, while eating?	3	2	1
13. Avoid the negative influence of friends and peers on your eating habits?	1	2	3
14. Take 20 minutes or longer to eat your meals?	1	2	3
15. Exercise regularly?	1	2	3
16. Leave your food on your plate?	1	2	3
17. Drink at least 6 glasses of water in a day?	1	2	3
18. Drink more than 2 alcoholic drinks in a day?	3	2	1
19. Drink at least 1 glass of water or other low-calorie fluid before each meal?	1	2	3
20. Eat in response to something other than hunger?	3	2	1

Add the numbers together that you circled.
Enter your score here _____

Interpretation

Interpret your score this way:

20-36	Very poor—Your eating habits need a lot of attention.
37-47	Average—You are doing all right, but there is room for improvement.
48-60	Very good—You have developed good consistent habits; however, do not reward yourself by overeating.

Laboratory Experience 9-2

Learning About Your Eating Habits

Name _____ Section _____ Date _____

To learn more about your eating habits, you need to keep a food diary for at least 2 days—a weekday and a weekend day (see Tables 9-3 and 9-4). Following are the instructions you will need to complete these food diary forms:

Time of Eating

For every meal or snack, record the time when you begin eating or drinking and when you finish.

Meal or Snack

Indicate whether it is a meal or a snack. Be sure to remember that everything you drink between meals is considered a snack. If it is a meal, indicate whether it is breakfast, lunch, or dinner.

Place of Eating

Record where you are when you eat that meal or snack or have that drink. If you are at home, record the room of the house you are in; otherwise, record whether you are in a restaurant, car, office, bar, etc.

Food and Amount

Indicate what you eat and the approximate amount. If you eat at home and you have a small scale, you will find it beneficial to measure the amount of the food that you eat so that you become more aware of portion sizes. If you do not know the exact amount, you will need to estimate this amount. If you estimate the amount of food, keep in mind that most people usually underestimate this amount.

Posture

Indicate your physical position while you are eating or drinking—lying down, sitting, standing, walking, etc.

Associated Activity

Record what else you are doing while you are eating or drinking. For example, preparing dinner, watching television, reading, driving a car, talking on the telephone, etc.

Social Situation

Indicate whether you are alone, with someone, or with a group of people each time you eat.

Mood

Record how you feel before you start to eat. Were you content? happy? sad? depressed? angry? bored? tired? rushed? lonely? tense? etc.

Hunger Level

Record how hungry you are before you start to eat. Rate your hunger level on a 10-point scale ranging from a score of 1, which would indicate that you were not hungry, to a score of 10, which would indicate that you were very hungry.

Evaluating Your Daily Food Recall Diary

By carefully evaluating your 3-day food diary, you will become aware of what you eat and how much you eat. You may find out that you are one of those people who do not realize how much they eat until they write everything down. You will also be able to see patterns as to when and why you eat.

Your food recall forms may also show that you eat too quickly without paying attention to your food or taking the time to enjoy it. If you eat frequently while standing up or while you are engaging in other activities, this is a good indication that you need to slow down and take the time to enjoy your food.

Analysis of the Three Food Recall Forms

By answering the following questions you may be able to identify some of these patterns:

- How many days did you skip at least one meal? _____
- How many times did you eat when you were not really hungry? _____
- How many times did you eat because you were bored? _____
- How many times did you eat because you were angry or depressed? _____
- How many days did you snack on foods that you know you should not have eaten? _____
- How many days did you drink more than one alcoholic beverage? _____
- How many days did you eat at least one dessert? _____
- How many times did other people trigger unwanted eating behavior? _____
- How many times did you eat a meal and when you were finished, you wished that you had not eaten so much? _____

| Table 9-3 | **Daily Food Recall Diary #1** |

Complete this form for at least 1 weekday and weekend day. Try to select typical days.

Time start-end	Meal or snack	Place	Food	Amount	Posture	Associated activity	Social situation	Mood	Hunger level

Name: Date:

| Table 9-4 | **Daily Food Recall Diary #2** |

Complete this form for at least 1 weekday and weekend day. Try to select typical days.

Time start-end	Meal or snack	Place	Food	Amount	Posture	Associated activity	Social situation	Mood	Hunger level

Name: Date:

Evaluating the Consistency of Your Eating and Exercise Habits

Name _____   Section _____   Date _____

To determine the consistency of your exercise and eating habits, it may be beneficial for you to evaluate your eating and exercise habits for a complete week. Simply use the weekly self-evaluation score sheet in Table 9-5 and score yourself each day. The procedures to follow have been given previously.

Calculating Your Score

To calculate your score for the week, total your score for each day. You then add the 7 daily totals and divide by 7 to determine your average score for the week.

Interpretation of Score

To have the consistency you need to be successful at losing weight or simply to have good consistent eating and exercise habits, you need to average 70 or more points. This score is based on the premise that you exercise no more than 5 times each week. If you exercise 6 times, you need to average 75 points, or if you exercise all 7 days, your average needs to be 80 points.

Table 9-5   Weight-Management/Exercise Program–Weekly Scoresheet

Rate yourself on the following 11 guidelines each day and record your score for each of them. At the end of each day, add up all 11 scores to determine your daily total.

	Day: Date:	Mon	Tues	Wed	Thu	Fri	Sat	Sun
Name: _____								

1. Eat a nutritious breakfast within an hour of when you wake up.
   - 3 points—if your breakfast includes a full glass of either skim milk, 1% milk, low-fat yogurt or ½ cup low-fat cottage cheese
   - 2 points—if your breakfast includes cereal or whole grain toast
   - 2 points—if your breakfast includes fruit or fruit juice
   - 2 points—if you eat breakfast and it does not include bacon, eggs, or hash browns

   MAXIMUM 7 points ☐ ☐ ☐ ☐ ☐ ☐ ☐

2. Eat at least 3 planned meals spaced regularly throughout the day.
   - 0 points—if you eat less than 3 meals a day

   MAXIMUM 3 points ☐ ☐ ☐ ☐ ☐ ☐ ☐

3. Eat your evening meal as early as possible.
   - 4 points—if you eat before 6 PM
   - 2 points—if you eat before 7 PM
   - 0 points—if you eat after 7 PM

   MAXIMUM 4 points ☐ ☐ ☐ ☐ ☐ ☐ ☐

4. Drink water frequently throughout the day (1 glass = 8 oz.)
   - 4 points—if you drink 8 or more glasses
   - 3 points—if you drink 6 or 7 glasses
   - 2 points—if you drink 4 or 5 glasses
   - 1 point—if you drink 2 or 3 glasses
   - 0 points—if you drink less than 2 glasses

   MAXIMUM 4 points ☐ ☐ ☐ ☐ ☐ ☐ ☐

5. Limit your alcoholic beverages each day.
   - 5 points—if you have 0 drinks
   - 3 points—if you have 1 or 2 drinks
   - 0 points—if you have 3 drinks
   - −2 points—for each drink above 3 (maximum—10 points)

   MAXIMUM 5 points

   MINIMUM −10 points ☐ ☐ ☐ ☐ ☐ ☐ ☐

6. Limit your between-meal snacks to fruit, vegetables, nonfat yogurt, pretzels, or air-popped popcorn (no butter or salt).
   - 3 points—if you do not snack or limit your snacks to the above foods
   - 1 point—if you have one snack other than the above (<150 cal)

   MAXIMUM 3 points ☐ ☐ ☐ ☐ ☐ ☐ ☐

Table 9-5   **Weight-Management/Exercise Program-Weekly—cont'd**

Rate yourself on the following 11 guidelines each day and record your score for each of them. At the end of each day, add up all 11 scores to determine your daily total.

Name: _____	Day: Date:	Mon	Tue	Wed	Thu	Fri	Sat	Sun

7. Limit your intake of simple sugars from sources other than fruit.
  2 points—if you do not eat jelly, jam, honey, or candy and you do not drink soda (you may drink <0 diet sodas).
  2 points—if you do not eat baked foods such as cookies, doughnuts, twinkies, cakes, pies, or desserts (you may record 1 point if these foods contain <100 cal).
	MAXIMUM
	4 points
		☐	☐	☐	☐	☐	☐	☐

8. Limit your intake of sodium and salt.
  2 points—if you do not add salt to your food or cook with salt.
  1 point—if you consistently select foods low in sodium
	MAXIMUM
	3 points
		☐	☐	☐	☐	☐	☐	☐

9. Limit the amount of fat that you eat each day.
  2 points—if you eat no butter or margarine
  2 points—if all your dairy products are low fat
  3 points—if you eat no cheese
  3 points—if your meat intake consists only of fish, turkey, chicken without skin, or 4 oz or less of lean red meat
  2 points—if you eat no food cooked in oil, no fried food, and no products with tropical oils
	MAXIMUM
	12 points
		☐	☐	☐	☐	☐	☐	☐

10. Increase your intake of dietary fiber.
  1 point—for each serving of fruit and vegetables (maximum–5 pts)
  1 point—for each serving from grain products and legumes (maximum–5 pts)
  1 point—for each 4 g of fiber from breakfast cereals (maximum–3 pts)
	MAXIMUM
	10 points
		☐	☐	☐	☐	☐	☐	☐

11. Exercise regularly.
  1 point—for each minute of organized continuous aerobic exercise where you are on your feet and supporting your body weight and moving
  ½ point—for each minute of organized continuous exercise that does not meet the above criteria
	MAXIMUM
	45 points
		☐	☐	☐	☐	☐	☐	☐

TOTAL POINTS PER DAY	MAXIMUM 100 points	☐	☐	☐	☐	☐	☐	☐

TOTAL POINTS FOR THE WEEK (add total points for all 7 days) ——————

AVERAGE POINTS/DAY (divide the total points for the week by 7) ——————

Chapter Ten **Stress Management**

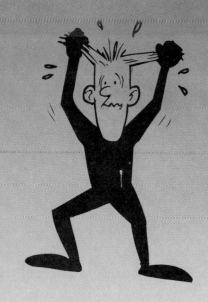

CHAPTER OBJECTIVES

Check off each objective you achieve.

- ❏ Define stress, and know the difference between too much stress, too little stress, and optimal stress.
- ❏ Discuss the way in which your body reacts to stress, and identify the three stages of stress.
- ❏ Discuss the problems associated with too much stress.
- ❏ Identify stressful situations, and determine how much stress is too much.
- ❏ Differentiate clearly between Type A and Type B behaviors.
- ❏ Discuss the role of exercise in stress reduction.
- ❏ Identify strategies you can use to effectively deal with stress.
- ❏ Determine your level of stress.

Stress is a normal part of everyday living—something we cannot avoid. It is necessary if we are to be productive, but it can be harmful if it occurs too frequently, is too intense, or lasts too long. Stress may be defined simply as our reaction to a specific situation or event. It is not the event that causes the stress but the reaction to it. The following case study illustrates this.

Case Study

ANNEMARIE

Annemarie is an 18-year-old who has just graduated from high school in a small rural community where she has many friends. She has lived at home with her parents all her life and has been "going steady" with the same boy for nearly 2 years. She is preparing to leave this environment to attend college in a large city 700 miles away.

She is very happy to be the first person in her family to attend college, but she is very apprehensive about some of the adjustments she now must make. Some of her anxiety is caused by the following:

- Her parents want her to do well in college.
- Her boyfriend does not want her to leave.
- She has to live on campus and share a room, and she is worried about whether she will get along with her roommate.
- She is concerned about having to eat on campus and is afraid she will gain weight like most other freshmen.
- She does not know which classes she should take.
- She has never had to worry about grades in high school, but now she knows that she will have to "compete" for good grades.

This is a typical college situation that many freshmen face, and it is obvious that such situations cause different reactions from different people. It is important to learn to balance stress with the demands placed on you with everyday living. To do this, you will need to do the following:

- Become more knowledgeable about stress.
- Determine the amount of stress in your life.
- Learn to identify the specific situations that cause stress for you.
- Develop effective ways of dealing with stress and reducing your stress level.

DEFINITION OF BASIC TERMS

Stress has been defined as your reaction to a specific situation or event. This reaction can be either positive or negative and would include such responses as anger,

joy, rejection, frustration, and happiness. It is obvious that stress is associated with both unpleasant and pleasant situations.

Distress is a term used to refer to high level of stress resulting in negative responses such as tension and frustration. Constant distress can negatively affect your health and performance.

Eustress is a term used to refer to a "good" stress that results in what is perceived as a positive reaction such as joy and happiness. It is usually associated with pleasurable situations such as getting married, graduation, promotion, and successfully completing a difficult task. Despite the fact that these types of events are viewed as "positive," they can also negatively influence your level of stress.

For example, getting married means that you must often make some major lifestyle adjustments. These may include buying or renting a house or apartment, buying furniture, moving, and having added financial responsibilities. These can all cause distress.

A **stressor** is any situation or event that initiates the stress response. The same stressor may result in two entirely different responses. For example, many people play golf for the enjoyment and relaxation that they get from playing. For others who are usually very competitive, it creates so much frustration that they have a hard time controlling the stress that it creates for them.

QUANTIFYING STRESS

It may be beneficial to find a way to quantify stress. A logical approach might be to consider stress as existing on a scale or continuum (Figure 10-1).

An optimal level of stress is defined as the level at which you perform most efficiently without encountering any harmful side effects. An optimal level of stress can help you to concentrate better on the job at hand and reach peak efficiency. You are likely to be able to think more clearly, your motivation level will be higher, and you will be in total control of the situation.

An extremely high level of stress is often referred to as negative stress. Many people perform their best work under extreme pressure. However, if high stress levels cannot be relieved by relaxation, you will not be

---

Distress: A high level of stress associated with negative responses such as anxiety, tension, and frustration.

Eustress: A positive reaction to stress, resulting in responses such as joy and happiness.

Stressor: Any change that causes a person to react in a stressful situation.

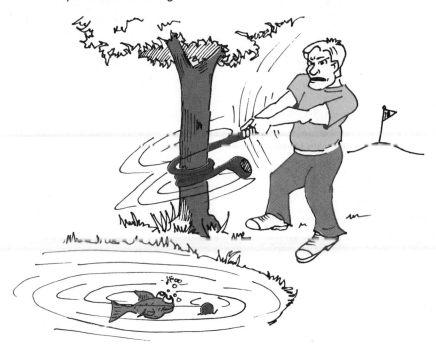

Some activities create stress for participants.

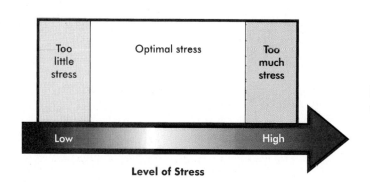

Figure 10-1   Stress should be viewed as existing on a continuum or scale.

able to function efficiently. Negative stress has also been associated with increased risk of coronary heart disease, hypertension, diabetes, and many other physical ailments.

A low level of stress is usually detrimental also. It may result in decreased motivation and performance, irritability, and boredom. We need a certain level of stress to be productive.

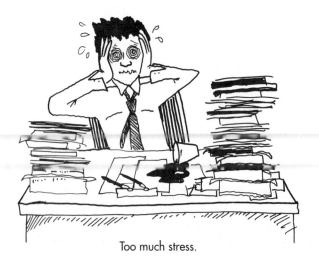

Too much stress.

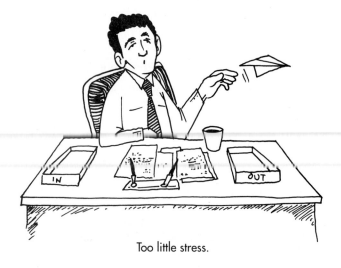

Too little stress.

THE NATURE OF STRESS

Your body has a built-in response to stress that occurs automatically, without conscious thought. Your natural reaction in response to a stressor is to prepare for physical activity.

Our bodies react the same way as in ancient times, when people had two choices on finding themselves face-to-face with physical stress: either they could fight or they could try to run away from it. This is referred to as the "fight or flight" response. Both of these responses require the body to quickly perform more physical work than normal.

Your physiological response to stressors may occur in three stages.

Stage I: These are immediate physiological changes that occur within the body to prepare for high-intensity physical activity. These are identified below:

> Your heart rate increases to circulate more blood to the muscles.
> Your blood pressure rises.
> Your breathing rate increases to provide more oxygen to the blood.
> Your muscles tense in anticipation of increased activity.
> Additional energy is automatically made available from stored carbohydrates.
> Perspiration increases in an attempt to control your body temperature.

Stage II: The second stage is often referred to as the resistance stage. In this stage the body reacts to the stressor, and most functions within the body return to normal. The body adjusts to the increased level of stress by secreting various hormones that have a calming effect on the body and that help you to adjust to the stressful situation.

Stage III: If the stress continues over an extended period of time or is extremely intense, the body may enter the third stage, where exhaustion and disease may occur.

The problem is that the majority of today's stressors are not physical in nature but are primarily emotional. Rarely is it appropriate to "attack" our problems or to "run away from them." However, our bodies still react in the same way. They are primed for action, and this just does not occur. The result is a prolonged state of tension that often results in irritability, depression, anger, anxiety, hostility, apathy, and fatigue.

In an attempt to cope with this prolonged state of tension, many people turn to such things as alcohol, drugs, smoking, overeating, or some other unhealthful practice. These do not relieve stress; in fact, in most cases they add to the problem. When your level of stress becomes extremely high and ongoing, your physical and emotional health are adversely affected. The more intense the stress or the longer it lasts, the more serious the consequences.

PROBLEMS ASSOCIATED WITH TOO MUCH STRESS

It has been estimated that more than 50% of all diseases in the United States have a stress-related origin. The diseases most frequently mentioned include cardiovascular disease, cancer, **hypertension, migraine headaches,** ulcers, allergies, and asthma.

- The incidence of cardiovascular disease is much higher in those who are characterized by a high stress level than those who experience very little stress.
- The hormones secreted in the body in abundance as part of the "fight or flight" response tend to remain in the body and may lessen the body's ability to fight infection.
- Stress is the cause of certain muscular problems. For example, many headaches are caused by continued contraction of certain muscles in the head and neck.
- Stress can contribute to high blood pressure, which is a risk factor associated with cardiovascular disease. It can also contribute to problems with the liver and kidneys.
- Constant levels of high stress can make you confused and may make it difficult for you to concentrate. This may make you more accident prone.

The relationship between stress and illness is summarized in Figure 10-2.

IDENTIFYING STRESSFUL SITUATIONS

It is important to be able to recognize and identify the situations in your life that cause stress.

Fitness Flash

Nearly one third of all Americans feel under "great stress" just about every day or several days per week.

Hypertension: Consistently elevated blood pressure.

Migraine headache: Intense pain in the head, usually confined to one side of the head. It may be preceded by changes in vision.

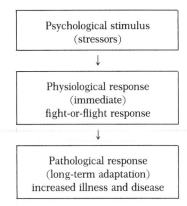

Figure 10-2   Short-term and long-term effects of stress. (Modified from Delin MM. *Well on the way to optimal health and fitness,* Irving, TX, 1987, Health Management Consultants.)

Stress may be caused by minor day-to-day events

Each day we encounter a variety of situations that in themselves are insignificant but that collectively can accumulate to negatively affect your level of stress. The following self-assessment lists some examples of day-to-day events that may increase your level of stress.

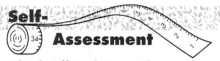

Self-Assessment

Check Off Each Item That Applies to You:

- Waiting in line
- Misplacing your keys or glasses
- Hosting a party
- Being late for an appointment
- Being caught in a traffic jam
- Not hearing your alarm and sleeping in
- Having a disagreement with a friend
- Not having sufficient time to complete an examination or assignment

Note that it is not the event that causes stress but your response to the specific situation. If you become impatient, irritated, frustrated, or apprehensive in response to any of these situations, or situations similar to these, your stress level will increase.

When you experience situations such as those mentioned previously, before you react negatively and let them bother you, you need to ask yourself, "Will this situation have an effect on my life tomorrow or next week?" In most cases it will not. Despite this, it is still often difficult to change the way you react to "minor" everyday stressors such as these.

Stress may be caused by lifestyle changes

Both positive and negative lifestyle changes require you to adjust to a new or different situation and can therefore be stressful. Following are some examples of lifestyle changes:

- Getting married
- Taking a vacation
- Starting a family
- Buying a new house
- Getting fired
- Relocating to a different city
- Experiencing the death of a close friend
- Getting promoted

Some lifestyle changes are completely out of your control, but many are controllable. If you are adjusting to many changes within a short period, you are much more likely to have a high level of stress. You should take your time and plan your changes gradually. It could be stressful to graduate from college, start a career, get married, buy a house, and start a family all within the first year of graduation.

Many people tend to overreact to change. For example, some people worry so much about what appears to be an unpleasant event that the worrying causes as much stress or even more than actually experiencing the event.

Let's Get Started

Coping with stress

Try to focus on those factors that you can control rather than on those over which you have no control.

Stress may be caused by overload

Overload occurs when you find yourself faced with demands that have accumulated to an unmanageable level and that exceed your capacity to meet them. These demands may be related to work, school, or home.

When you become overloaded, you try to do too many things at the same time, with the result that you have too many deadlines to meet and not enough hours in the day to accomplish all that needs to be done.

When this occurs, you often have trouble deciding which task to attempt first.

Some people become totally involved in their work and thrive on overload. They are usually remarkably satisfied with their lives and are willing to make sacrifices in other areas so that they have time to complete their work. These people are often referred to as "workaholics."

This situation is far too stressful for most people, and it often results in the following:

- Lack of motivation, despite the fact that they are overloaded
- A feeling of frustration and helplessness
- Decreased productivity
- Inability to sleep soundly
- Chronic fatigue
- Reduced judgment and recall

When this situation occurs, it is important to sit down, try to relax, and get things in perspective. You need to decide on priorities and then complete one step at a time. Added stress associated with work can also result from the following:

- Having to meet deadlines
- Being forced to make important decisions
- Having high levels of expectation relating to job performance

- Lacking confidence in your ability
- Having too much responsibility

In Summary

Being aware of what causes your stress is the first step involved in finding a solution to the problem.

HOW MUCH STRESS IS TOO MUCH?

People react differently to potentially stressful situations. However, there are certain signs and symptoms that could indicate that you are under too much stress. Your first step in trying to cope with stress is to learn to recognize some of these early signs and symptoms. The self-assessment below may help you to determine some of these early signs and symptoms that relate to your mood and disposition.

There are also other internal signs and symptoms or particular responses that may indicate a potentially high stress level. By completing the self-assessment on p. 236, you should be able to identify which of these symptoms apply to you.

By evaluating your response to these early signs of excess stress, you should be able to identify situations that may create problems for you. With regard to the two sets of signs and symptoms, if several of your responses are "often" or "sometimes," then you could be

Self-Assessment

Check the Frequency with Which the Following Responses Apply to You:

How Frequently Do You Feel:	Rarely	Sometimes	Often
Insecure: You think the worst possible outcome.			
Irritable: You may be short-tempered or impatient.			
Depressed: You are easily upset—you may eat or drink in response to how you feel.			
Angry: You may be hostile, violent, or irrational.			
Overly aggressive: You may be demanding, selfish, or insensitive.			
Easily distracted: You find it difficult to concentrate—you may be preoccupied or may experience decreased productivity.			
Forgetful: You may be absentminded or suffer from insomnia.			
Anxious: You may be frequently worried or nervous.			
Reckless: You may act violently, or you may be careless or self-destructive.			

Self-Assessment

Check Off the Frequency with Which the Following Apply to You:

Response	Rarely	Sometimes	Often
Pain or tension in back of your neck			
Increased frequency of eating			
Increased smoking			
Tension headaches			
Easily startled by unexpected sounds			
Profuse sweating			
Pounding of heart or irregular heartbeat			
Hands feel moist and/or cold			
Upset stomach			
Increased blood pressure			
Difficulty standing still			
Reduced attention span			
Difficulty sitting quietly			

considered as either having a high level of stress or else you are a high-risk candidate for developing a high level of stress. You need to avoid or confront the specific stressors that create problems for you. The following case study will show you how to do this:

Case Study

SCOTT

Scott is a very "competitive" college student who likes to excel. He never seems to have enough time and is constantly rushing to meet specific guidelines. Today he has a test at 9:30 AM. He overslept and missed his first class because he stayed up until 5:00 AM studying for the test. Not only did he miss his first class, but he did not have time to eat breakfast or to review his notes for the test. His stress level is extremely high as he rushes out the door and barely makes it in time for his examination.

By analyzing the events that happen in a stressful situation such as in the case study above, you should be able to come up with a plan in an attempt to avoid this situation in the future. Scott could have begun studying for the test several days in advance so that he did not have to "cram" everything into one night. He could have then gotten a good night's rest, had a leisurely breakfast while he reviewed his notes, attended his first class, and made it to the examination refreshed without the extra stress caused by rushing, missing a class, and not eating breakfast.

You need to analyze specific events such as these that create high levels of stress for you and plan how you can modify your behavior and reduce your level of stress.

In Summary

If you are to be successful at controlling your level of stress, you need to:
- Confront a specific problem
- Identify the causes
- Plan so that you can avoid such a problem in the future

PERSONALITY FACTORS

Your attitude and your perception of the stressor will determine your reaction to each specific stressful situation. Those who see problems as worse than they really are will be likely to reach a higher level of stress and maintain this level for a longer period. Basically, people can be classified into two groups according to how they perceive specific situations.

The first class, **Type A,** is associated with a high level of stress. Type A personalities rate high on the following criteria:

Ambition—An intense, sustained drive to achieve self-selected but usually poorly defined goals

Competitiveness—A profound inclination and eagerness to compete

Aggressiveness—Persistent desire for recognition and advancement

Chronic sense of time urgency—Continuous involvement in multiple functions while constantly subject to restrictions

Drive—Persistent efforts to accelerate the rate of execution of many physical and mental functions

These traits are normally present in most individuals, but the Type A person possesses them to an excessive degree. Individuals in this group include those who cannot stand to have unscheduled time on their hands, who are impatient with the world, who become very upset when they are kept waiting, and who always walk, talk, and eat rapidly.

Those who rate low on these traits are classified as **Type B.** These people usually are able to relax easily. Very seldom do they let outside factors adversely influence their emotional state. The level of anxiety and tension of a Type B person is therefore very low.

There are some short-term benefits associated with being a Type A person. However, more often than not, in the long run it impairs efficiency and creates definite health problems. It is also interesting to note that Type A people have a lower than average self-esteem. This may explain why they feel that they must attempt to do more and to work at a faster pace.

If you have a Type A personality, it is very difficult to change. You will need to work hard at learning to adjust differently to given situations. You need to become less competitive, to concentrate on one task at a time, and to slow down. Specific lifestyle changes that may be beneficial to you are found in the following section on stress management.

STRESS MANAGEMENT

The first step in coping with stress is to be aware that stress exists and that, if it persists, its effects can be detrimental to your health and wellness. Some people simply refuse to accept the fact that they are under too much stress and fail to recognize the signs and symptoms associated with excess stress.

The next step is to identify the environmental situations that cause your stress. We have seen that much of our stress is caused by the following:

- Minor day to day hassles
- Significant lifestyle changes
- Too many responsibilities and deadlines

In many cases we cannot change the nature of the stressors, but we can learn new skills so that we can control the effects that stressors have on us.

Lifestyle changes

By intentionally changing those aspects of your lifestyle and environment that create stress, you can reduce your level of frustration, anxiety, hostility, and irritability. Making these changes may not be as difficult as it may at first appear. Following are some suggestions that may be helpful.

- When a major change occurs in your life, you can minimize the amount of stress by reducing the number of other changes made. Continue to engage in familiar and enjoyable activities that help you to relax.

- Try to slow down and allow yourself more time to do the things that need to be done. If you are always rushed in the morning, get up earlier so that you have more time. Establish a routine that becomes automatic and that allows plenty of time. When traveling, try to leave 10 to 20 minutes earlier than normal so that you do not have to rush from one place to the next. Try to eliminate the things you do hurriedly that don't save you much time, such as changing lanes on the freeway or running a red light because you are in a hurry.

- Plan each day by listing the tasks that need to be accomplished in their order of importance so that the most important ones can be completed first. If a task appears to be long and complicated and you become frustrated at even getting started, break it down into a series of smaller tasks. Work on each of these, one at a time. As each task is completed, check it off. This will give you a sense of satisfaction and will increase your level of motivation instead of increasing your level of stress.

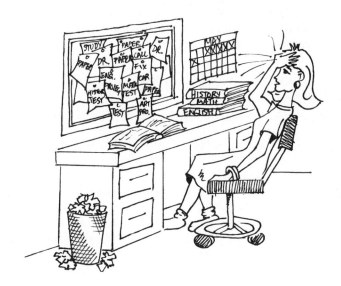

Type A: A person who is aggressive, anxious, and impatient and who frequently works excessively.

Type B: A person who is relaxed, not rushed, and not affected by deadlines or demands.

- Use a good time-management technique by matching things that need to be accomplished with the time you have available. Do not accept additional responsibilities if you do not have time to complete the tasks you are presently working on. Learn to assign work and additional responsibility to others. Do not plan too many things close together or at the same time. Avoid taking work home with you; learn to leave unfinished work from day to day.

- If you experience a time when you feel unproductive and have difficulty completing a task, take a short break to stretch, walk, relax, or simply get away from it for awhile.

- Make your work environment as relaxing as possible. Such things as soft music, healthy plants, and nice furniture may help.

Personality changes

By intentionally changing the stressful aspects of your personality, you can improve the way you react to stressful situations. How you react to a given situation is usually a habit that has been learned and developed over a period of time and possibly maintained in your lifestyle for a number of years. You need to realize that these habits will be extremely difficult to change; it will take time, effort, and discipline. However, keep in mind that with determination it can be done.

If you are to be successful, the following may be important:

- You may need to realize that you will not get the same satisfaction with new experiences as you did with old ones. However, with time, how you feel will fall in line with what you do.

- Evaluate each positive change. Each time you make different choices, old bonds will loosen and new behaviors will become easier.

- Be as objective as possible. Do not underestimate what you can achieve.

- Reinforce positive outcomes.

If you are to be successful in changing your habits, the following may be important considerations.

Improving your self-concept   You must believe in your ability to succeed. This is important because it determines how much effort you will expend in trying to change your habits, how long you will persist, and how much stress you will experience while you are changing your lifestyle. You need to develop a positive attitude by making up your mind that you can make specific changes and then by working hard to meet the challenge at hand. You will need to change your negative self-talk and irrational thinking and work on raising your self-esteem.

Improving your relationships with others   When changing your habits, the support and encouragement you get from other people are very important. It will be beneficial to you at this time to try to improve your relationship with your fellow workers, your friends, and your family. You need to be understanding and tolerant toward them, to be willing to understand their viewpoints, and to realize that this may be different from how you feel. Your social life at this time can be extremely important. You need to get together with your friends regularly, keep in touch with your family members, and try to become involved with church, club, or organizational activities or projects.

Taking care of yourself   You can adapt better to changes if you take good care of your body. This can be achieved by following a few simple guidelines.

- Get sufficient sleep so that you feel awake and refreshed each morning.

- Participate regularly in an aerobic exercise program.

- Eat regular, healthful meals.

- Maintain normal weight.

- Moderate your use of alcohol and caffeine.

- Refrain from smoking or inhaling the smoke of others.

Relaxation techniques for stress management

Physiologically, relaxation is the opposite response to the stress response and is the key to balancing stress. Several different relaxation techniques are available that allow you to regulate body processes. By using these techniques, you become more aware of your body and how it responds to stress.

Deep breathing technique   One of the "fight or flight" responses to stress is an increased respiration rate—you breathe more rapidly. Deep breathing is simply a technique where you consciously breathe slowly and deeply in an attempt to relieve tension in the body. With this technique, you inhale slowly through your nose; your stomach should expand at this time. You then hold your breath for a few seconds before exhaling through your mouth.

Meditation   Meditation is another relaxation technique that can help to reduce your stress by "clearing your mind" and blocking out any thoughts that might be responsible for increased tension. When your mind is clear, you then try to concentrate on a pleasant thought or situation.

Progressive muscle relaxation   This relaxation technique consists basically of a series of exercises designed to contract and relax the major muscle groups of the body. The objective is to reduce the tension in the muscles. You begin by tightening the muscle and then releasing the tension while you concentrate on how different the two tension levels feel. This technique can be used with the stretching exercises described in Chapter 6 and can provide an excellent form of relaxation.

Listening to music   Sitting or lying and listening to music can be an excellent way to relax and to cope with stress.

Stretching   If stress persists over an extended period, muscle tension is likely to develop in certain parts of the body. This situation can often be alleviated by simply performing stretching exercises for the part or parts of your body affected.

GUIDELINES FOR REDUCING STRESS

The following guidelines may be helpful to you in reducing your level of stress.

1. Exercise regularly

We have seen that the natural reaction of the body to stress is the "fight or flight" response, as your body prepares for an increased level of physical activity. However, most of the stressors we encounter in today's world are mental in nature rather than physical. Because of this, a natural reaction would be to undertake some form of physical activity to use this extra energy as you attempt to accelerate the dissipation of the by-products of stress.

It has also clearly been shown that those people who are physically fit and who exercise regularly can handle stress more easily than those who are unfit. Exercise has a "calming" effect on the body. As a result of exercise, you will not only look better but you will feel better, and you should be more relaxed and better able to deal with the stress in your life.

In addition, if you exercise regularly, you are likely to have a lower resting heart rate and lower blood pressure, and you should be able to handle better the negative effects of stress on your body relative to these two responses.

It should be realized, however, that for some people, exercise can increase their level of stress. This is particularly true where competition is involved. Those people who have a high level of stress and who are very competitive should not select a competitive form of exercise.

2. Improve your personal appearance

By exercising and eating right, you can often improve your personal appearance. When you look better, you usually feel better. By feeling better, you will have a much more positive attitude and outlook and will be in a position to react more favorably in certain stressful situations.

3. Adopt good eating habits

A healthful eating plan can increase your resistance to stress. By eating well, you can increase your energy level and help your body to resist illness and infection. Skipping meals and getting too few complex carbohydrates and too much simple refined sugar can trigger a drop in your blood glucose level, resulting in irritability and fatigue.

4. Learn to think clearly

If you are to schedule time effectively, establish realistic goals, and determine priorities, you need to be able to think clearly. To do this, you must get a sufficient amount of sleep. Lack of sleep often results in poor decisions.

5. Think positively

No matter what you are trying to achieve, you must believe that you can be successful and you must think positively rather than always coming up with negative thoughts. You need to make up your mind that you can achieve your goal and then plan how you are going to do it.

6. Learn how to make decisions for yourself

You need to be in control and make sure that you decide what you need to do each day. You are going to have to learn how to say no to other people when they ask you to do something that you will not have time to if you are struggling to complete the tasks and activities that you are already doing.

7. Learn to listen to other people

If you listen more and talk less, you will probably be able to cope with stress better.

8. Schedule time to relax

Try to plan your schedule so that you have time to sit or lie down and relax by listening to music, reading a book, or watching television. Getting outdoors and enjoying nature is also an excellent way to relax. Positive and negative coping skills are included in Laboratory Experience 10-2.

9. Express your feelings openly

Many of the everyday problems that contribute to a high level of stress are caused by lack of communication. People who tend to keep their feelings inside frequently "blow up" and take out their anger and frustration on others. By not discussing problems and resolving them, they often get out of control.

10. Do your best

The adage "Do your best, and leave the rest" is probably the best advice anyone could give you for reducing and coping with stress.

Chapter Summary

The following summary will help you to identify some of the important concepts covered in this chapter:

- Stress is something we cannot avoid—a certain level of stress is necessary if we are to be productive.
- Our responses to stressful situations may be either positive or negative.
- The body's natural response to stress is to prepare for physical activity.
- Stress that is prolonged and intense contributes to many physical and mental disorders.
- Stress can be caused by simple everyday events.
- Changes in our lifestyle can significantly affect our level of stress.
- Trying to do too much can negatively affect our level of stress.
- Improving our self-concept and our relationships with others can help us to cope with stress better.
- Exercise can have a very positive effect on stress.
- By eating right, we can increase our resistance to stress.

References

1. Althoff SA, Svoboda M, Girdano DA: *Choices in health and fitness for life*, ed 2, Scottsdale, Ariz, 1991, Gorsuch Scarisbrick.
2. Anspaugh DJ, Hamrick MH, Rosato FD: *Wellness: concepts and applications*, ed 2, St Louis, 1994, Mosby.
3. Benson H: *Beyond the relaxation process*, New York, 1984, Berkley.
4. Cooper CL, Payne R: *Causes, coping and consequences of stress at work*, New York, 1988, Wiley.
5. Cooper KH, Gallman JS, McDonald JL: Role of aerobic exercise in reduction of stress, *Dent Clin North Am* 30:4-6, 1986.
6. Dehn MM: *Well on the way to optimal health and fitness*, Irving, Tex, 1987, Health Management Consultants.
7. *Fit to win: your handbook*, The Army's Health Promotion Program, Washington, DC, 1987, US Government Printing Office.
8. Floyd PA et al: *Wellness: a lifetime commitment*, Winston-Salem, NC, 1991, Hunter.
9. Forman JW, Myers D: *The personal stress reduction program*, Englewood Cliffs, NJ, 1987, Prentice Hall.
10. Johannson N: Effectiveness of a stress management program in reducing anxiety and depression in nursing students, 1991, *College Health* 40:129-139, 1991.
11. Miller A: Stress on the job, *Newsweek*, pp. 40-45, April 25, 1988.
12. Murphy P: Stress and the athlete: coping with exercise, *The Physician and Sportsmedicine* 14(4):141-146, 1986.
13. Randall Sports/Medical Products, *Wellness Newsletter* 2:2, 1990, Kirkland, Wash.
14. Roth DL, Holmes DS: Influence of physical fitness in determining the impact of stressful life events on physical and psychological health, *Psychosom Med* 47:2, 1985.
15. Selye H: *The stress of life*, ed 2, New York, 1976, McGraw-Hill.

Determining Your Stress Level

Name	Section	Date

To evaluate your level of stress and to help you identify changes that you need to make, circle the number under the appropriate response to each question.

Use the following guidelines in making your decisions:

Rarely—Almost never
Sometimes—Once or twice each week
Often—Four or more times each week

How Frequently Do You:	RARELY	SOMETIMES	OFTEN
1. Experience one or more of the symptoms of excess stress such as tension, pain in the neck or shoulders, or headaches?	1	3	5
2. Find it difficult to concentrate on what you are doing because of deadlines or other tasks that must be completed?	1	3	5
3. Become irritable when you have to wait in line or get caught in a traffic jam?	1	3	5
4. Eat, drink, or smoke in an attempt to relax and/or relieve tension?	1	3	5
5. Worry about your work or other deadlines at night and/or on weekends?	1	3	5
6. Wake up in the night thinking about all the things you must do the next day?	1	3	5
7. Feel impatient at the slowness with which many events take place?	1	3	5
8. Find yourself short of time to complete everything that needs to be done?	1	3	5
9. Become upset because things have not gone *your* way?	1	3	5
10. Tend to lose your temper and get irritable?	1	3	5
11. Wake up in the night and have a hard time getting back to sleep?	1	3	5
12. Drive over the speed limit?	1	3	5
13. Interrupt people while they are talking or complete their sentences for them?	1	3	5
14. Forget about appointments and/or lose objects or forget where you put them?	1	3	5
15. Take on too many responsibilities?	1	3	5

Add the numbers together that you circled.

Enter your score here _____

Evaluate your score according to the following criteria:

Potential level of stress

Low	<35
Moderate	35-42
High	43 50
Very high	>50

Laboratory Experience 10-2

Positive and Negative Coping Skills

Name _____   Section _____   Date _____

People react differently to stressful situations. Following is a list of what would be considered "positive" responses.

Check off the appropriate response for each of these. If there are other positive ways that you deal with stress, please list them at the bottom of the list.

Response	NEVER	SOMETIMES	OFTEN
Meditate	_____	_____	_____
Stretch	_____	_____	_____
Engage in progressive muscle relaxation	_____	_____	_____
Listen to music	_____	_____	_____
Exercise aerobically	_____	_____	_____
Watch television	_____	_____	_____
Go to the movies	_____	_____	_____
Read	_____	_____	_____
Work on puzzles or play games	_____	_____	_____
Go for a leisurely walk	_____	_____	_____
Go to a health club	_____	_____	_____
Relax in a steam room or sauna	_____	_____	_____
Spend time alone	_____	_____	_____
Go fishing or hunting	_____	_____	_____
Participate in some form of recreational activity such as golf	_____	_____	_____
Do some work in the yard	_____	_____	_____
Socialize with friends	_____	_____	_____
Sit outside and relax	_____	_____	_____
Engage in a hobby	_____	_____	_____
Other responses—list	_____	_____	_____
_____	_____	_____	_____
_____	_____	_____	_____
_____	_____	_____	_____

Listed below are some negative ways of reacting to stress. Check off the appropriate column for each of these. If there are other negative ways you react to stress, list these at the bottom of the list.

Response	NEVER	SOMETIMES	OFTEN
Act violently	_____	_____	_____
Yell at someone	_____	_____	_____
Overeat	_____	_____	_____
Do not eat for long periods	_____	_____	_____
Drink an excessive amount of alcohol	_____	_____	_____
Drink lots of coffee	_____	_____	_____

Response	NEVER	SOMETIMES	OFTEN
Smoke tobacco	_____	_____	_____
Kick something	_____	_____	_____
Throw something	_____	_____	_____
Drive fast in a car	_____	_____	_____
Swear	_____	_____	_____
Pace up and down	_____	_____	_____
Bite your fingernails	_____	_____	_____
Take tranquilizers	_____	_____	_____
Take valium or other drugs	_____	_____	_____
Other responses—list	_____	_____	_____
_____	_____	_____	_____
_____	_____	_____	_____
_____	_____	_____	_____

You should compare the number of positive and negative responses. If your negative responses outnumber your positive responses, you have reason to be concerned about your stress level. You will need to try some of the positive responses in an attempt to reduce your level of stress.

Modified from Anspaugh DJ, Hamrick MH, Rosato FD: *Wellness: concepts and applications*, St. Louis, 1991, Mosby.

Chapter Eleven **Exercise and Cardiovascular Disease**

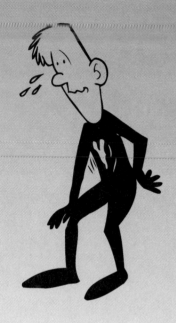

CHAPTER OBJECTIVES

Check off each objective you achieve.

- ❑ Identify the diseases that affect the cardiovascular system.
- ❑ Define atherosclerosis, and explain why it is the underlying cause of most cardiovascular disease.
- ❑ Discuss the lifestyle behaviors that contribute to the development of cardiovascular disease.
- ❑ Identify the primary and contributing risk factors associated with cardiovascular disease.
- ❑ Explain why the number of deaths from cardiovascular disease has decreased significantly in the last 10 years.
- ❑ Identify the two important lipoproteins, and differentiate clearly between them.
- ❑ Explain why the cholesterol/HDL ratio is a better indicator of cardiovascular disease than simply using the total cholesterol level.
- ❑ Differentiate clearly between Type I and Type II diabetes.
- ❑ Explain how exercise can positively influence other cardiovascular risk factors.
- ❑ Evaluate your lifestyle, and identify changes you can make to reduce your chances of cardiovascular disease.
- ❑ Determine your risk of cardiovascular disease.

The word **cardiovascular** refers to the heart and blood vessels that make up the life stream of the human body. Basic information about the circulation of the blood in the body and the changes that occur with regular aerobic exercise is presented in Chapter 3. Before reading this chapter, you may want to review the material contained in that chapter.

Although the death rate from cardiovascular disease has declined significantly in the United States in the past 20 years (Figure 11-1), this group of disorders is still the leading cause of death; it accounts for more than 720,000 deaths each year, which is approximately 40% of all deaths. Deaths from cancer total approximately 510,000 each year.

Facts and Figures

Consider the following facts relative to cardiovascular disease:

- Each American has a 50% chance of developing some form of cardiovascular disease.

- Over 40% of all Americans die from some form of cardiovascular disease.

- In America there are more than 1.5 million heart attacks each year.

- Approximately one third of all heart attacks result in death.

- Cardiovascular diseases are not just a threat to elderly persons—nearly one fifth of all persons who die from cardiovascular disease are under the age of 65, and 45% of all heart attacks occur to persons in this age group.

CARDIOVASCULAR DISEASE

Diseases affecting the cardiovascular system may be inherited; they also can be caused by various personal habits or by infection or injury. The major cause of cardiovascular disease is the buildup of fatty substances along the inside walls of blood vessels. These blood vessels then narrow to create a condition known as **atherosclerosis.** Blood may not be supplied in a sufficient quantity to various parts of the body; those areas are thus deprived of a sufficient supply of oxygen.

The heart, which is composed of muscular tissue, also requires its own continuous blood supply. This supply is delivered through a special set of arteries known as the coronary arteries.

With cardiovascular disease, damage may occur in the heart itself, in the coronary arteries, or in other blood vessels throughout the body. Thus cardiovascular disease is not a single disorder but rather comprises several specific diseases.

Atherosclerosis

Atherosclerosis is the underlying cause of more than 85% of all cardiovascular disease. It is the more common form of **arteriosclerosis,** or hardening of the arteries. With atherosclerosis the arterial walls thicken and harden.

The process may start with several lipids present in the bloodstream, including cholesterol, triglycerides, phospholipids, and fatty acids. It is believed that atherosclerosis usually begins with a deposit of some form of fatty material on the inner layer of the arterial wall. Such a deposit is known as **plaque.** After a time, these deposits may become embedded in the intima, the inner layer of the artery. The lumen—or opening—through which the blood must pass gradually narrows with each deposit, and the blood flow may be seriously impaired. This is illustrated in Figure 11-2.

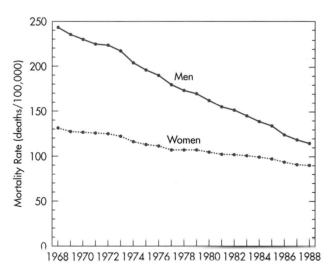

Figure 11-1 Decline in mortality rates for heart attacks in men and women from 1968-1988. Data from the National Center for Health Statistics.[9]

Cardiovascular: Pertaining to the heart and blood vessels.

Atherosclerosis: A narrowing of the arteries as fatty substances build up on arterial walls.

Arteriosclerosis: A hardening of the arteries that causes the arterial walls to thicken and lose elasticity.

Plaque: A deposit of fatty substances on the inner lining of the artery wall.

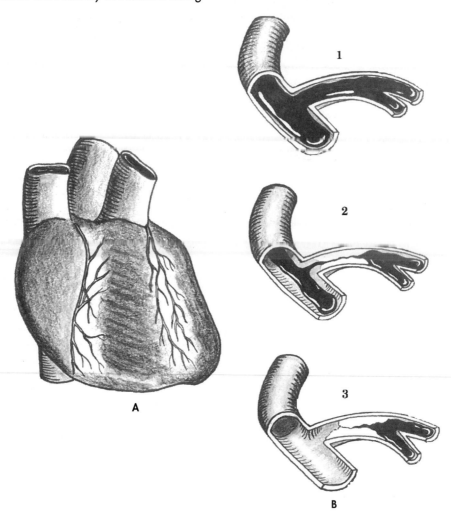

Figure 11-2 **A,** The heart showing the right and left coronary arteries. **B,** The development of artherosclerosis: *1,* normal blood flow; *2,* restricted blood flow; *3,* completely blocked coronary artery.

Atherosclerosis may begin developing early in life, yet the symptoms may not appear until much later. A person can have the condition for 50 years or more and not die from it. However, many people are not so fortunate; each year approximately 700,000 people in the United States die from diseases caused by atherosclerosis.

Coronary heart disease

Coronary heart disease, often referred to as a heart attack, causes almost 480,000 deaths in the United States each year. A heart attack occurs when a section of the heart muscle is deprived of its blood supply. The gradual narrowing of the coronary arteries sets the stage for this development. Most heart attacks occur when a blood clot lodges in one of the narrowed arteries, cutting off or limiting the blood supply to a particular area of the heart. Although such an attack is usually sudden, it commonly stems from slowly developing atherosclerosis in the coronary arteries.

When part of the heart is deprived of sufficient oxygen, certain damage may occur. This damage is referred to as **myocardial infarction.** *Myocardium* is the Latin name of the heart muscle. The word *infarction* means death to tissue by loss of its normal supply of oxygenated blood. Thus the term *myocardial infarction* means that a small portion of the heart muscle has died because an artery or branch of an artery that formerly supplied it with oxygenated blood has been closed.

With regular aerobic exercise, not only is the incidence of coronary heart disease much lower, but the survival rate is much higher. This is possibly due to the development of a system of smaller blood vessels that detour the blood around a blockage in a coronary artery. This secondary system is called **collateral circulation,** and these vessels are much more extensively developed in active people than in individuals who are not active.

Signs of a heart attack A common initial symptom of coronary heart disease is chest pain, called **angina pectoris,** which results when the heart muscle does not receive enough blood. The pain can be described as a pressing or squeezing sensation, and it usually lasts for a few minutes. It is focused in the center of the chest below the sternum, although it may spread to the shoulders and may also be felt in one or both arms. Immediate rest usually provides relief. This condition usually occurs when the heart's need for oxygen increases, such as during physical exertion or as a result of stress.

Angina pectoris may be accompanied by one or more of the following: dizziness, fainting, shortness of breath, and excessive sweating. If you have chest pain and discomfort lasting for more than 2 minutes, you need to seek emergency medical help immediately. It should be noted, however, that sharp, short twinges of pain that last for only a few seconds are not usually signals of a heart attack.

Stroke

A stroke occurs when a part of the brain is deprived of its blood supply, leaving the nerve cells in that part of the brain unable to function properly. When this happens, the parts of the body controlled by these nerve cells also cannot function.

The importance of a regular supply of oxygen to the brain is clearly demonstrated during prolonged vigorous exercise, when the body demands additional oxygen for the working muscles to use. Blood is diverted from various parts of the body to the working musculature. The brain is the only area where the blood supply does not change, which demonstrates the importance of a steady supply of blood to the brain. The blood supply to the brain may be impaired by clotting, compression, or hemorrhage.

The most common cause of a stroke is a **thrombus** lodged in one of the arteries leading to the brain. If such a blockage occurs, the blood supply to part of the brain is impaired, and the person has suffered from cerebral thrombosis. In the case of a stroke, as with a heart attack, atherosclerosis is an important underlying cause. A stroke also can be caused by a brain tumor or by excess pressure on the brain or on an artery supplying blood to the brain. A fourth cause of stroke is bleeding, or hemorrhage, in an artery supplying blood to the brain, which reduces the supply of blood available to the brain.

IDENTIFICATION OF RISK FACTORS ASSOCIATED WITH CARDIOVASCULAR DISEASE

Preventive medicine is the key to reducing the chances of having a heart attack. It is obvious that what we eat and how we live largely determine our susceptibility. In a recent survey in the United States, more than 92% of the participants agreed with the following statement: "If we lived more healthful lives, ate more nutritious foods,

smoked less, maintained our proper weight, and exercised regularly, it would do more to improve our health than anything doctors or medicine could do for us."[30]

During the past 30 years, attempts have been made to determine the basic cause or causes of heart disease. Large populations have been observed over long periods and their living habits and medical records carefully analyzed in relation to the incidence of coronary heart disease. The Framingham heart study[30] began in 1949 under the direction of the National Heart, Lung, and Blood Institute. Over 5000 participants started in this program, and of these almost 3000 still remain. These subjects are monitored each year, and the information obtained relative to heart disease and lifestyle habits has contributed greatly to our knowledge of cardiovascular disease. Another large study involved more than 17,000 Harvard alumni who were studied for more than 20 years.[32] These studies have helped to identify several factors associated with an increased risk of cardiovascular disease.

Risk factors that cannot be changed

Four of the risk factors associated with cardiovascular disease cannot be altered by the individual:

1. *Heredity:* Evidence supports the hypothesis that a history of heart disease in the immediate family increases the possibility of cardiovascular illness.
2. *Gender:* Research indicates that the incidence of heart attacks is lower in women under 45 years of age than in men of a comparable age.
3. *Race:* Hypertension, accompanied by a higher incidence of heart attack deaths and stroke, is much more prevalent among black Americans than among whites.
4. *Age:* The incidence of heart attack and the death rates attributable to it increase with age. For example, for those who are 65 years of age or older, 60% of all deaths are caused by cardiovascular disease. This figure is only 11% for those aged 15 to 24 years and 27% for the age group 35 to 44 years.

Myocardial infarction: Damage to the heart when it is deprived of sufficient oxygen.

Collateral circulation: A system of small arteries that may carry blood to part of the heart when a coronary artery is blocked.

Angina pectoris: A chest pain caused by insufficient blood supply to the heart.

Thrombus: A blood clot.

Risk factors that can be changed

Fortunately, many of the risk factors associated with premature death from cardiovascular disease can be reduced by an adjustment in living habits. It is interesting to note that the 40% decrease in deaths associated with cardiovascular disease in the past two decades has coincided with the following:

- A reduction in cigarette smoking
- A decrease in the average serum cholesterol level
- A decrease in the consumption of foods high in fat
- An increase in the number of people controlling hypertension
- An increase in the number of people exercising regularly

The risk factors that can be changed are identified in Figure 11-3.

Notice that not only do each of these factors contribute directly to cardiovascular disease, but many of them interact to intensify the risk. An arrow pointing from one factor to another indicates that that factor has a negative influence on the one to which it points. Arrows pointing in both directions between two factors (such as with overweight and high blood pressure) indicate that the two factors have a negative influence on each other.

The American Heart Association suggests that the risk factors be grouped into two classifications: major risk factors and contributing risk factors.

Major risk factors are those that the research has shown to be directly associated with an increase in the risk of cardiovascular disease. They are sometimes referred to as primary risk factors. They are identified in Figure 11-4.

Contributing risk factors are also associated with an increased risk of cardiovascular disease but not as directly, and their significance has not yet been as clearly determined. They are often referred to as secondary risk factors and are identified in Figure 11-5.

MAJOR RISK FACTORS

Cigarette Smoking

Cigarette smoking is the single most preventable cause of premature death in the United States, accounting for one out of every six deaths.[11] Figures released by the Department of Health and Human Services ranks the

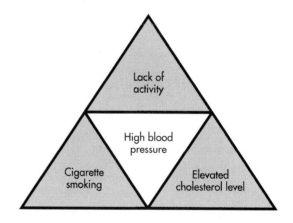

Figure 11-4 Major risk factors associated with cardiovascular disease.

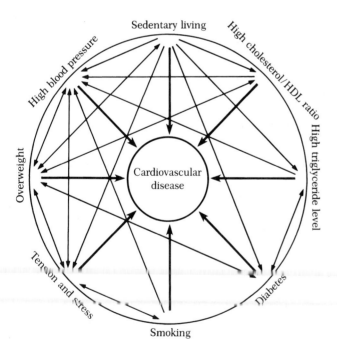

Figure 11-3 Modifiable factors associated with cardiovascular disease.

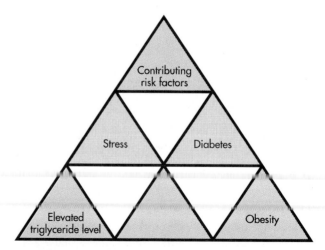

Figure 11-5 Contributing risk factors associated with cardiovascular disease.

use of tobacco as the leading cause of death in the United States, with over 400,000 deaths each year from diseases caused by smoking. These figures were presented in Table 1-2.

Surprisingly, smoking is associated with more deaths associated with cardiovascular disease than with cancer[5] (Figure 11-6).

From 1970 to 1990 the number of Americans who smoke cigarettes has decreased by almost 30%. However, since 1990 the number of smokers has remained fairly stable, with approximately 50 million Americans continuing to smoke. This represents about 26% of the adult population. Over 70% of those who smoke have been smoking for more than 10 years. Information pertaining to the number of cigarettes smoked daily by those who smoke is summarized below.

Cigarettes Smoked Per Day	Percent of Smokers
Less than 1 pack	46
Approximately 1 pack	35
More than 1 pack	19

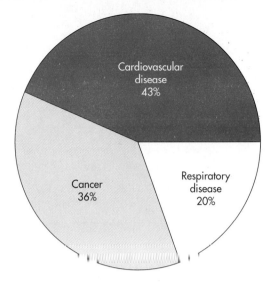

Figure 11-6 Smoking-related deaths. Smoking accounts for over 400,000 deaths per year, with over 40% attributable to cardiovascular disease. *(From cigarette smoking—attributable mortality and years of potential life lost—United States, 1990. MMWR 42(33):645-648, 1993.)*

Facts and Figures

Consider the following statistics relative to smoking:

- Cigarette smoking is responsible for an estimated 21% of all coronary heart disease deaths.
- The risk of dying from lung cancer is 22 times higher for men and 12 times higher for women who smoke compared with lifetime nonsmokers.
- Cigarette smoking is responsible for 87% of all lung cancer deaths.
- Cigarette smokers have a 70% higher rate of early death from all causes compared with nonsmokers.

Summarized from material from the American Heart Association and reports from the Surgeon General of The United States.

Cigarette smoking and cardiovascular disease

The following is a summary of the research available on cigarette smoking and cardiovascular disease.

- Cigarette smoking is directly responsible for 21% of all deaths from coronary heart disease. This accounts for approximately 110,000 deaths annually.[18]
- The greater the number of cigarette smoked daily, the higher the incidence of coronary heart disease[29] (Figure 11-7).
- The incidence of sudden death after a heart attack is much greater in those who smoke compared with those who do not smoke.

- Pipe and cigar smokers rate only slightly higher than nonsmokers with regard to the incidence of cardiovascular disease.[12]
- For those who quit smoking, there is a 50% to 70% decrease in the risk of cardiovascular disease within 5 years of quitting. Even after one year the excess risk of heart disease is reduced by half.[18]

Fitness Flash

Of those who successfully quit smoking, 95% do so on their own, and those who quit all at once are more successful than those who try to quit in steps.

Successful quitters give the following reasons for stopping:

- Health concerns
- Wanting to set an example for others, particularly family members
- Desire for self-control
- Aesthetic reasons, such as breath odor and loss of taste for food

Most people who smoke regularly are aware of smoking's detrimental effects on overall health and wellness. In summary, these effects are the following:

- Smoking releases nicotine and other toxic substances into the blood, adversely affecting the inner linings of the blood vessels. This makes it eas-

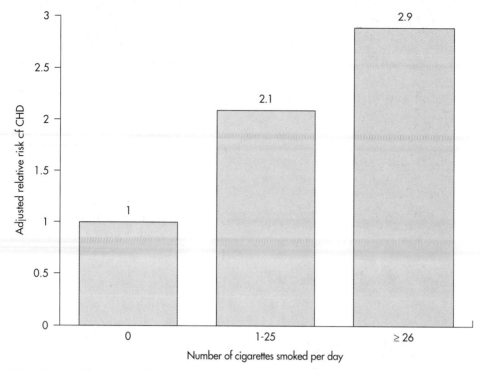

Figure 11-7 Cigarette smoking and coronary heart disease (CHD).[29] Modified from Nieman.[30]

ier for cholesterol and triglycerides to be deposited on the arterial walls and for plaques to form.

■ Smoking makes red blood cells more cohesive, thus increasing the formation of blood clots.

■ Smoking reduces the body's level of high-density lipoprotein (HDL) and increases the low-density lipoprotein (LDL) level.

■ Smoking increases the heart rate.

■ Smoking constricts blood vessels and may increase blood pressure.

Smoking and other health-related habits

It is interesting to note that those who smoke cigarettes also tend to have poor health habits. Following is a summary of data from a recent nationwide survey comparing the percentage of smokers with nonsmokers for selected health practices.[34]

Health Habit	Percentage of Smokers	Percentage of Nonsmokers
Limit the amount of fat in diet	40	58
Exercise at least 3 days each week	33	39
Try to limit salt and sodium intake	39	50
Feel under great stress	48	33
Know their cholesterol level	45	55
Wear their seat belt regularly	63	76

Smoking and exercise

Several studies have shown that the percentage of smokers among those people who exercise regularly is much lower than for the general population and that smokers tend to exercise less than nonsmokers. Possibly this is why many smokers try to quit smoking when they start a serious exercise program.

Smoking also has a negative effect on your aerobic capacity. There is a direct inverse relationship between the number of cigarettes smoked and also the number of years a person has smoked[21] (Figure 11-8).

If you quit smoking and you are trying to lose weight, it is important that you make some adjustments in your eating and/or exercise habits. The reason for this is that smoking speeds up your metabolism. Studies show that smoking one pack of cigarettes per day can increase your metabolism by approximately 250 calories. So if you quit smoking, you would have to either eat 250 calories less per day or exercise so that you burn 250 more calories simply to maintain your present weight. In terms of exercise, this is equivalent to walking 2 to 2½ miles for most people. You can determine the equivalent amount of food by consulting Appendix B.

HIGH BLOOD PRESSURE

Blood pressure is the amount of force that blood exerts against the walls of the arteries. Blood pressure is generated by the heart as it contracts and is maintained by the elasticity of the arterial walls.

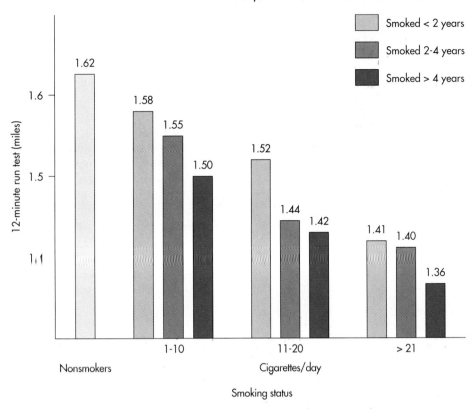

Figure 11-8 Performance on 12-minute run test in relation to smoking status.[21]

Blood pressure changes constantly during each cardiac cycle. Each time the heart contracts, blood pressure goes up as more blood is forced from the heart into the arterial system. The contraction phase of the cardiac cycle is called systole; thus the upper blood pressure figure is referred to as systolic blood pressure. The relaxation phase of the cardiac cycle is called diastole, hence the lower blood pressure figure is known as diastolic blood pressure. Additional information about blood pressure and the procedures for measuring it are included in Chapter 3.

Consistently high blood pressure is called **hypertension,** one of the risk factors of cardiovascular disease. The higher the blood pressure, the greater the risk. Although it is difficult to define the limits of "normal" blood pressure, there seems to be general agreement that a systolic reading of 140 mm Hg (systolic hypertension) or a diastolic reading of 90 mm Hg (diastolic hypertension) would form the lower limits for a person to be classified as borderline hypertensive. Standards for various classifications of blood pressure are presented in Table 11-1.

The incidence of hypertension by age is presented in Figure 11 9.

The risk of death from cardiovascular disease increases significantly with an increase in systolic blood pressure (Figure 11-10) and also with an increase in diastolic blood pressure (Figure 11-11).

Let's Get Started

Lifestyle modifications to control hypertension

If you have high blood pressure, the following recommendations may be of help:

- If you are overweight, your primary goal should be weight reduction. Losing as little as 10 lb has been shown to have a significant effect on your blood pressure.
- Reduce your sodium intake—excessive sodium intake contributes to approximately 25% of the cases of high blood pressure.
- Learn to relax so that you can minimize the effects of stress in your life.
- Participate regularly in a good aerobic exercise program.
- Stop smoking (if you are a cigarette smoker).
- Decrease your alcohol intake.
- Be careful about taking high doses of nose drops or over-the-counter sinus medicines. These may raise your blood pressure.

Hypertension: Blood pressure that is consistently higher than normal.

Facts and Figures

Sodium Intake

Sodium may be obtained from three sources:

- Small amounts occur naturally in some foods
- It is added to foods during processing
- It is added to foods during cooking or at the table

NOTE: 1 teaspoon of salt contains over 2000 mg of sodium.

You need only approximately 1000 mg of sodium per day, yet the average American gets almost 7500 mg.

The National Research Council recommends between 1100 and 3300 mg per day and that those with high blood pressure or a history of hypertension should limit their intake to 2000 mg or less per day.

Table 11-1	Classification of Systolic and Diastolic Blood Pressure Scores	
Category	**Systolic (mm Hg)**	**Diastolic (mm Hg)**
Normal	<130	<85
High Normal	130-139	85-89
Hypertension		
Mild	140-159	90-99
Moderate	160-179	100-109
Severe	>179	>109

Modified from Anspaugh DJ, Hamrick MH, Rosato FD: *Wellness: concepts and applications,* ed 2, St Louis, 1994, Mosby.

Statistics indicate that ideal blood pressure for longevity is approximately 110 mm Hg for systolic and 70 mm Hg for diastolic and that even moderate increases above these figures place you at an increased risk for cardiovascular disease.

Lifestyle modification—does it work?

Results from a 1-year study involving lifestyle modification showed that those with mild hypertension were able to reduce their systolic blood pressure by an average of 11 mm Hg and their diastolic pressure by 8 mm Hg. During this study, participants doubled the amount of physical activity they were engaging in previous to the study and they were able to decrease their sodium intake by an average of 23%. These two changes also resulted in an average weight loss of 10 lb.[39]

If you have high blood pressure and lifestyle modification does not result in a decrease in your blood pressure, it may be necessary for you to take medication. If so, you should follow your doctor's recommendations.

Fitness Flash

Although most adults with high blood pressure are aware of it, only about 30% of them are successful at controlling it.

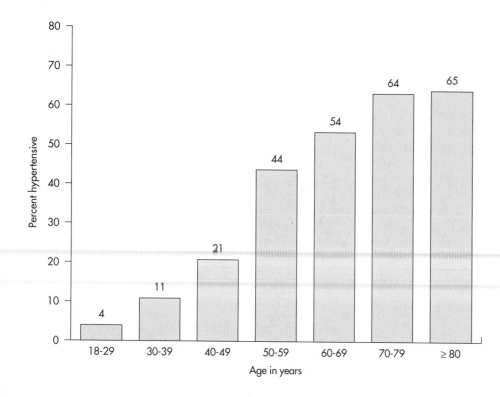

Figure 11-9 The incidence of hypertension increases drastically with age. (From Neaton JD, Wentworth D: Serum blood cholesterol, blood pressure, cigarette smoking, and death from coronary heart disease, *Arch Int Med* 152:56 64, 1992.)

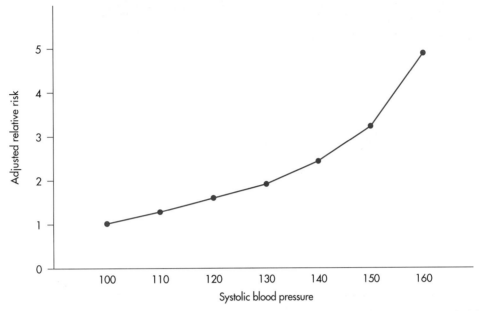

Figure 11-10   Systolic blood pressure and cardiovascular mortality. The risk of mortality rises sharply as systolic blood pressure increases. (From Stamler J, Stamler R, Neaton J: Blood pressure, systolic and diastolic, and cardiovascular risks: US population data, *Arch Int Med* 153:598-615, 1993.)

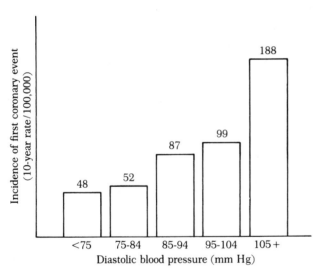

Figure 11-11   The relationship of the diastolic blood pressure to the incidence of coronary heart disease. (From *Heart book: a guide to prevention and treatment of cardiovascular disease,* New York, 1980, American Heart Association.)

ELEVATED CHOLESTEROL LEVEL

Cholesterol is an odorless, white, fatlike substance found in the body and in all foods of animal origin. It performs several crucial functions:

- It is an important constituent of all cell walls.
- It is important for conducting nerve impulses.
- It is used to make various hormones, such as estrogen and testosterone.

- It is used to make bile, which aids in the process of breaking up fat.

Research indicates that the amount of cholesterol in the blood—referred to as serum cholesterol—is one of the most important risk factors associated with the development of atherosclerosis. Atherosclerosis occurs when the inner lining of the artery is damaged in some way. Such damage is usually caused by a toxic substance, such as nicotine. Under these conditions, cholesterol can penetrate the inner lining of the artery and a plaque (fatty deposit) can form. Once the arterial lining has been damaged, the extent of the buildup within the artery wall depend largely on the amount of cholesterol in the blood stream. That in turn will be influenced by three factors:

- The amount of cholesterol manufactured by the liver
- The amount of cholesterol and saturated fat in the food eaten
- The efficiency with which the body breaks down and excretes cholesterol

The production and breaking down of cholesterol occur primarily in the liver, and usually the two are balanced such that the amount of cholesterol in the blood is maintained within safe limits. However, some people have an inherited tendency for a very high choles-

> **Cholesterol:** A fatlike substance that is obtained only from foods from animal origin and that may be manufactured by the body.

terol level, whereas others seem to have a very low level regardless of what they eat. In general, however, a person's cholesterol level apparently is influenced most by how much saturated fat and cholesterol he or she eats. Other contributing factors include excess body fat, high level of stress, and lack of exercise.

Research has shown that people with a high level of serum cholesterol have a greater chance of developing coronary heart disease (Figure 11-12). Note that with a total blood cholesterol level of less than 200 mg/dl, the incidence of coronary heart disease is relatively low.

The risk levels for total blood cholesterol proposed by the National Heart, Lung, and Blood Institute are presented in Table 11-2.

The ideal values for adults would appear to be somewhere between 120 and 160 mg/dl. The incidence of cardiovascular disease is lowest when the serum cholesterol level is below 160 mg/dl.

Table 11-3 compares the fat and cholesterol content of several foods and gives the saturated fat content for each. This information can help you to identify the total amount of fat in each food listed, as well as the amount of saturated fat in these foods. You should also

look closely at the information pertaining to fast foods, which is included in Appendix C. When selecting foods, you should try to pick low-fat items and pay particular attention to the amount of saturated fat.

Cholesterol/HDL ratio

The total amount of cholesterol in the blood is an excellent measurement for predicting your risk of developing coronary heart disease. However, you can get an even better indication of your risk with a more sophisticated measurement of cholesterol.

Let's Get Started

Strategies for reducing your cholesterol level

The following changes are recommended for people whose blood cholesterol level is too high:

- Decrease your total fat intake to less than 30% of your total calories.
- Reduce saturated fat to less than 10% of your total calories.
- Decrease your dietary cholesterol to less than 300 mg/day or ideally to less than 200 mg/day.
- Increase your intake of water-soluble fiber—found mainly in fruits, vegetables, grains, and legumes.
- Lose weight or fat if you are overweight or obese.
- Participate regularly in aerobic exercise.
- Reduce your stress level.

Table 11-2	**Total Cholesterol and Risk Level for Cardiovascular Disease**	
Risk	**Cholesterol Level**
Low	<200 mg/dl
Borderline to high	200-239 mg/dl
High	>240 mg/dl

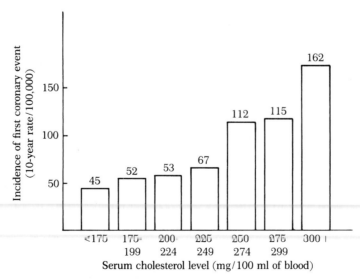

Figure 11-12 The relationship of the serum cholesterol level to the incidence of the first coronary event. (From *Heart book: a guide to prevention and treatment of cardiovascular disease,* New York, 1980, American Heart Association.)

Table 11-3	**Fat and Cholesterol Content of Selected Foods***			
Food	Serving Size	Saturated Fat (g)	Total Fat (g)	Cholesterol (mg)
Beef				
Top round lean (broiled)	3½ oz	2.2	6.2	84
Ground lean (broiled)	3½ oz	7.3	18.5	87
Prime rib (broiled)	3½ oz	14.9	35.2	86
Processed meats				
Link sausage, smoked (pork and beef)	3½ oz	10.6	30.3	71
Bologna (beef)	3½ oz	11.7	28.4	56
Frankfurter (beef)	3½ oz	12.0	29.4	48
Salami (pork or beef)	3½ oz	12.2	34.4	79
Pork				
Ham (extra lean)	3½ oz	1.4	4.2	45
Pork-center loin (lean)	3½ oz	4.7	13.7	111
Pork spareribs (braised)	3½ oz	11.8	30.3	121
Poultry				
Chicken (roasted)				
White meat without skin	3½ oz	1.3	4.5	85
White meat with skin	3½ oz	3.1	10.9	84
Dark meat without skin	3½ oz	2.7	9.7	93
Dark meat with skin	3½ oz	4.4	15.8	91
Fish				
Cod	3½ oz	0.1	0.7	58
Perch	3½ oz	0.2	1.2	115
Snapper	3½ oz	0.4	1.7	47
Rockfish	3½ oz	1.6	6.3	49
Mackerel	3½ oz	4.2	17.8	75
Crustaceans				
Crab	3½ oz	0.2	1.8	100
Lobster	3½ oz	0.1	0.5	72
Shrimp	3½ oz	0.3	1.1	195
Liver meats				
Chicken	3½ oz	1.8	5.5	631
Beef	3½ oz	1.9	4.9	389
Eggs				
Egg yolk	1	1.7	5.7	272
Egg white	1	0	Trace	0
Whole egg	1	1.7	5.6	272
Nuts				
Almonds (dry roasted)	3½ oz	4.9	51.6	0
Pistachios (dry)	3½ oz	6.1	48.4	0
Peanuts (dried)	3½ oz	6.8	49.2	0
Cashews	3½ oz	9.2	46.4	0
Brazil nuts	3½ oz	16.2	66.2	0

*From *Facts about blood cholesterol*, US Department of Health and Human Services, 1986, National Institute of Health.

Continued

Table 11-3	**Fat and Cholesterol Content of Selected Foods*—cont'd**			
Food	Serving Size	Saturated Fat (g)	Total Fat (g)	Cholesterol (mg)
Milk and cream				
Skim milk	1 cup	0.3	0.4	4
Low-fat milk (1% fat)	1 cup	1.6	2.6	10
Whole milk (3.7% fat)	1 cup	5.6	8.9	35
Light cream	1 cup	28.8	46.3	159
Heavy cream	1 cup	54.8	88.1	326
Yogurt and sour cream				
Plain yogurt (skim milk)	1 cup	0.3	0.4	4
Plain yogurt (low-fat)	1 cup	2.3	3.5	14
Plain yogurt (whole milk)	1 cup	4.8	7.4	29
Sour cream	1 cup	30.0	48.2	102
Soft cheeses				
Cottage cheese (low-fat)	1 cup	1.5	2.3	10
American (processed spread)	1 cup	30.2	48.1	125
Cream cheese	1 cup	49.9	79.2	250
Hard cheeses				
Mozzarella (part skim)	8 oz	22.9	36.1	132
Mozzarella (whole)	8 oz	29.7	49.0	177
Provolone	8 oz	38.8	60.4	157
Swiss	8 oz	40.4	62.4	209
Muenster	8 oz	43.4	68.1	218
American (processed)	8 oz	44.7	71.1	213
Cheddar	8 oz	47.9	75.1	238
Vegetable oils and shortening				
Safflower oil	1 cup	19.8	218.0	0
Sunflower oil	1 cup	22.5	218.0	0
Corn oil	1 cup	27.7	218.0	0
Olive oil	1 cup	29.2	216.0	0
Soybean oil	1 cup	31.4	218.0	0
Margarine, soft	1 cup	32.2	182.6	0
Margarine, stick or brick	1 cup	34.2	182.6	0
Peanut oil	1 cup	36.4	216.0	0
Household vegetable shortening	1 cup	51.2	205.0	0
Cottonseed oil	1 cup	56.4	218.0	0
Palm oil	1 cup	107.4	218.0	0
Coconut oil	1 cup	188.5	218.0	0
Animal Fats				
Chicken fat	1 cup	61.2	205.0	175
Lard	1 cup	80.4	205.0	195
Beef fat	1 cup	102.1	205.0	223
Butter	1 cup	114.4	183.9	496

Lipids (fats) are insoluble in water and cannot be transported in the blood by themselves. They combine with protein to form **lipoproteins.** There are three major lipoproteins:

- **High-density lipoproteins** (HDLs)
- **Low-density lipoproteins** (LDLs)
- **Very low-density lipoproteins** (VLDLs)

The amounts of protein and lipids present in each of these is summarized in Figure 11-13.

The HDLs are the smallest and most dense—they contain approximately 50% proteins and about 18% cholesterol. HDLs are very stable and tend to attract loose particles of cholesterol in the blood and remove them from the bloodstream. Research has shown that people with a high HDL level have a lower incidence of heart disease. For this reason, these lipoproteins have become known as "good" cholesterol.

LDLs, on the other hand, contain large amounts of cholesterol (43%) and relatively small amounts of protein (25%). Their poor stability often allows cholesterol to break away from the protein, making people more susceptible to coronary heart disease. Increased LDL levels are associated with an increased incidence of cardiovascular disease. For this reason, LDLs are often referred to as "bad" cholesterol. VLDLs contain mainly triglycerides and only very small amounts of cholesterol.

The ratio of total cholesterol to HDL cholesterol is probably the best single measurement for predicting cardiovascular disease. The lower the **cholesterol/HDL ratio,** the less is your chance of having coronary heart disease. To determine your ratio, simply divide your total cholesterol value by your HDL value.

> **example:**
> If your total cholesterol is 200 and your HDL is 50, you can calculate your ratio as follows:
> Total cholesterol/HDL ratio = 200/50
> = 4.0

The risk levels for the total cholesterol/HDL ratio are presented in Table 11-4. Because the HDL level differs significantly between men and women, a separate set of scores is necessary for each gender.

Table 11-4	**Cholesterol/HDL Ratio and Risk of Cardiovascular Disease**	
Risk	**Men**	**Women**
Low	<5.0	<4.4
Borderline to high	5.0-5.7	4.4-5.1
High	>5.7	>5.1

Also of importance are your HDL and LDL levels. Your desirable LDL level is less than 130 mg/dl. Between 130 and 160 mg/dl is borderline, and above 160 mg/dl, you are at high risk for cardiovascular disease. With regard to HDL, men whose level is less than 25 mg/dl and women whose level is less than 40 mg/dl are at three times the normal risk for developing cardiovascular disease.

Your total cholesterol/HDL ratio is influenced primarily by what you eat and what you do. To lower this ratio and thereby reduce your chance of coronary heart disease, you must lower your LDL level and increase your HDL level.

Let's Get Started

To lower your LDL level, you should:

- Reduce your intake of foods high in cholesterol.
- Reduce your intake of foods high in saturated fat.
- Exercise regularly in a good aerobic exercise program.
- Maintain a desirable weight and a desirable percentage of body fat.

Aerobic exercise can contribute more to increasing your HDL level than any other single factor. Studies show that people who exercise regularly have a higher HDL level than do people who do not exercise. An extremely high level of exercise is associated with an extremely high level of HDL.

Research also has pinpointed three substances that lower your HDL level. When possible, these should be avoided.

Lipoprotein: The combination of a lipid with protein so that lipids can be transported in the blood.

High-density lipoprotein (HDL): A lipoprotein that contains the highest proportion of protein—often referred to as "good" cholesterol.

Low-density lipoprotein (LDL): A lipoprotein that contains the highest proportion of cholesterol—high levels of LDL have been associated with increased incidence of cardiovascular disease. Also referred to as "bad" cholesterol.

Very low-density lipoprotein (VLDL): A lipoprotein that contains mainly triglycerides together with a small amount of cholesterol.

Cholesterol/HDL ratio: The ratio of total cholesterol to high-density lipoprotein (HDL) cholesterol.

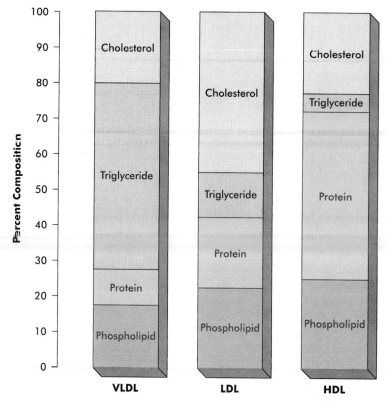

Figure 11-13   The percentage of protein and lipids present in HDL, LDL, and VLDL.

Cigarette smoking: One pack of cigarettes per day will reduce your HDL level by 5 points or more.

Birth control pills: Regular use of birth control pills will also reduce your HDL level by 5 points or more.

Prescription medications: Several medications used for blood pressure or heart disease have a detrimental effect on your HDL level.

Amount of exercise necessary to change blood lipids

Considerable research has been done on the effects of exercise on blood lipids. These studies show that men and women who participate regularly in aerobic exercise generally have a slightly lower total cholesterol level and a much higher HDL level.

It appears that the minimum amount of exercise needed to precipitate these changes corresponds closely to the amount prescribed for the development of aerobic fitness—30 minutes of continuous activity performed three to five times per week with the heart rate sustained in the target zone. In a walking or running program, this would mean approximately 10 to 15 miles per week. Several studies have shown, however, that even greater changes occur in blood lipid levels if the amount of activity is increased substantially above this level.

Benefits of reduced cholesterol

Several recent studies have demonstrated conclusively that lowering the cholesterol level in the blood helps to reduce the incidence of coronary heart disease. A 12-year study costing $150 million—performed by the National Heart, Lung, and Blood Institute—showed conclusively that reducing the serum cholesterol level results in a decrease in heart disease. The research concluded that for those who reduce their blood cholesterol levels by 25%, there will be a 49% reduction in the incidence of cardiovascular disease. Other research shows the following:

- A diet with moderate fat intake reduced the level of cholesterol by 3% to 4% for all participants. People on a much stricter diet had a decrease of 10% to 15%.

- People who took cholestyramine, a cholesterol-lowering drug, had cholesterol levels reduced by as much as 25%.

- Overall, people whose cholesterol levels were lowered an average of 8% had a 19% lower rate of fatal and nonfatal heart attacks.

- Cholesterol reduction is also associated with lower rates of atherosclerosis and coronary bypass surgery.

Multiple risk factors

With regard to the three primary risk factors, the incidence of heart disease increases in proportion to the number of risk factors present. This is illustrated in Figure 11-14.

Notice that when none of the risk factors are present, the risk of cardiovascular disease is less than that for the average American. A person who smokes and has a high cholesterol level and high blood pressure has a risk of 3.84. This means that he or she is 3.84 times more likely to have a heart attack than is the average American.

LACK OF ACTIVITY

A [illegible] of America's sedentary lifestyle. It was shown that automobiles, elevators, television sets, home computers, and many other mechanical devices have reduced expenditure of physical effort. Indisputably, these changes have had a detrimental effect on the fitness level of Americans.

Numerous studies have shown that physical inactivity and lack of exercise are associated with a significantly higher rate of cardiovascular disease with the sedentary person, at almost twice the risk as the more active person.[18]

The quality of the recent research was such that in 1993 the American Heart Association finally listed inactivity as a major risk factor associated with cardiovascular disease.[1]

Fitness Flash

A comprehensive review of the research shows that more active or fit people develop less coronary heart disease than those who are inactive and for active people who do develop coronary heart disease, it occurs at a later age and tends to be less severe.

Data from a 16-year study of nearly 17,000 Harvard alumni are summarized in Table 11-5.[32]

Table 11-5	Death Rates/10,000 Among 16,936 Harvard Alumni, 1962-1978, Classified According to Physical Activity		
	Physical Activity Level (Calories/Week)		
Causes of Death	**<500**	**500-2000**	**>2000**
All causes	84.8	66.0	52.1
Cardiovascular disease	39.5	30.8	21.4

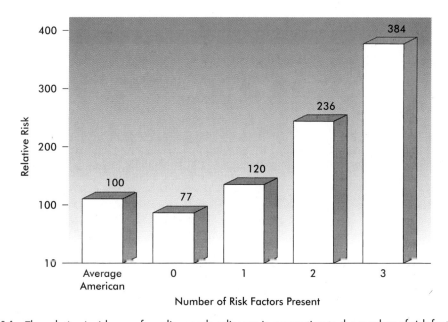

Figure 11-14 The relative incidence of cardiovascular disease in proportion to the number of risk factors present.

This study clearly shows an inverse relationship between the amount of physical activity and the incidence of death from all causes and death from cardiovascular disease. In this study, as in several others that show similar findings, other potential risk factors—such as smoking, obesity, and hypertension—also were analyzed. They did not appear to account for the relationship between physical inactivity and the risk of coronary heart disease.

Notice in the study cited in Table 11-5 that the amount of exercise associated with the lowest death rate (from cardiovascular disease and from all causes) is the amount required to burn 2000 or more calories per week. This is more exercise than is prescribed for the development of aerobic fitness. For example, a 154-lb person running at a speed of 12 minutes per mile would have to run for approximately 40 minutes five times per week to burn 2000 calories. You can use the caloric expenditure values for selected physical activities in Table 8-4 to determine the calories you burn in your exercise program.

The information in Figure 11-3 shows that sedentary living contributes to each of the other risk factors except smoking. Regular exercise can positively influence each of these factors and can reduce your risk of cardiovascular disease.

This relationship between aerobic fitness level and selected risk factors can clearly be seen in the data on more than 3000 men from the Aerobics Clinic in Dallas. These data are summarized in Table 11-6.

Notice that an increase in the aerobic fitness level is associated with a positive change in each of the cardiovascular risk factors. The changes include the following:

■ Reduced level of cholesterol and triglycerides

■ Lower body weight and lower percentage of body fat

■ Lower resting blood pressure (both systolic and diastolic)

■ Higher level of HDL cholesterol

These factors would explain, at least in part, why several studies have shown that physically active people have a much lower incidence of coronary heart disease than do inactive people.

Several studies have now been completed and published that evaluate the level of fitness directly rather than looking at the physical activity habits as reported by the participants.[3] The data from one of these studies is summarized in Figure 11-15.

This study classified individuals into 5 groups according to their fitness level ranging from low (group 1) to high (group 5). This data suggests that moderate intensity exercise such as walking briskly for 20 to 30 minutes several times each week can significantly reduce the death rate risk.

Of particular interest, a recent follow-up study showed that unfit men who became fit quickly reduce their risk of death from all causes by 44% and from cardiovascular disease by 64%. This study involved almost 10,000 men who were studied over a 20-year period of time and who were given at least two maximal treadmill tests to determine their level of fitness.[4]

The fact that inactivity ranked essentially the same as hypertension, cigarette smoking, and elevated cholesterol actually placed physical inactivity as a much greater heart disease risk because many more people lead sedentary lives than possess one or more of the other three primary risk factors (Table 11-7).

Many heart attacks occur during sudden bursts of vigorous activity, such as during the first snowstorm of the season, when shoveling is necessary, or during the hunting season, when the body is called on to do more work than it is accustomed. People who exercise regularly show a lower incidence of cardiovascular disease at these times, and they are much more likely to survive a heart attack if one occurs.

There are several possible explanations for this. Regular exercise increases the efficiency of the circulatory system, so the same amount of work can be performed with less stress on the heart. There may also be an increase in the diameter of the coronary arteries, ac-

Table 11-6	**Aerobic Fitness Level and Selected Cardiovascular Risk Factors**					
Aerobic Fitness Level	Body Weight (kg)	Percent Body Fat	Blood Pressure (mm Hg)	Cholesterol (mg/dl)	Triglyceride (mg/dl)	HDL Cholesterol (mg/dl)
Poor	90.0	29.3	133/87	238	182	37
Fair	86.3	26.9	127/84	237	172	40
Average	82.8	24.0	125/83	228	140	42
Good	79.4	20.8	123/81	222	114	45
Excellent	76.4	18.2	122/80	217	87	50

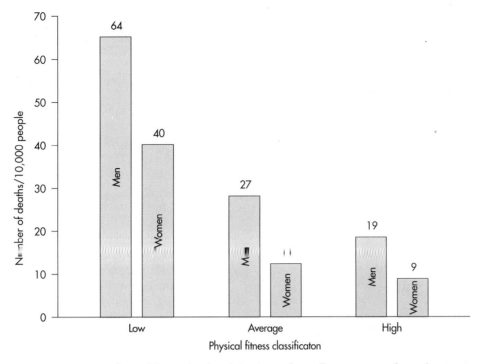

Figure 11-15 Physical fitness level and death rate from all causes. Data from Blair.[3]

Table 11-7	**Incidence of Selected Cardiovascular Disease Risk Factors**	
Risk Factor	**Estimated number of Americans (millons)**	**Percent of adult population**
Cigarette smoking	52.9	27
Elevated cholesterol level >240 mg/dl	38.4	20
Hypertension—>140 mm Hg systolic or >90 mm Hg diastolic	50.00	26
Overweight—>20% above desirable weight	63.3	33
Inactivity—less than 3 days of exercise/week	132.2	69
Completely sedentary	61.0	
Irregular activity	71.2	

companied by the development of additional capillaries (collateral circulation), so that blood may actually be able to bypass a partially obstructed artery. Remember also that exercise places stress on the body, and it is therefore accustomed to working at a higher level than is the body of a sedentary person.

INFORMATION ON CONTRIBUTING RISK FACTORS

Even though these risk factors may not have a "direct" relationship to cardiovascular disease, they are still very important factors. The following information is relative to each of these factors.

Elevated triglyceride level

Triglycerides are another form of fat circulating in the bloodstream. Most people know quite a bit about cho-

lesterol but very little about triglycerides. High levels of triglycerides also contribute to the high incidence of cardiovascular disease.

Of the fat we eat, 95% is in the form of triglycerides; this is also the type of fat that is stored under the skin in the fat cells. Triglycerides in the blood either come from the food we eat or are manufactured by the liver. A high intake of refined sugar and/or alcohol often causes the liver to overproduce triglycerides. Therefore high sugar and/or alcohol consumption usually raises triglyceride levels significantly.

A high level of triglycerides is also associated with increased development of atherosclerosis and is therefore classified as a risk factor. High triglyceride levels

Triglycerides: Fats consisting of three fatty acids and glycerol.

are particularly dangerous for people with a high cholesterol level.

The level of risk associated with different triglyceride readings is identified in Table 11-8. To be at a low risk for cardiovascular disease, you need to keep your triglyceride level below 140 mg/dl.

Let's Get Started

Strategies for reducing your triglyceride level

If your triglyceride level is high, the following suggestions may be of value to you:

- Reduce your body weight and/or body fat. If you are overweight or obese, a reduction in weight and/or fat usually results in a decrease in your triglyceride level.

- Reduce your intake of refined sugars and alcohol.

- Participate regularly in a good aerobic exercise program. (A recent study showed that people with a high triglyceride level who exercised for 1 hour three times a week reduced their triglyceride level by 25% over a 4-month period.)

- Reduce your fat intake to less than 30% of your total calories.

- Reduce your intake of saturated fat to less than 10% of your total calories.

- Increase your intake of polyunsaturated fat, particularly from fish.

- Increase your intake of complex carbohydrates.

HIGH LEVEL OF TENSION OR STRESS

Stress is defined as a physical or emotional factor that causes tension. It is an important part of living, and if you handle it properly, you can learn to relax and cope with your anger, fear, tension, and external pressure.

People react differently to specific situations that occur daily; how a person reacts to a situation will determine his or her stress level. Each person can be classified as one of two types. The first is Type A—people exhibiting a high stress level and rating high on the five criteria mentioned in Chapter 10.

These traits are normally present in most individuals, but the Type A person possesses them to an excessive degree. People in this group include those who cannot stand to have unscheduled time on their hands and who become very upset when they are kept waiting.

Those who rate low in these traits are classified as Type B. This is the type of person who usually is able to relax easily. Very seldom does this individual let outside factors adversely influence his or her emotional

Table 11-8	**Triglyceride Level and Risk of Cardiovascular Disease**
Risk	**Triglyceride Level**
Low	<140 mg/dl
Borderline to high	140-180 mg/dl
High	>180 mg/dl

state. A Type B person's level of anxiety and tension is therefore very low.

The relationship between the level of stress and cardiovascular disease has been evaluated, and research clearly shows the following:

- Cardiovascular disease is much more prevalent in the high-stress group (Type A) than in the low-stress group (Type B).

- Those with a high stress level also have a higher cholesterol level compared with those with a low stress level.

- The incidence of cigarette smoking is higher in those with a high stress level than in those with a low stress level.

Many people who have a high stress level and have difficulty coping with this stress turn to drugs, alcohol, smoking, and overeating. These are all unhealthful, and they help to increase the incidence of cardiovascular disease. Many people turn to exercise as a means of coping with this stress. Chapter 10 deals with stress, especially the role exercise plays in preventing and controlling it.

OBESITY AND EXCESS WEIGHT

Most people are familiar with the health hazards associated with excess fat and excess weight. These are identified in Chapter 8. The conclusion is that it is clearly more healthy to keep body fat and body weight within acceptable limits.

The procedures for measuring body fat and for determining ideal weight also are clearly identified in Chapter 8. If you do not have the opportunity to conduct these tests, if possible you may be able to think back to a time when you looked and felt good; try to recall what your weight probably was then.

Obesity and/or excess weight are risk factors associated with cardiovascular disease. For example, in the Framingham study, people who were 20 lb or more overweight suffered three times as many heart attacks as those of normal weight. The link between obesity and cardiovascular disease may possibly be caused by the following:

- Extra stress is placed on the heart because of the added workload.

- People who are obese or overweight tend to exercise less.

- Obesity is closely associated with increased blood pressure. (One study showed that successful weight reduction reduced hypertension by 41%.)

- Obesity is usually accompanied by increased levels of cholesterol and triglycerides.

- Diabetes occurs more frequently in people who are overweight and/or obese.

DIABETES

Glucose is a simple sugar we get by digesting carbohydrates. It is transported in the blood throughout the body and serves as the main source of energy for each of the body's cells. A high blood glucose level is the primary characteristic of diabetes.

Insulin, a hormone secreted by the pancreas, is responsible for controlling your blood glucose level. Normally, when the blood glucose level rises, more insulin is secreted and most of the body's cells respond by "taking up" glucose from the blood. This excess glucose is stored as glycogen in the muscles or liver or converted to fat and stored in the body. Usually the blood glucose level then quickly returns to normal. However, this process breaks down in the more than 11 million Americans who have diabetes; their bodies cannot maintain a normal blood glucose level.

There are basically two types of diabetes. **Type I diabetes** accounts for fewer than 10% of the cases. With this type of diabetes, the body cannot produce enough insulin. For this reason, this type is often referred to as insulin-dependent diabetes. **Type II diabetes** is known as non–insulin-dependent diabetes. Sufficient insulin is available, but for some reason the body does not react to it and is unable to control the blood glucose level. More than 90% of all diabetic patients are non–insulin-dependent. This disorder usually occurs in people over the age of 40, and almost 90% of the patients can be classified as obese at the time of onset of the disease.

An elevated fasting blood glucose level may be an early sign of diabetes. If you know your blood glucose level, you can evaluate your score by consulting Table 11-9.

It has been shown that people who have diabetes not only have excess glucose in the blood, they may also have difficulty metabolizing fat. This often causes increased atherosclerosis throughout the body and contributes to a high incidence of cardiovascular disease. More than 80% of all people who have diabetes die from some form of cardiovascular disease.

Exercise is the key to controlling diabetes. Research shows that sedentary people have a much higher incidence of diabetes than do active people and that this result occurs independently of the differences in obesity.

The results from a recent 5-year study involving 22,000 male subjects are presented in Table 11-10.

Note that the risk of Type II diabetes was reduced by 23% in those men who exercised vigorously only once per week, and for those who exercised 5 or more times a week, there was a 42% reduction.[19] Similar results were also found in a study involving women.[20]

There appear to be several reasons why exercise is important in controlling Type II diabetes:

- Exercise promotes the use of glucose for energy. Diabetic patients who exercise regularly thus can control their blood glucose levels better and require less insulin than those who do not exercise.

- Exercise increases the number of insulin receptors in the cells and therefore contributes to insulin's effectiveness in removing glucose from the bloodstream.

- Exercise can contribute to the reduction or prevention of obesity. Regular aerobic activity of the correct intensity and duration can prevent the loss of lean body mass and can reduce the amount of body fat. The role that exercise plays is described in detail in Chapter 8.

There is no known cure for diabetes, so it is extremely important to control this disease. This can be done most effectively through diet and exercise and, in extreme cases, by the administration of insulin.

Table 11-9	Classification of Blood Glucose Level (Fasting)
Classification	**Level**
Normal	<115 mg/dl
Borderline to high	115-140 mg/dl
High	>140 mg/dl

Table 11-10	Vigorous Exercise and Risk of Type II Diabetes
Frequency of Exercise	**Reduction in Risk (%)**
Once a week	23
2-4 times a week	38
5 or more times a week	42

From *Medical World News*, July 1992.

Type I diabetes: A type of diabetes in which the body is unable to produce sufficient insulin.

Type II diabetes: A type of diabetes in which insulin is ineffective in controlling the blood sugar level.

Chapter Summary

The following summary will help you to identify some of the important concepts covered in this chapter:

- Despite the fact that the death rate from cardiovascular disease has decreased by 25% in the last 10 years, cardiovascular disease is still by far the leading cause of death in the United States.
- This decrease in deaths from cardiovascular disease has been associated with many positive lifestyle changes.
- The three major risk factors associated with cardiovascular disease are cigarette smoking, high blood pressure, and an elevated cholesterol level.
- Cigarette smokers also tend to have poorer health habits than those who do not smoke.
- Reducing your sodium intake and your body weight may significantly reduce your blood pressure.
- With regard to cholesterol, you will be at a very low risk for cardiovascular disease if your cholesterol level is less than 160 mg/dl, your ratio of cholesterol/HDL is less than 5.0 (men) or less than 4.4 (women), and your LDL is less than 130 mg/dl.
- The more major risk factors that apply to you, the greater your chances of cardiovascular disease.
- Contributing risk factors associated with cardiovascular disease include elevated triglyceride level, high level of stress or tension, obesity or excess weight, and diabetes.
- Despite the fact that many of the risk factors associated with cardiovascular disease have decreased significantly in recent years, there are still far too many Americans who place themselves at high risk.

References

1. American Heart Association: *Heart and stroke facts: 1994 statistical supplement,* Dallas, 1994, the Association.
2. Anspaugh DJ, Hamrick MH, Rosato FD: *Wellness: concepts and applications,* ed 2, St Louis, 1994, Mosby.
3. Blair SN et al: Physical fitness and all-cause mortality: a prospective study of healthy men and women, *JAMA* 162:2395-2401, 1989.
4. Blair SN et al: Changes in physical fitness and all-cause mortality: a prospective study of healthy men and women, *JAMA* 273:1093-1098, 1995.
5. Cigarette smoking—attributable mortality and years of potential life lost—United States, 1990. *MMWR* 42(33):645-648, 1993.
6. Duncan JJ, Gordon NF, Scott CB: Women walking for health and fitness, *JAMA* 266(23):3295-3299, 1991.
7. Egan B: Nutritional and lifestyle approaches to the prevention and management of hypertension, *Compr Ther* 11(8):15-20, 1985.
8. *Facts about blood cholesterol,* Pub No 882696, US Department of Health and Human Services, November 1987.
9. Fuster V et al: The pathogenesis of coronary heart disease and the acute coronary syndromes, *N Engl J Med* 314:488-500, 1992.
10. Haskell WL et al: Cardiovascular benefits and assessment of physical activity and physical fitness in adults, *Med Sci Sports Exerc* 24(6):S201-S220, 1992.
11. *Healthy People 2000,* National Health Promotion and Disease Prevention Objectives, Pub No PH591-50213, US Department of Health and Human Services, Public Health Service, Washington, DC, 1991, US Government Printing Office.
12. *Heart book: a guide to prevention and treatment of cardiovascular disease,* New York, 1980, American Heart Association.
13. Hubert HB et al: Lifestyle correlates of risk factor change in young adults—an eight year study of coronary heart disease risk factors in the Framington offspring, *Am J Epidemiol* 125:812-831, 1987.
14. Kann el WG: Meaning of the downward trend in cardiovascular mortality, *JAMA* 247(6):877-881, 1982.
15. Kuczmarski RJ et al: Increasing prevalence of overweight among US adults: The national health and nutrition examination survey, 1960 to 1991, *JAMA* 272(3):205-211, 1994.
16. Lakka TA et al: Relation of leisure-time physical activity and cardiorespiratory fitness to the risk of acute myocardial infarction in men, *N Engl J Med* 330(22):1549-1554, 1994.
17. Lechere S et al: High density lipoprotein cholesterol, habitual physical activity and physical fitness, *Atherosclerosis* 57:43-51, 1985.
18. Manson JE et al: The primary prevention of myocardial infarction, *N Engl J Med* 326(21):1406-1416, 1992.
19. Manson JE et al: A prospective study of exercise and incidence of diabetes among US male physicians, *JAMA* 268(1):63-67, 1992.
20. Manson JE et al: Physical activity and incidence of non-insulin dependent diabetes mellitus in women, *Lancet* 338:774-778, 1991.
21. Marti B et al: Smoking, alcohol consumption, and endurance capacity: an analysis of 6,500 19-year-old conscripts and 4,100 joggers, *Prev Med* 17:79-92, 1988.

22. McArdle WD, Katch FI, Katch VL: *Essentials of exercise physiology*, Philadelphia, 1994, Lea & Febiger.

23. McCunney RJ: Fitness, heart disease, and high density lipoprotein: a look at the relationship, *The Physician and Sportsmedicine* 15(2):67-79, 1987.

24. Miller RW: On being too rich, too thin and too cholesterol laden, *FDA Consumer*, pp 31-34, July/August 1981.

25. Min Lee I, Hsieh CC, Paffenberger RS: Exercise intensity and longevity in men—the Harvard alumni study, *JAMA* 273(15):1179-1184, 1995.

26. Morgan DW et al: HDL concentrations in weight-trained, endurance trained and sedentary females, *The Physician and Sportsmedicine* 14:3, 1986.

27. Morris JN et al: Vigorous exercise in leisure time: protection against coronary heart disease, *Lancet* 8206:1207-1210, 1980.

28. National High Blood Pressure Education Program: *Working group report on primary prevention*, Hyattsville, MD, 1992, National Heart, Lung, and Blood Institute.

29. Neaton JD, Wentworth D: Serum cholesterol, blood pressure, cigarette smoking, and death from coronary heart disease, *Arch Intern Med* 152:56-64, 1992.

30. Nieman DC: *Fitness and sports medicine*, ed 3, Palo Alto, Calif, 1995, Bull Publishing.

31. Nieman DC et al: *Nutrition*, Dubuque, Ia, 1990, Wm C Brown.

32. Paffenberger RS et al: Physical activity, all-causes mortality and longevity of college alumni, *N Engl J Med* 314:605-613, 1986.

33. Powell KE et al: Physical activity—the incidence of coronary heart disease, *Annu Rev Public Health* 8:254-287, 1987.

34. *Prevention index—1995 summary report*, 1995, Emmaus, Penn, Rodale Press.

35. Siscovick DS, LaPorte RE, Newman JM: The disease-specific benefits and risks of physical activity and exercise, public health reports, *Journal of the US Public Health Service* 100(2):122-126, 1985.

36. Stamler J, Stamler R, Neaton JD: Blood pressure, systolic and diastolic, and cardiovascular risks: US population data, *Arch Intern Med* 153:598 615, 1993.

37. Stamler R et al: Nutrition therapy for high blood pressure, *JAMA* 257:1484-1491,1987.

38. Storer TW, Ruhling RO: Essential hypertension and exercise, *The Physician and Sportsmedicine* 9(6):59, 1981.

39. Treatment of Mild Hypertension Research Group: The treatment of mild hypertension, *Arch Intern Med* 151:1413-1423, 1991.

40. US Department of Health and Human Services: *The health consequences of smoking*, Washington, DC, 1988, US Government Printing Office.

41. Wood PD et al: Distribution of plasma lipoproteins in middle age male runners, *Metabolism* 25:1249,1976.

Laboratory Experience 11-1

Arizona Heart Institute Cardiovascular Risk Factor Analysis

Name _____ Section _____ Date _____

Directions: Indicate the points that you have scored in the column on the right for each of the following risk factors. When you finish, total your points and compare that with the results at the end of the activity.

Risk factors	Score		
1. Age	Age 56 or over	1	
	Age 55 or under	0	_____
2. Gender	Male	1	
	Female	0	_____
3. Family history	If you have:		
	Blood relatives who have had a heart attack or stroke at or before age 60	12	
	Blood relatives who have had a heart attack or stroke after age 60	6	
	No blood relatives who have had a heart attack or stroke	0	_____
4. Personal history	50 or under: If you had either a heart attack, a stroke, heart or blood vessel surgery	20	
	51 or over: If you had any of the above	10	
	None of the above	0	_____
5. Diabetes	Diabetes before age 40 and now on insulin	10	
	Diabetes at or after age 40 and now on insulin or pills	5	
	Diabetes controlled by diet, or diabetes after age 55	3	
	No diabetes	0	_____
6. Smoking	Two packs per day	10	
	Between one and two packs per day or quit smoking less than a year ago	6	
	If you smoke six or more cigars a day or inhale a pipe regularly	6	
	Less than one pack per day or quit smoking more than 1 year ago	3	
	Never smoked	0	_____
7. Cholesterol (if cholesterol count is not known, answer 8)	Cholesterol level—276 or above	10	
	Cholesterol level—between 225 and 275	5	
	Cholesterol level—224 or below	0	
8. Diet (If you have answered 7, do not answer 8)	Does your normal eating pattern include:		
	One serving of red meat daily, more than seven eggs a week, and daily consumption of butter, whole milk, and cheese	8	
	Red meat 4-6 times a week, 4-7 eggs a week, margarine, low fat dairy products, and some cheese	4	
	Poultry, fish, little or no red meat, three or fewer eggs a week, some margarine, skim milk, and skim milk products	0	_____

From Anspaugh DJ, Hamrick MH, Rosato FD: *Wellness*, St. Louis, 1991, Mosby.

Risk factors	Score	
9. High blood pressure	If either number is:	
	160 over 100 (160/100) or higher	10
	140 over 90 (140/90) but less than 160 over 100 (160/100)	5
	If both numbers are less than 140 over 90 (140/90)	0 _____
10. Weight	Ideal Weight Formula:	
	Men = 110 lb plus 5 lb for each inch over 5 feet	
	Women = 100 lb plus 5 lb for each inch over 5 feet	
	25 lb overweight	4
	10 to 24 lb overweight	2
	Less than 10 lb overweight	0 _____
11. Exercise	Do you engage in any aerobic exercise (brisk walking, jogging, bicycling, racketball, swimming) for more than 15 minutes:	
	Less than once a week	4
	1 to 2 times a week	2
	3 or more times a week	0 _____
12. Stress	Are you:	
	Frustrated when waiting in line, often in a hurry to complete work or keep appointments, easily angered, irritable	4
	Impatient when waiting, occasionally hurried, or occasionally moody	2
	Comfortable when waiting, seldom rushed, and easygoing	0 _____

TOTAL POINTS   _____

Score results

PLEASE NOTE: A high score does not mean you will develop heart disease. It is merely a guide to make you aware of a potential risk. Since no two people are alike, an exact prediction is impossible without further individualized testing.

With answer to question 9		Without answer to question 9	
High risk	40 and above	High risk	36 and above
Medium risk	20-39	Medium risk	19-35
Low risk	19 and below	Low risk	18 and below

Chapter Twelve **Personalizing Your Fitness Program**

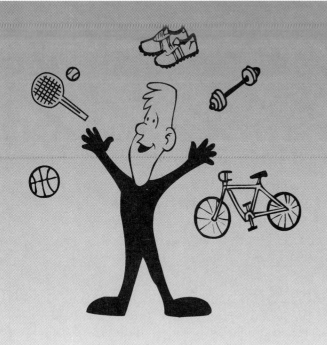

CHAPTER OBJECTIVES

Check off each objective as you achieve it.

- ❏ Evaluate the importance of regular exercise, and decide whether to make a commitment to exercise regularly.
- ❏ Discuss the reason it is important to carefully and systematically plan an exercise program.
- ❏ Explain why overload and progression are important in a good exercise program.
- ❏ List appropriate objectives for yourself, and plan an exercise program to achieve these objectives.
- ❏ Initiate this exercise program, and participate regularly.

In the preceding chapters, we have done the following:

- Discussed the importance of regular physical activity
- Defined physical fitness and identified each of the health-related components
- Presented the reasons for achieving and maintaining an optimal level of physical fitness
- Included simple tests that allow you to determine your present status in each of the physical fitness components
- Presented norms so that you can evaluate your test results
- Identified the principles and procedures for the development of each of the health-related physical fitness components
- Summarized several existing programs that can be used for developing physical fitness

This information has been presented in the hope that you will recognize the importance of and do something about your own physical fitness. Knowing about physical fitness and even recognizing its importance are not enough; more than 90% of college students indicate that exercise and fitness are important, but fewer than 40% of these same students exercise on a regular basis.

CHANGING YOUR EXERCISE HABITS

Most people are aware that exercise makes them healthier and more attractive, makes them feel better and function more efficiently, and helps them deal with stress—in fact, that exercise is an ideal way to cope with stress. Yet many of these same people do not exercise on a regular basis, and many who start an exercise program have a hard time sticking with it.

Changing our daily living habits is a difficult task. Even though we realize that we need to make changes, we often lack the necessary motivation or discipline to do so, and we often come up with seemingly valid excuses for not exercising. To succeed in changing your daily habits to positively influence your health, you must develop a positive way of thinking and believe in your ability to succeed. Without confidence and a positive attitude, you are unlikely to succeed.

Following is a list of excuses for not exercising. These excuses have no place in the minds of people who want to be physically fit.

EXCUSES FOR NOT EXERCISING

- **I work hard and I'm too tired.** This is actually an argument *for* exercise. It has been shown conclusively that regular exercise increases, not decreases, your level of energy. People who participate regularly in a good exercise program can attest to its value after a stressful day at work.

- **I don't have the time.** As stated previously, people will make time for things they consider to be important. A recent survey showed that this was true for exercise. People who exercised regularly had the same amount of leisure time available as those who did not exercise regularly. The difference between the two groups was in the priorities that determined how the time was to be used.

- **I get all the exercise I need each day without doing anything extra.** People who are active each day at work or around the house might burn up calories, but the activity is either not strenuous enough or not continuous enough in most cases to promote cardiovascular fitness.

- **If I exercise, I will automatically eat more.** This is clearly not true. A person who exercises for 1 hour per day will actually eat less than does a person who does not exercise at all. Exercise tends to suppress your appetite.

- **When I exercise, I always get sore muscles.** Muscle soreness can be reduced to a minimum by warming up correctly, starting gradually, and progressing slowly. If a person exercises regularly and muscle soreness does occur, it does so only at the start of the program and lasts for only a few days.

- **It is too late to change the way I live.**
- **I know I should exercise, but ...**
- **I don't like to exercise.**

It's never too late to change your habits, and if exercise is important enough to you, you will take the time to apply the knowledge you now have to designing a program for yourself. You must follow this program on a regular basis. Your good intentions must be turned into action.

REVIEW OF THE PRINCIPLES OF EXERCISE

Before you start your program, it might be beneficial to review some of the important principles of exercise. Cardiovascular fitness, which is also referred to as *aerobic fitness,* is the most important type of fitness. It involves the efficient functioning of the heart, lungs, and circulatory system, so there are many advantages associated with an optimum level of cardiovascular fitness. Your fitness program should include the following:

A 5- to 10-minute warm-up, as the body gradually moves from a state of minimum activity to a much higher level of activity. Many people drop out of an exercise program during the first few weeks because of muscle soreness. Much of this discomfort can be avoided by taking time to warm up and by starting gradually and progressing slowly in your program.

Twenty to 30 minutes of continuous activity at an intensity that keeps your heart rate in your target zone. Remember that your target zone can be calculated by taking 70% to 85% of your predicted maximum heart rate, which is determined by subtracting your age from 220. Any continuous activity that involves the use of large muscle groups can fulfill this purpose. Suitable activities include walking, jogging, bicycling, swimming, cross-country skiing, aerobic dancing, basketball, and racquetball.

Activities for the development of strength and muscular endurance. Many people prefer some type of weight training for this part of their program.

A 5- to 10-minute cool-down session. It is important to slow down gradually, and depending on the type of activities you have selected, it may be equally important to again stretch the various muscle groups that have been used.

Frequency. For aerobic fitness, you need to exercise a minimum of 3 times and a maximum of 5 times each week. If your main objective for exercise is to lose weight and fat, you need to make a commitment to exercise for 45 minutes, 5 days each week.

OTHER CONSIDERATIONS

In planning your program, it is also important to remember the following:

- Exercise sessions must be scheduled regularly 3 to 5 times each week.

- **Overload** must be built into the program. Overload involves subjecting the body to a task slightly beyond its normal level, so that enough stress is placed on the body to stimulate the desired response. In the development of strength and cardiovascular and muscular endurance, improvement occurs only if the body is subjected to a workload greater than that to which it is accustomed.

- **Progression** is another important part of every exercise program. The body will adapt to the increased level of resistance as improvement takes place. For this reason, it is necessary to measure progress and to increase the workload frequently. Progress is greatest and most apparent at the start of a program, particularly if you have been inactive. In aerobic activities, progression can be incorporated by carefully checking the heart rate each day and adjusting the intensity to ensure that the heart rate remains in the desired target zone.

- An exercise program will result in **specificity of improvement.** Each exercise program is specific and results in improvement only in the area or areas it is designed to develop. For example, a person who lifts weights regularly develops strength and muscular endurance in those muscle groups for which exercises are included. Similarly, unless you include an aerobic exercise that keeps your heart rate in the target zone for an extended period, you should not expect a significant improvement in cardiovascular endurance.

The activities making up the program determine the results attained.

STARTING A SUCCESSFUL EXERCISE PROGRAM

Beginning a successful exercise program involves several steps.

Make a commitment to exercise

We have seen that the first step in beginning an exercise program is to commit yourself to the idea that exercise and fitness are important to you. Having made this commitment, you must now put into practice the principles you have learned, and exercise must become a permanent part of your life.

It is important to realize that it will take time and effort to achieve your objectives and experience significant changes. It requires discipline and determination. There are no shortcuts or easy methods. However, this does not mean that exercise cannot be enjoyable. It is very important to select an activity that you enjoy and that will contribute to your objectives. You must then participate at a level that is comfortable but of sufficient intensity to produce the desired changes. If you become bored with an activity, vary your program and include other activities.

Physical examination

If you are less than 35 years of age and starting a serious exercise program and you have no medical problems, you do not need a physical examination. Just make sure that if you are out of shape that you gradually ease into your program and do not do too much too soon.

If you are over 35 years of age and out of shape and haven't exercised regularly for some time, it is important to find out whether it is safe for you to exercise. The demand placed on your heart while you exercise is much greater than the effort required for most everyday activities.

A good physical examination will include a graded exercise test that will evaluate your blood pressure, heart rate, and electrocardiogram responses while you are exercising. These data can also be used to evaluate your aerobic fitness level. The examination should also include measurements of strength, muscular endurance, flexibility, and body fat.

By taking such tests, you will not only know if it is safe for you to exercise, you will have baseline figures to use in planning your program. This will allow you to establish realistic objectives and measure your progress. This should increase your motivation.

Define your goals

You can waste much time and energy if you don't establish certain goals for your program. These goals should be based on your individual needs. They should be both challenging and realistic. You must allow yourself a reasonable amount of time to reach them. Do not expect too much too soon.

In determining your goals, you should think about why you want to exercise. For example, your exercise program will be different if your major objective is to lose weight than if it is simply to develop an optimal level of aerobic fitness. Of course, an exercise program can be designed for both of these objectives.

What are realistic objectives? Knowing what realistic objectives are is very important when you start an exercise program. You need to set your objectives so that you can attain some degree of success. Losing 20 lb in a month or running 10 miles in an hour are unrealistic goals for most people. These are not the types of objectives to be set if you follow the procedures outlined in the previous chapters.

A realistic objective for the development of cardiovascular fitness might be to average four exercise sessions for 15 consecutive weeks and accumulate from 12 to 16 miles per week by jogging at an intensity sufficient to maintain your heart rate in the desired target zone. A realistic goal for weight control might be to average 20 miles per week walking and to reduce your caloric intake so that in 12 weeks you will lose 12 lb. Often it is advantageous to write out your objectives in the form of a contract. In this way, you can periodically evaluate your progress to determine how effective and consistent your exercise program is and whether you need to make any adjustments in your program (see Laboratory Experience 12-1).

In Summary

You need to define objectives that are important to you, are realistic and challenging, and will require discipline, determination, and effort.

Have a plan of action

Your exercise program must be systematic and carefully planned. All too frequently, exercise is performed irregularly, with little thought given to the objectives or to the reasons for including specific exercises. In designing your program you need to know how much exercise is enough for you, and you must set weekly goals as you move toward your objectives. Remember that consistency from week to week will determine your degree of success.

The first few weeks are very important; it is during this time that a large number of people become disheartened and give up. It should be emphasized that you cannot start out at too low of a level. It has probably taken you a long time to get out of shape, and it will take you more than a few days to get back into shape. You need patience and determination.

It will take at least 8 weeks for you to experience many of the major changes that take place. However, during the first few weeks you should be able to see definite progress as you become more skilled at adjusting the intensity of the exercise to match your level of fitness. Activities that initially appear difficult become much easier, and you will quickly find out how much work you can do.

The personal checklist in the box may help you identify some of your preferences for an exercise program. The decisions you make will help you plan your program.

Personal Checklist

Check off one response to each of the following:
1. I would prefer to exercise
   - ❏ on my own
   - ❏ with a friend
   - ❏ with a group of people
2. In scheduling my program
   - ❏ I have the motivation to exercise regularly on my own or with others
   - ❏ I need to participate in an organized program at a set time and place each day
3. I prefer to exercise
   - ❏ indoors
   - ❏ outdoors
4. I prefer to work out regularly
   - ❏ early in the morning
   - ❏ at noon
   - ❏ immediately after work
   - ❏ later in the evening
5. I feel that I am best suited to
   - ❏ competitive activities
   - ❏ noncompetitive activities
6. As far as expense is concerned
   - ❏ I am willing to spend money and join a health club or YMCA
   - ❏ I am willing to spend money to buy equipment of my own, such as an exercise bike or weight-training set
   - ❏ I want a program with little or no expense
7. I am interested in
   - ❏ the same activity year around
   - ❏ a variety of activities

Modified from Fitness: the facts, Book 6, *The final ingredient,* Participation, Canada, 1979, Ministry of Culture and Recreation.

Overload: Subjecting the body to a task slightly more difficult than that to which it is accustomed.

Progression: Increasing the amount of exercise from time to time so that the body must work harder.

Specificity of improvement: Improvement occurs only in the area or areas that each exercise is designed to develop.

Activity selection

You must select activities that you enjoy and that will enable you to achieve your objectives for the program. You may wish to exercise on your own, where you are in complete control of what you do. This way you do not have to worry about or rely on anyone else, and you can get away from everyone and be by yourself. Another advantage is that you can decide when and where you exercise. Exercises such as walking, jumping rope, bicycling, jogging, swimming, and skating are examples of activities you can do alone.

If you thrive on competition, you may wish to participate against a person of equal ability in a sport such as racquetball or one-on-one basketball. These activities can be enjoyable and very good for cardiovascular fitness. For those who are competitive and lack the skill or interest to participate in individual sports, team sports may be the answer. They are equally enjoyable and beneficial. Basketball, water polo, ice hockey, soccer, rugby, and field hockey are examples of sports that make a major contribution to the development of cardiovascular fitness.

The objective is to find an activity that is both enjoyable and strenuous enough to contribute to cardiovascular fitness and/or weight loss. If you enjoy what you are doing and it is challenging and satisfying, exercise is much more likely to become a regular part of your daily routine.

Regularity of exercise

Choose a regular time for exercise. To achieve your specific objectives, you must participate on a regular basis. Those who wait until they "find" time to exercise do not exercise very often. If you believe strongly enough in the importance of exercise, you will make time available on a regular basis and exercise will become a habit. A good exercise program requires less than 5 hours per week. This is very little time to spend, considering all the benefits you will receive.

If you are trying to lose weight, exercising in the late afternoon might be advantageous because it will help you decrease your caloric intake. By exercising you may be able to avoid the temptation to stop at a local hotel, restaurant, or bar for a happy hour, where you tend to consume a large number of extra calories. Also, a vigorous workout late in the day will often suppress your appetite.

Be willing to work at it

In any endeavor, people who are successful work hard. Nothing comes easy. Many people who do not exercise use the excuse that they just do not have enough energy. You should not let the grind of your daily routine keep you from exercising. Regular exercise will actually increase your energy level and enable you to be more productive in your everyday tasks. You should feel refreshed after a good workout.

Monitor your progress

It is important to monitor your progress on a regular basis, which you can do by keeping a record of your workouts. This enables you to chart your progress and get some immediate feedback on the total time spent each week, number of calories burned, aerobic points earned, and changes in body weight. Many different computer programs are available that can be used on home computers for this purpose.

An exercise logging program is part of the computer software package available for use with this textbook. A sample printout similar to the one from this program appears in Figure 12-1.

This example is a monthly printout. It clearly shows the following:

- The number of exercise days for the month
- Changes in body weight from the beginning to the end of the month
- The total miles accumulated in running, bicycling, and swimming
- The total calories burned for the month
- The total number of aerobic points earned for the month
- Corresponding totals for the previous month, which allows you to compare the 2 months to see whether you are making any progress

COMMON-SENSE PRECAUTIONS

Get an adequate amount of rest

Your muscles, as well as your entire body, need an adequate amount of rest if you are to get the most out of your exercise program. You can't expect to have a good workout if you stayed up for most of the night with only 2 or 3 hours of sleep.

We also know that most muscle injuries are caused by overuse—it is not reasonable to expect to work out vigorously each day, particularly in a weight-bearing activity, and not get injured. If you exercise 5 days each week, make sure that you do not exercise for 5 consecutive days and then take the next 2 days off. This is a poorly planned program. Your body will react much better if you split up the days off and take one at the weekend and one in the middle of the week.

Take good care of your feet

Make sure that you have the correct shoes for the activity in which you participate, so that you get adequate support and cushioning. This will help you to avoid injuries such as shin splints and bone bruises. Wearing a thick pair of socks can help to prevent blisters.

Date: 10/31/1983 Height: 72 in   Name: Joe Jock SSN: 345-67-8901   Sex: Male
                                                                                              Age: 30 yr

Session	Date	Mode	Weight (lb)	Duration (min)	Run/Walk Distance (mi)	Bicycle Distance (mi)	Swim Distance (mi)	Calories Burned	Aerobic Points
1	10/01/1983	Warm-up activities	175	20				115.5	0.5
		Walking/running treadmill	175	45	4.5			630.0	21.5
2	10/02/1983	Walking/running	175	50	5.0			700.0	24.0
3	10/03/1983	Basketball	173	55				428.2	8.3
4	10/05/1983	Racquetball	173	60				685.1	9.0
5	10/06/1983	Stationary bicycle riding	173	40		8.3		379.8	9.5
6	10/09/1983	Bicycle riding	172	30		7.5		361.2	9.8
7	10/10/1983	Swimming	170	20			0.7	530.4	19.5
8	10/12/1983	Aerobic dance	170	55				467.5	5.8
9	10/15/1983	Racquetball	170	45				504.9	6.8
		Walking/running	170	45	4.0			573.8	16.3
10	10/20/1983	Racquetball	169	60				669.2	9.0
11	10/22/1983	Walking/running	169	50	6.0			760.5	33.8
12	10/26/1983	Walking/running treadmill	168	45	4.5			604.8	21.5
13	10/27/1983	Aerobic dance	168	30				252.0	3.1
		TOTALS	650		24.0	15.8	0.7	7662.9	198.4
		AVERAGE (PER EXERCISE DAY)		50	4.8	7.9	0.7	589.5	15.3

Activity	Totals Last Month	Lifetime
⫿⫿⫿ ⫿ ⫿ ⫿⫿	⫿⫿⫿ ⫿⫿⫿⫿ ⫿	⫿ ⫿ ⫿ ⫿⫿⫿⫿⫿
Bicycle riding	13.0 miles	96.4 miles
Swimming	1.3 miles	12.4 miles
Raquetball	6 hours 30 min.	45 hours 20 minutes
Aerobic dance	22 hours 36 min.	42 hours 10 minutes

Data from the Department of Health, Physical Education, and Athletics, Trinity University—Exercise Physiology Laboratory.

Figure 12-1 Sample printout of computer program for summary of physical activity.

Maintain proper muscle balance

Frequently we neglect specific muscle groups at the expense of others, and this creates an imbalance. This often contributes to muscle injuries. An aerobic program combined with a good weight-training program should result in good muscle balance.

Listen to signals from your body

Most people pay close attention to some signals from their body but completely disregard others. If you experience tightness or pain in the chest and you feel faint or light-headed, you would probably stop exercising immediately and seek medical help to find out the extent of the problem.

On the other hand, many people who are constantly fatigued and/or experience nagging muscle injuries will continue exercising and disregard these signals. These signals are your body's way of telling you that something is wrong. You need to also find out what is causing the problems.

Vary your workouts

Since most muscle injuries are caused by overuse, if you are prone to muscle injuries or want to try to avoid them, you may need to vary your activities when you work out on consecutive days. Include nonimpact activities such as swimming and bicycling on alternate days.

STICKING WITH YOUR PROGRAM

Several different studies show that 60% or more of adults who start an exercise program drop out within the first month. You must be patient. It will take some time to develop your fitness level to the point where you function most efficiently. When you have achieved an optimal level of fitness, you should feel so much better that you will need little or no motivation to continue. Achieving this much has involved a lot of hard work and discipline, and you should be proud of your accomplishments. However, it is very important to continue to exercise on a regular basis to maintain this level of fitness. Exercise must become a lifetime commitment. By now you will realize that the benefits far outweigh the effort.

Chapter Summary

The following summary will help you to identify some of the important concepts covered in this chapter:

- Knowledge concerning exercise and fitness is important if you are to design an exercise program that best fits your individual needs.
- Your exercise program must be systematic and well-planned, and you must participate in it regularly if you are to be successful.
- Because your body will adapt, progression and overload must be built into your program.
- Specific goals and a plan of action will increase your chances of sticking with your program.
- If you have a very busy lifestyle, you will need to schedule a time to exercise if you are to develop the consistency that is necessary to be successful.

References

1. Fisher GA: *Your heart rate: the key to real fitness,* Provo, Utah, 1976, Brigham Young University Press.
2. Fitness: the facts, Book 4, *The activities,* Participation, Canada, 1979, Ministry of Culture and Recreation.
3. Fitness: the facts, Book 6, *The final ingredient,* Participation, Canada, 1979, Ministry of Culture and Recreation.
4. Kusinitz I, Fine M: *Your guide to getting fit,* ed 2, Mountain View, Calif, 1991, Mayfield.
5. *Nutrition exercise health lifestyle,* 1987, Pritikin Resource Book.
6. Rosenstein AH: The benefits of health maintenance, *Physician and Sports Medicine* 15:4, April 1987.
7. Wellness Newsletter, Randall Sports/Medical Products, Kirkland, Wash, 3:1, 1991.

Laboratory Experience 12-1

Personal Fitness Contract

Name _____   Section _____ Date _____

By writing a personal fitness contract, you will formulate some specific objectives and you will be more likely to make a lasting commitment to exercise. The example at the end of this section may be of help to you.

Step 1. State the overall objectives that you would like to achieve:

Step 2: State specifically what you will do to achieve these objectives: (You need to state which activities you will participate in, and you will need to determine goals for these in terms of frequency, duration, and so on.)

Step 3: State the specific time you will allow yourself to attain these objectives:

Contract:

I, _____ , *am making a contract with myself to regularly follow an exercise program as specified above, as I work toward achieving the specified objectives.*

I will begin my program on _____

I will achieve all my objectives by _____

Signed _____ *Date* _____

Witness _____

Example: Jill Jock

Step 1: Overall objectives:
1. To develop consistent exercise habits
2. To improve my aerobic fitness level to where I can jog slowly and complete 3 miles in 30 minutes
3. To reduce my percentage of body fat from 24% to 20%

Step 2: Specific objectives:
1. To develop consistent exercise habits, I need to make a commitment to exercise at least 3 times each week. I will initially exercise for a minimum of 30 minutes on each of the exercise days.
2. To improve my aerobic fitness level, I need to check my intensity level each time I exercise to make sure that my heart rate remains in my target zone.
3. Every 3 weeks I will test myself to see how far I can run in 30 minutes. I will need to see gradual improvement until I can run my 3 miles in 30 minutes.
4. I plan on walking and/or jogging each exercise session, depending on my initial level of fitness.
5. After 4 weeks of exercise, I will increase the duration of each exercise session to 45 minutes and will increase the frequency from 3 to 5 times each week.

Step 3: Time schedule:
1. By the start of the third week, I will have met my first overall objective and each week thereafter, this will continue to be met.
2. I will allow myself 12 additional weeks to meet the other two overall objectives.

Contract:

I, _____Jill Jock_____ , *am making a contract with myself to regularly follow an exercise program as specified above, as I work toward achieving the specified objectives.*

I will begin my program on _September 1, 1995_

I will achieve all my objectives by _December 15, 1995_

Signed _____ *Date* _9/01/95_

Witness _____

Food Exchange Lists

MILK LIST

The milk list contains various types of milk and milk products. It does not include cheeses, which are on the meat list or other dairy fats such as butter, which are on the fat list. The milk list is divided into three categories based on fat content. The categories are as follows:

Skim and very low-fat milk
Low-fat milk
Whole milk
One cup equals 8 fluid oz.

Skim and very low-fat milk

Each serving of milk or milk product on this list contains approximately 12 g of carbohydrates, 8 g of protein, and 0 to 3 g of fat (approximately 90 calories).

Skim milk	1 cup
½% milk	1 cup
1% milk	1 cup
Nonfat or low-fat buttermilk	1 cup
Evaporated skim milk	½ cup
Nonfat dry milk	⅓ cup
Plain or fruit-flavored nonfat yogurt	1 cup

Low-fat milk

Each serving of milk or milk product on this list contains approximately 12 g of carbohydrates, 8 g of protein, and 5 g of fat (approximately 125 calories).

2% milk	1 cup
Plain or fruit-flavored low-fat yogurt	1 cup

Whole milk

Each serving of milk or milk product on this list contains approximately 12 g of carbohydrates, 8 g of protein, and 8 g of fat (approximately 150 calories).

Whole milk	1 cup
Evaporated whole milk	½ cup
Whole plain or fruit-flavored yogurt	1 cup

FRUIT LIST

The fruit list contains fresh, frozen, canned and dried fruits, and fruit juices. Each item on the list contains approximately 15 g of carbohydrates (approximately 60 calories). Portion sizes for each food item are indicated.

Fruits

Apple (2-inch diameter)	1 apple
Apricots (fresh)	4 whole
Apricots (dried)	8 halves
Banana (4 oz)	1 small
Blackberries	¾ cup
Blueberries	¾ cup
Cantaloupe (small)	⅓ melon or 1 cup
Cherries (fresh)	12 large
Cherries (canned)	½ cup
Dates	3 dates
Figs (fresh)	2 medium
Grapefruit	½ large
Grapes	15 large
Honeydew melon	1 cup cubes
Kiwi	1 large
Mango (small)	½ mango
Nectarine	1 small
Orange	1 small
Peach (fresh)	1 medium
Peaches (canned)	½ cup
Pear	½ large
Pineapple (fresh)	¾ cup
Pineapple (canned)	½ cup
Plums	2 small
Prunes (dried)	3 small
Raisins	2 tbsp
Raspberries	1 cup
Strawberries	1¼ whole berries
Tangerines	2 small
Watermelon	1¼ cup cubes

Fruit juices

Apple juice/cider	½ cup
Cranberry juice	⅓ cup
Grape juice	⅓ cup
Grapefruit juice	½ cup
Orange juice	½ cup
Pineapple juice	½ cup

VEGETABLE LIST

This list contains vegetables that contain small amounts of carbohydrates and very few calories. Other vegetables are on the starch list. Each serving on this list contains approximately 5 g of carbohydrates and 2 g of protein (approximately 25 calories). Unless otherwise specified, the serving size is ½ cup of cooked vegetable or vegetable juice or 1 cup of raw vegetables.

Artichokes	Celery
Asparagus	Cucumbers
Beans (green)	Eggplants
Bean sprouts	Green onions
Broccoli	Greens (mixed green vegetables)
Brussels sprouts	Mushrooms
Cabbage	Okra
Carrots	Onions
Cauliflower	Peppers (all varieties)
Radishes	Turnips
Spinach	Water chestnuts
Summer squash	Zucchini
Tomatoes	

STARCH LIST

This list contains cereals, grains, pasta, breads, crackers, snacks, and starchy vegetables. Each item on the list contains approximately 15 g of carbohydrates, 3 g of protein, and 0 to 1 g of fat (approximately 80 calories). Portion sizes for each item are indicated.

Bread

Bagel	½
Bread (reduced calorie)	2 slices
Bread (white, whole-wheat, rye, etc.)	1 slice
English muffin	½
Hamburger bun	½
Hot dog roll	½
Pita bread (6 inches across)	1
Tortilla (corn - 6 inches across)	1
Tortilla (flour - 7 to 8 inches across)	1

Cereals and grains

Bran cereals (flaked)	½ cup
Bran cereals (concentrated, e.g., All Bran)	⅓ cup
Cooked cereals	½ cup
Grape Nuts	¼ cup
Other unsweetened cereals	¾ cup
Pasta (cooked)	½ cup
Rice (cooked)	⅓ cup
Shredded wheat	½ cup

Starchy vegetables

Baked beans	⅓ cup
Beans and peas (cooked)	½ cup
Corn	½ cup
Corn on cob (6 inches long)	1 piece
Mixed vegetables with corn, peas, or pasta	1 cup
Potato (baked or boiled)	1 small
Potato (mashed)	½ cup
Squash (winter)	1 cup
Yam	½ cup
Sweet potato	½ cup

Crackers and snacks

Animal crackers	8 crackers
Graham crackers (2½ sq. inches)	3 crackers
Melba toast	5 slices
Oyster crackers	24 crackers
Popcorn (no fat added)	3 cups
Pretzels	¾ oz
Rice cakes (4-inch diameter)	2 cakes
Saltine-type crackers	6 crackers
Fat-free chips (tortilla, potato)	15 to 20 chips
Whole-wheat crackers (no fat added)	2 to 5 crackers

Starchy foods prepared with fat

Count as 1 starch and 1 fat exchange.

Corn bread (2-inch cube)	1 (2 oz)
Crackers (round - butter type)	6 crackers
Croutons	1 cup
Granola	¼ cup
Muffin (1½ oz)	1 small
Pancakes (4-inch diameter)	2 pancakes
Popcorn (microwave)	3 cups
Stuffing (bread)	⅓ cup
Taco shell (6 inches across)	2 shells
Waffle (4 1/2 sq. inches)	1 waffle

OTHER CARBOHYDRATES LIST

You can substitute items from this list for a starch, fruit, or milk. Note that some choices will also count as one or more fat choices. One exchange on this list contains 15 g of carbohydrates (approximately 60 calories).

Food	Serving Size	Exchanges Per Serving
Angel-food cake (unfrosted)	1/12 cake	2 carbohydrates
Brownie, small (unfrosted)	2 sq. inches	1 carbohydrate, 1 fat
Cake (unfrosted)	2 sq. inches	1 carbohydrate, 1 fat
Cake (frosted)	2 sq. inches	2 carbohydrates, 1 fat
Cookie (fat free)	2 small	1 carbohydrate
Cupcake (frosted)	1 small	2 carbohydrates, 1 fat
Cranberry sauce (jellied)	¼ cup	2 carbohydrates
Doughnut (plain cake)	1 medium	1½ carbohydrates, 2 fats
Doughnut (glazed)	3¾ inches across	2 carbohydrates, 2 fats
Fruit juice bars (frozen)	1 bar	1 carbohydrate
Gingersnaps	3 gingersnaps	1 carbohydrate
Granola bar	1 bar	1 carbohydrate, 1 fat
Granola bar (fat free)	1 bar	2 carbohydrates
Ice cream	½ cup	1 carbohydrate, 2 fats
Ice cream (light)	½ cup	1 carbohydrate, 1 fat
Ice cream (fat free, no sugar added)	½ cup	1 carbohydrate
Jam or jelly	1 tbsp	1 carbohydrate
Pie (fruit)	⅙ pie	3 carbohydrates, 2 fats
Pie (pumpkin or custard)	⅛ pie	1 carbohydrate, 2 fats
Potato chips	1 oz (12 to 18)	1 carbohydrate, 2 fats
Salad dressing (fat free)	¼ cup	1 carbohydrate
Spaghetti or pasta sauce (canned)	½ cup	1 carbohydrate, 1 fat
Sweet roll or danish	1 item	2½ carbohydrates, 2 fats
Syrup (light)	2 tbsp	1 carbohydrate
Syrup (regular)	1 tbsp	1 carbohydrate
Tortilla chips	1 oz (6 to 12 chips)	1 carbohydrate, 2 fats
Yogurt (frozen low fat, fat free)	⅓ cup	1 carbohydrate, 0 to 1 fat
Yogurt frozen (fat free, no sugar)	½ cup	1 carbohydrate
Yogurt (low fat with fruit)	1 cup	3 carbohydrates, 0 to 1 fat
Vanilla wafers	5 wafers	1 carbohydrate, 1 fat

MEAT AND MEAT SUBSTITUTE LIST

This list contains meat and meat substitutes that contain both protein and fat. This list is divided into four categories based on the fat content. The categories are as follows:

- Very lean
- Lean
- Medium fat
- High fat

Very lean meat and meat substitute list

Each item on this list contains 7 g protein and 0 to 1 g fat (approximately 35 calories).

Poultry (chicken or turkey, white meat no skin)	1 oz
Fish (fresh or frozen cod, flounder, haddock, halibut, trout, tuna)	1 oz
Shellfish (clams, crab, lobster, scallops, shrimp)	
Game (duck, pheasant, venison, buffalo, ostrich)	1 oz
Cottage cheese (nonfat or low fat)	¼ cup
Cheese (fat free with less than 1 g fat per ounce)	1 oz
Other	
Egg whites	2 whites
Egg substitutes (plain)	¼ cup
Hot dogs (1 g fat or less per ounce)	1 oz

Lean meat and substitute list

Each item on this list contains approximately 7 g protein and 3 g fat (approximately 55 calories).

Beef (USDA select or choice grades of lean beef, e.g., round, sirloin, flank tenderloin)	1 oz
Pork (lean—fresh ham, Canadian bacon, tenderloin)	1 oz
Lamb (roast, chop, leg)	1 oz
Veal (lean chop, roast)	1 oz
Poultry (chicken/turkey dark meat with no skin or white meat with skin)	1 oz
Fish (herring, salmon, sardines)	1 oz
Cheese (3 g fat or less per ounce)	1 oz
Other (hot dogs, processed sandwich meats with 3 g fat or less per ounce)	1 oz

Medium-fat meat and substitute list

Each item on this list contains 7 g protein and 5 g fat (approximately 75 calories).

Beef (most beef products in this category—ground beef, meat loaf, corned beef, short ribs, prime grades of meat trimmed of fat)	1 oz
Pork (top loin, chop, Boston butt, cutlet)	1 oz
Lamb (rib roast, ground)	1 oz
Veal (cutlet, ground, unbreaded)	1 oz
Poultry (chicken dark meat with skin, ground chicken or turkey, fried chicken)	1 oz
Fish (any fried fish product)	1 oz
Cheese (4 or 5 g fat per ounce)	1 oz
Egg	1 medium

High-fat meat and substitute list

Each item on this list contains approximately 7 g protein and 8 g fat (approximately 105 calories). Most foods on this list are high in saturated fat, cholesterol, and calories. You need to limit your intake of items on this list.

Pork (spareribs, ground pork, pork sausage)	1 oz
Cheese (common cheeses such as American, cheddar, Monterey Jack, Swiss with more than 5 g fat per ounce)	1 oz
Processed sandwich meats (salami, bologna, etc.)	1 oz
Bacon	3 slices

FAT LIST

Each serving on this list contains approximately 5 g of fat (approximately 45 calories). Limit your fat intake and, where possible, try to select unsaturated fats.

Unsaturated fats

Safflower oil	1 tsp
Corn oil	1 tsp
Sunflower oil	1 tsp
Sesame oil	1 tsp
Olive oil	1 tsp
Olives	10 small/5 large
Peanut oil	1 tsp
Peanuts	20 small/10 large
Peanut butter	2 tsp
Avocados	⅛ medium
Margarine	1 tsp
Mayonnaise (low calorie)	1 tbsp
Almonds (dry roasted)	6 whole
Pecans	2 whole
Walnuts	2 whole
Salad dressing (low calorie)	2 tbsp

Saturated fats

Butter	1 tsp
Bacon	1 slice
Coffee whitener	4 tsp
Sour cream	2 tbsp
Cream cheese	1 tbsp
Salad dressing (mayonnaise type)	2 tsp
French dressing	1 tbsp
Italian dressing	1 tbsp

Appendix B **Nutritional Information for Selected Foods**

Food Item	Serving size	Grams	Calories	Protein (g)	Carbohydrate (g)	Fat (g)	Cholesterol (mg)	Sodium (mg)
Beverages								
Alcoholic								
Beer								
Regular	12 fl oz	360	150	1	13	0	0	18
Light	12 fl oz	355	95	1	5	0	0	11
Gin, rum, vodka whiskey								
80-proof	1½ fl oz	42	95	0	Tr	0	0	Tr
86-proof	1½ fl oz	42	105	0	Tr	0	0	Tr
90-proof	1½ fl oz	42	110	0	Tr	0	0	Tr
Wines								
Dessert	3½ fl oz	103	140	Tr	8	0	0	9
Table								
Red	3½ fl oz	102	75	Tr	3	0	0	5
White	3½ fl oz	102	80	Tr	3	0	0	5
Carbonated								
Club soda	12 fl oz	355	0	0	0	0	0	78
Cola type								
Regular	12 fl oz	369	160	0	41	0	0	18
Diet, artificially sweetened	12 fl oz	355	Tr	0	Tr	0		32[a]
Ginger ale	12 fl oz	366	125	0	32	0	0	29
Grape	12 fl oz	372	180	0	46	0	0	48
Lemon lime	12 fl oz	372	155	0	39	0	0	33
Orange	12 fl oz	372	180	0	46	0	0	52
Pepper type	12 fl oz	369	160	0	41	0	0	37
Root beer	12 fl oz	370	165	0	42	0	0	48
Fruit drinks, noncarbonated								
Canned								
Fruit punch drink	6 fl oz	190	85	Tr	22	0	0	15
Grape drink	6 fl oz	187	100	Tr	26	0	0	11
Pineapple-grapefruit juice drink	6 fl oz	187	90	Tr	23	Tr	0	24
Frozen lemonade concentrate, diluted with 4⅓ parts water by volume	6 fl oz	185	80	Tr	21	Tr	0	1

Tr, Trace amount.

[a]Blend of aspartame and saccharin; if only saccharin is used, sodium is 75 mg; if only aspartame is used, sodium is 23 mg. Information summarized from *Nutritive value of foods*, Superintendent of Documents, US Government Printing Office, Washington, DC, Revised 1981.

Food Item	Serving size	Grams	Calories	Protein (g)	Carbohydrate (g)	Fat (g)	Cholesterol (mg)	Sodium (mg)
Dairy products								
Butter. See Fats and oils								
Cheese								
Cheddar								
Cut pieces	1 oz	28	115	7	Tr	9	30	176
	1 in	17	70	4	Tr	6	18	105
Shredded	1 cup	113	455	28	1	37	119	701
Creamed (cottage cheese, 4% fat):								
Large curd	1 cup	225	235	28	6	10	34	911
Small curd	1 cup	210	215	26	6	9	31	850
With fruit	1 cup	226	280	22	30	8	25	915
Low fat (2%)	1 cup	226	205	31	8	4	19	918
Cream	1 oz	28	100	2	1	10	31	84
Feta	1 oz	28	75	4	1	6	25	316
Mozzarella, made with								
Whole milk	1 oz	28	80	6	1	6	22	106
Part-skim milk (low moisture)	1 oz	28	80	8	1	5	15	150
Muenster	1 oz	28	105	7	Tr	9	27	178
Parmesan, grated	1 oz	28	130	12	1	9	22	528
Provolone	1 oz	28	100	7	1	8	20	248
Swiss	1 oz	28	105	8	1	8	26	74
Pasteurized process cheese								
American	1 oz	28	105	6	Tr	9	27	406
Swiss	1 oz	28	95	7	1	7	24	388
Pasteurized process cheese food, American	1 oz	28	95	6	2	7	18	337
Pasteurized process cheese spread, American	1 oz	28	80	5	2	6	16	381
Cream, sweet								
Half-and-half (cream and milk)	1 cup	242	315	7	10	28	89	98
	1 tbsp	15	20	Tr	1	2	6	6
Light, coffee, or table	1 cup	240	470	6	9	46	159	95
	1 tbsp	15	30	Tr	1	3	10	6
Cream, sour	1 cup	230	495	7	10	48	102	123
	1 tbsp	12	25	Tr	1	3	5	6
Ice cream. See Milk desserts, frozen								
Milk								
Whole (3.3% fat)	1 cup	244	150	8	11	8	33	370
Low fat (2%)	1 cup	244	120	8	12	5	18	377
Low fat (1%)	1 cup	244	100	8	12	3	10	381
Nonfat (skim)	1 cup	245	85	8	12	Tr	4	406
Chocolate milk (commercial)								
Regular	1 cup	250	210	8	26	8	31	149
Low fat (2%)	1 cup	250	180	8	26	5	17	151
Low fat (1%)	1 cup	250	160	8	26	3	7	152

Tr, Trace amount.

Food Item	Serving size	Grams	Calories	Protein (g)	Carbohydrate (g)	Fat (g)	Cholesterol (mg)	Sodium (mg)
Dairy products—cont'd								
Milk beverages								
Cocoa and chocolate-flavored beverages								
Prepared (8 oz whole milk plus ¾ oz powder)	1 serving	265	225	9	30	9	33	176
Eggnog (commercial)	1 cup	254	340	10	34	19	149	138
Malted milk								
Chocolate	¾ oz	21	85	1	18	1	1	49
Prepared (8 oz whole milk plus ¾ oz powder)	1 serving	265	235	9	29	9	34	168
Shakes, thick								
Chocolate	10-oz container	283	335	9	60	8	30	314
Vanilla	10-oz container	283	315	11	50	9	33	270
Milk desserts, frozen								
Ice cream, vanilla								
Regular (about 11% fat)	1 cup	133	270	5	32	14	59	116
Yogurt								
Made with low-fat milk								
Fruit flavored[b]	8-oz container	227	230	10	43	2	10	133
Plain	8-oz container	227	145	12	16	4	14	159
Made with nonfat milk	8-oz container	227	125	13	17	Tr	4	174
Made with whole milk	8-oz container	227	140	8	11	7	29	105
Eggs								
Eggs, large (24 oz per dozen):								
Fried in margarine	1 egg	46	90	6	1	7	211	162
Hard-cooked, shell removed	1 egg	50	75	6	1	5	213	62
Poached	1 egg	50	75	6	1	5	212	140
Scrambled (milk added) in margarine	1 egg	61	100	7	1	7	215	171
Fats and oils								
Butter (4 sticks per lb)								
Stick	½ cup	113	810	1	Tr	92	247	933[c]
Tablespoon (⅛ stick)	1 tbsp	14	100	Tr	Tr	11	31	116[c]
Pat (1-in square, ⅓-in high; 90 per lb)	1 pat	5	35	Tr	Tr	4	11	41[c]

Tr, Trace amount.

[b]Carbohydrate content varies widely because of amount of sugar added and amount of added flavoring. Consult the label if more precise values for carbohydrate and calories are needed.

[c]For salted butter; unsalted butter contains 12 mg sodium per stick, 2 mg per tbsp, or 12 mg per pat.

Food Item	Serving size	Grams	Calories	Protein (g)	Carbohydrate (g)	Fat (g)	Cholesterol (mg)	Sodium (mg)
Fats and oils—cont'd								
Margarine								
Regular (about 80% fat)								
Stick	½ cup	113	810	1	1	91	0	1066[d]
Tablespoon (⅛ stick)	1 tbsp	14	100	Tr	Tr	11	0	132
Pat (1-in square, ⅓-in high; 90 per lb)	1 pat	5	35	Tr	Tr	4	0	47[d]
Oils, salad or cooking								
Corn	1 tbsp	14	125	0	0	14	0	0
Olive	1 tbsp	14	125	0	0	14	0	0
Peanut	1 tbsp	14	125	0	0	14	0	0
Safflower	1 tbsp	14	125	0	0	14	0	0
Sunflower	1 tbsp	14	125	0	0	14	0	0
Salad dressings								
Blue cheese	1 tbsp	15	75	1	1	8	3	164
French								
Regular	1 tbsp	16	85	Tr	1	9	0	188
Low calorie	1 tbsp	16	25	Tr	2	2	0	306
Italian								
Regular	1 tbsp	15	80	Tr	1	9	0	162
Low calorie	1 tbsp	15	5	Tr	2	Tr	0	136
Mayonnaise								
Regular	1 tbsp	14	100	Tr	Tr	11	8	80
Thousand island								
Regular	1 tbsp	16	60	Tr	2	6	4	112
Low calorie	1 tbsp	15	25	Tr	2	2	2	150
Fish and shellfish								
Crab meat, canned	1 cup	135	135	23	1	3	135	1350
Fish sticks, frozen, reheated (stick, 4 by 1 by ½ in)	1 fish stick	28	70	6	4	3	26	53
Flounder or sole, baked, with lemon juice								
With butter	3 oz	85	120	16	Tr	6	68	145
Ocean perch, breaded, fried[e]	1 fillet	85	185	16	7	11	66	138
Salmon								
Baked (red)	3 oz	85	140	21	0	5	60	55
Smoked	3 oz	85	150	18	0	8	51	1700
Scallops, breaded, frozen, reheated	6 scallops	90	195	15	10	10	70	298
Shrimp, French fried (7 medium)[f]	3 oz	85	200	16	11	10	168	384
Trout, broiled, with butter and lemon juice	3 oz	85	175	21	Tr	9	71	122

Tr, Trace amount.
[d]For salted margarine.
[e]Dipped in egg, milk, and bread crumbs; fried in vegetable shortening.
[f]Dipped in egg, milk, and bread crumbs; fried in vegetable shortening.

Food Item	Serving size	Grams	Calories	Protein (g)	Carbohydrate (g)	Fat (g)	Cholesterol (mg)	Sodium (mg)
Fish and shellfish—cont'd								
Tuna, canned, drained solids								
Oil pack, chunk light	3 oz	85	165	24	0	7	55	303
Water pack, solid white	3 oz	85	135	30	0	1	48	468
Tuna salad[g]	1 cup	205	375	33	19	19	80	877]
Fruits and fruit juices								
Apples								
Raw								
Unpeeled, without cores 3¼-in diameter (about 2 per lb with cores)	1 apple	212	125	Tr	32	1	0	Tr
Peeled, sliced	1 cup	110	65	Tr	16	Tr	0	Tr
Apple juice, bottled or canned	1 cup	248	115	Tr	29	Tr	0	7
Apricots								
Raw, without pits (about 12 per lb with pits)	3 apricots	106	50	1	12	Tr	0	1
Bananas, raw, without peel								
Whole (about 2½ per lb with peel)	1 banana	114	105	1	27	1	0	1
Sliced	1 cup	150	140	2	35	1	0	2
Blueberries, raw	1 cup	145	80	1	20	1	0	9
Cherries, sweet, raw, without pits and stems	10 cherries	68	50	1	11	1	0	Tr
Grapefruit, raw, without peel, membrane and seeds (3¾-in diameter 1 lb 1 oz, whole, with refuse)	½ grapefruit	120	40	1	10	Tr	0	Tr
Grapes, European type (adherent skin) raw, Thompson seedless	10 grapes	50	35	Tr	9	Tr	0	1
Melons, raw, without rind and cavity contents								
Cantaloupe, orange fleshed (5-in diameter, 2⅓ lb, whole, with rind and cavity contents)	⅙ melon	267	95	2	22	1	0	24

Tr, Trace amount.
[g]Made with drained, chunk light tuna, celery, onion, pickle relish, and mayonnaise-type dressing.

Food Item	Serving size	Grams	Calories	Protein (g)	Carbohydrate (g)	Fat (g)	Cholesterol (mg)	Sodium (mg)
Fruits and fruit juices—cont'd								
Honeydew (6½-in diameter, 5¼ lb, whole, with rind and cavity contents)	¹⁄₁₀ melon	129	45	1	12	Tr	0	13
Nectarines, raw, without pits (about 3 per lb with pits)	1 nectarine	136	65	1	16	1	0	Tr
Oranges, raw, whole, without peel and seeds (2⅝-in diameter, about 2½ per lb, with peel and seeds)	1 orange	131	60	1	15	Tr	0	Tr
Orange juice								
Raw, all varieties	1 cup	248	110	2	26	Tr	0	2
Canned, unsweetened	1 cup	249	105	1	25	Tr	0	5
Peaches								
Raw								
Whole, 2½-in diameter, peeled, pitted (about 4 per lb with peels and pits)	1 peach	87	35	1	10	Tr	0	Tr
Sliced	1 cup	170	75	1	19	Tr	0	Tr
Pears, raw, with skin, cored, Bartlett, 2½-in diameter (about 2½ per lb with cores and stems)	1 pear	166	100	1	25	1	0	Tr
Pineapple, raw, diced	1 cup	155	75	1	19	1	0	2
Pineapple juice, unsweetened, canned	1 cup	250	140	1	34	Tr	0	3
Plums, without pits, raw, 2⅛-in diameter (about 6½ per lb with pits)	1 plum	66	35	1	9	Tr	0	Tr
Raisins, seedless, cup, not pressed down	1 cup	145	435	5	115	1	0	17
Raspberries, raw	1 cup	123	60	1	14	1	0	Tr
Strawberries, raw, capped, whole	1 cup	149	45	1	10	1	0	1
Watermelon, raw, without rind and seeds, piece (4- by 8-in wedge with rind and seeds; ¹⁄₁₆ of 32⅔-lb melon, 10 by 16 in)	1 piece	482	155	3	35	2	0	10

Tr, Trace amount.

Food Item	Serving size	Grams	Calories	Protein (g)	Carbohydrate (g)	Fat (g)	Cholesterol (mg)	Sodium (mg)
Grain products								
Bagels, plain or water, enriched, 3½-in diameter[h]	1 bagel	68	200	7	38	2	0	245
Breads								
French or vienna bread, enriched[i]								
Slice								
French, 5 by 2½ by 1 in	1 slice	35	100	3	18	1	0	203
Vienna, 4¾ by 4 by ½ in	1 slice	25	70	2	13	1	0	145
Italian bread, enriched								
Slice, 4½ by 3¼ by ¾ in	1 slice	30	85	3	17	Tr	0	176
Mixed grain bread, enriched[i]								
Slice (18 per loaf)	1 slice	25	65	2	12	1	0	106
Pita bread, enriched, white, 6½-in diameter	1 pita	60	165	6	33	1	0	339
Pumpernickel (⅔ rye flour, ⅓ enriched wheat flour)[i]:								
Slice, 5 by 4 by ⅜ in	1 slice	32	80	3	16	1	0	177
Rye bread, light (⅔ enriched wheat flour, ⅓ rye flour)[i]								
Slice, 4¾ by 3¾ by ⁷⁄₁₆ in	1 slice	25	65	2	12	1	0	175
Wheat bread, enriched[i]								
Slice (18 per loaf)	1 slice	25	65	2	12	1	0	138
Whole-wheat bread[i]								
Slice (16 per loaf)	1 slice	28	70	3	13	1	0	180
Breakfast cereals								
All Bran (about ⅓ cup)	1 oz	28	70	4	21	1	0	320
Cap'n Crunch (about ¾ cup)	1 oz	28	120	1	23	3	0	213
Cheerios (about 1¼ cup)	1 oz	28	110	4	20	2	0	307
Corn flakes (about 1¼ cup)								
Kellogg's	1 oz	28	110	2	24	Tr	0	351
Toasties	1 oz	28	110	2	24	Tr	0	297
40% bran flakes								
Kellogg's (about ¾ cup)	1 oz	28	90	4	22	1	0	264
Post (about ⅔ cup)	1 oz	28	90	3	22	Tr	0	260

Tr, Trace amount.
[h]Egg bagels have 44 mg cholesterol.
[i]Made with vegetable shortening.
[j]Made with vegetable shortening.

Food Item	Serving size	Grams	Calories	Protein (g)	Carbohydrate (g)	Fat (g)	Cholesterol (mg)	Sodium (mg)
Grain products—cont'd								
Fruit Loops (about 1 cup)	1 oz	28	110	2	25	1	0	145
Lucky Charms (about 1 cup)	1 oz	28	110	3	23	1	0	201
100% Natural cereal (about ¼ cup)	1 oz	28	135	3	18	6	Tr	12
Product 19 (about ¾ cup)	1 oz	28	110	3	24	Tr	0	325
Raisin bran Kellogg's (about ¾ cup)	1 oz	28	90	3	21	1	0	207
Post (about ½ cup)	1 oz	28	85	3	21	1	0	185
Special K (about 1⅓ cup)	1 oz	28	110	6	21	Tr	Tr	265
Sugar Frosted Flakes, Kellogg's (about ¾ cup)	1 oz	28	110	1	26	Tr	0	230
Wheaties (about 1 cup)	1 oz	28	100	3	23	Tr	0	354
Cakes prepared from cake mixes with enriched flour[k]								
Angel food, piece, ¹⁄₁₂ of cake	1 piece	53	125	3	29	Tr	0	269
Devil's food with chocolate frosting Piece, ¹⁄₁₆ of cake	1 piece	69	235	3	40	8	37	181
Cupcake, 2½-in diameter	1 cupcake	35	120	2	20	4	19	92
Cakes prepared from home recipes using enriched flour								
Carrot, with cream cheese frosting[l] Piece, ¹⁄₁₆ of cake	1 piece	96	385	4	48	21	74	279
Pound Slice, ¹⁄₁₇ of loaf	1 slice	30	120	2	15	5	32	96
Cheesecake Piece, ¹⁄₁₂ of cake	1 piece	92	280	5	26	18	170	204
Cookies made with enriched flour								
Brownies with nuts, commercial, with frosting, 1½ by 1¾ by ⅞ in	1 brownie	25	100	1	16	4	14	59
Chocolate chip commercial, 2¼-in diam, ⅜ in thick	4 cookies	42	180	2	28	9	5	140
Oatmeal with raisins, 2⅝-in diam, ¼ in thick	4 cookies	52	245	3	36	10	2	148

Tr, Trace amount.
[k]Excepting angel food cake, cakes were made from mixes containing vegetable shortening and frostings were made with margarine.
[l]Made with vegetable oil.

Food Item	Serving size	Grams	Calories	Protein (g)	Carbohydrate (g)	Fat (g)	Cholesterol (mg)	Sodium (mg)
Grain products—cont'd								
Peanut butter cookie, from home recipe, 2⅝-in diam[m]	4 cookies	48	245	4	28	14	22	142
Corn chips	1-oz package	28	155	2	16	9	0	233
Crackers[n]								
Graham, plain, 2½ in square	2 crackers	14	60	1	11	1	0	86
Melba toast, plain	1 piece	5	20	1	4	Tr	0	44
Saltines[o]	4 crackers	12	50	1	9	1	4	165
Wheat, thin	4 crackers	8	35	1	5	1	0	69
Croissants, made with enriched flour, 4½ by 4 by 1¾ in	1 croissant	57	235	5	27	12	13	452
Doughnuts, made with enriched flour								
Cake type, plain, 3¼-in diam, 1 in high	1 doughnut	50	210	3	24	12	20	192
Yeast—leavened, glazed, 3¾-in diam, 1¼ in high	1 doughnut	60	235	4	26	13	21	222
English muffins, plain, enriched	1 muffin	57	140	5	27	1	0	378
French toast, from home recipe	1 slice	65	155	6	17	7	112	257
Macaroni, enriched, cooked (cut lengths, elbows, shells), firm stage (hot)	1 cup	130	190	7	39	1	0	1
Muffins made with enriched flour, 2½-in diam, 1½ in high								
From home recipe								
Blueberry[m]	1 muffin	45	135	3	20	5	19	198
Bran	1 muffin	45	125	3	19	6	24	189
Corn	1 muffin	45	145	3	21	5	23	169
Noodles (egg noodles), enriched, cooked	1 cup	160	200	7	37	2	50	3
Noodles, chow mein, canned	1 cup	45	220	6	26	11	5	450
Pancakes, 4-in diam								
Buckwheat, from mix (with buckwheat and enriched flours), egg and milk added	1 pancake	27	55	2	6	2	20	125

Tr, Trace amount.
[m]Made with vegetable shortening.
[n]Crackers made with enriched flour except for rye wafers and whole-wheat wafers.
[o]Made with lard.

Food Item	Serving size	Grams	Calories	Protein (g)	Carbohydrate (g)	Fat (g)	Cholesterol (mg)	Sodium (mg)
Grain products—cont'd								
Plain								
From home recipe using enriched flour	1 pancake	27	60	2	9	2	16	115
From mix (with enriched flour), egg, milk, and oil added	1 pancake	27	60	2	8	2	16	160
Pies, piecrust made with enriched flour, vegetable shortening, 9-in diam								
Apple, piece, 1/6 of pie	1 piece	158	405	3	60	18	0	476
Blueberry, piece, 1/6 of pie	1 piece	158	380	4	55	17	0	423
Cherry, piece, 1/6 of pie	1 piece	158	410	4	61	18	0	480
Lemon meringue, piece, 1/6 of pie	1 piece	140	355	5	53	14	143	395
Pecan, piece, 1/6 of pie	1 piece	138	575	7	71	32	95	305
Popcorn, popped								
Air-popped, unsalted	1 cup	8	30	1	6	Tr	0	Tr
Popped in vegetable oil, salted	1 cup	11	55	1	6	3	0	86
Sugar syrup coated	1 cup	35	135	2	30	1	0	Tr
Pretzels, made with enriched flour								
Stick, 2¼ in long	10 pretzels	3	10	Tr	2	Tr	0	48
Twisted, dutch, 2¾ by 2⅝ in	1 pretzel	16	65	2	13	1	0	258
Rice								
Brown, cooked, served hot	1 cup	195	230	5	50	1	0	0
White, enriched cooked, served hot	1 cup	205	225	4	50	Tr	0	0
Instant, ready-to-serve, hot	1 cup	165	180	4	40	0	0	0
Rolls, enriched								
Commercial								
Dinner, 2½-in diam, 2 in high	1 roll	28	85	2	14	2	Tr	155
Frankfurter and hamburger (8 per 11½-oz pkg)	1 roll	40	115	3	20	2	Tr	241
Hard, 3¾-in diam, 2 in high	1 roll	50	155	5	30	2	Tr	313
Hoagie or submarine, 11½ by 3 by 2½ in	1 roll	135	400	11	72	8	Tr	683

Tr, Trace amount.

Food Item	Serving size	Grams	Calories	Protein (g)	Carbohydrate (g)	Fat (g)	Cholesterol (mg)	Sodium (mg)
Grain products—cont'd								
Spaghetti, enriched, cooked								
Firm stage, "al dente," served hot	1 cup	130	190	7	39	1	0	1
Tender stage, served hot	1 cup	140	155	5	32	1	0	0
Tortillas, corn	1 tortilla	30	65	2	13	1	0	1
Waffles, made with enriched flour, 7-in diam								
From home recipe	1 waffle	75	245	7	26	13	102	445
From mix, egg and milk added	1 waffle	75	205	7	27	8	59	515
Legumes, nuts, and seeds								
Almonds, shelled								
Whole	1 oz	28	165	6	6	15	0	3
Beans, dry								
Black	1 cup	171	225	15	41	1	0	1
Lima	1 cup	190	260	16	49	1	0	4
Pea (navy)	1 cup	190	225	15	40	1	0	13
Pinto	1 cup	180	265	15	49	1	0	3
Black-eyed peas, dry, cooked (with residual cooking liquid)	1 cup	250	190	13	35	1	0	20
Brazil nuts, shelled	1 oz	28	185	4	4	19	0	1
Cashew nuts, salted								
Dry roasted	1 oz	28	165	4	9	13	0	181[p]
Roasted in oil	1 oz	28	165	5	8	14	0	177[q]
Lentils, dry, cooked	1 cup	200	215	16	38	1	0	26
Mixed nuts, with peanuts, salted								
Dry roasted	1 oz	28	170	5	7	15	0	190[r]
Roasted in oil	1 oz	28	175	5	6	16	0	185[r]
Peanuts, roasted in oil, salted	1 oz	28	165	8	5	14	0	122[s]
Peanut butter	1 tbsp	16	95	5	3	8	0	75
Peas, split, dry, cooked	1 cup	200	230	16	42	1	0	26
Pistachio nuts, dried, shelled	1 oz	28	165	6	7	14	0	2
Refried beans, canned	1 cup	290	295	18	51	3	0	1228
Sesame seeds, dry, hulled	1 tbsp	8	45	2	1	4	0	3
Sunflower seeds, dry, hulled	1 oz	28	160	6	5	14	0	1

Tr, Trace amount.
[p]Cashews without salt contain 21 mg sodium per cup or 4 mg per oz.
[q]Cashews without salt contain 22 mg sodium per cup or 5 mg per oz.
[r]Mixed nuts without salt contain 3 mg sodium per oz.
[s]Peanuts without salt contain 22 mg sodium per cup or 4 mg per oz.

Food Item	Serving size	Grams	Calories	Protein (g)	Carbohydrate (g)	Fat (g)	Cholesterol (mg)	Sodium (mg)
Meat and meat products								
Beef, cooked[t]								
Cuts braised, simmered, or pot roasted								
Relatively fat such as chuck blade								
Lean and fat, piece, 2½ by 2½ by ¾ in	3 oz	85	325	22	0	26	87	53
Relatively lean, such as bottom round								
Lean and fat, piece, 4⅛ by 2¼ by ½ in	3 oz	85	220	25	0	13	81	43
Ground beef, broiled, patty, 3 by ⅝ in								
Lean	3 oz	85	230	21	0	16	74	65
Regular	3 oz	85	245	20	0	18	76	70
Roast, oven cooked, no liquid added								
Relatively fat, such as rib								
Lean and fat, 2 pieces, 4⅛ by 2¼ in	3 oz	85	315	19	0	26	72	54
Relatively lean, such as eye of round								
Lean and fat, 2 pieces, 2½ by 2½ by ⅜ in	3 oz	85	205	23	0	12	62	50
Steak								
Sirloin, broiled								
Lean and fat, piece, 2½ by 2½ by ¾ in	3 oz	85	240	23	0	15	77	53
Lamb, cooked								
Chops, (3 per lb with bone)								
Arm, braised								
Lean and fat	2.2 oz	63	220	20	0	15	77	46
Loin, broiled								
Lean and fat	2.8 oz	80	235	20	0	16	78	62
Leg, roasted								
Lean and fat, 2 pieces, 4⅛ by 2¼ by ¼ in	3 oz	85	205	22	0	13	78	57

Tr, Trace amount.

[t]Outer layer of fat was removed to within approximately ½ inch of lean. Deposits of fat within the cut were not removed.

Food Item	Serving size	Grams	Calories	Protein (g)	Carbohydrate (g)	Fat (g)	Cholesterol (mg)	Sodium (mg)
Meat and meat products—cont'd								
Rib, roasted								
Lean and fat, 3 pieces, 2½ by 2½ by ¼ in	3 oz	85	315	18	0	26	77	60
Pork, cured, cooked								
Bacon								
Regular	3 medium slices	19	110	6	Tr	9	16	303
Canadian-style	2 slices	46	85	11	1	4	27	711
Ham, light cured, roasted								
Lean and fat, 2 pieces, 4⅛ by 2¼ by ¼ in	3 oz	85	205	18	0	14	53	1009
Luncheon meat								
Canned, spiced or unspiced, slice, 3 by 2 by ½ in	2 slices	42	140	5	1	13	26	541
Chopped ham (8 slices per 6 oz pkg)	2 slices	42	95	7	0	7	21	576
Cooked ham (8 slices per 8-oz pkg)								
Regular	2 slices	57	105	10	2	6	32	751
Extra lean	2 slices	57	75	11	1	3	27	815
Pork, fresh, cooked								
Chop, loin (cut 3 per lb with bone)								
Broiled								
Lean and fat	3.1 oz	87	275	24	0	19	84	61
Ham (leg), roasted								
Lean and fat, piece, 2½ by 2½ by ¾ in	3 oz	85	250	21	0	18	79	50
Rib, roasted								
Lean and fat, piece, 2½ by ¾ in	3 oz	85	270	21	0	20	69	37
Shoulder cut, braised								
Lean and fat, 3 pieces, 2½ by 2½ by ¼ in	3 oz	85	295	23	0	22	93	75
Sausages								
Bologna	2 slices	57	180	7	2	16	31	581
Frankfurter	1 frank	45	145	5	1	13	23	504
Pork link	1 link	13	50	3	Tr	4	11	168
Salami								
Cooked type, slice (8 per 8-oz pkg)	2 slices	57	145	8	1	11	37	607

Tr, Trace amount.

Food Item	Serving size	Grams	Calories	Protein (g)	Carbohydrate (g)	Fat (g)	Cholesterol (mg)	Sodium (mg)
Meat and meat products—cont'd								
Veal, medium fat, cooked, bone removed								
Cutlet, 4⅛ by 2¼ by ½ in, braised or broiled	3 oz	85	185	23	0	9	109	56
Rib, 2 pieces, 4⅛ by 2¼ by ¼ in, roasted	3 oz	85	230	23	0	14	109	57
Mixed dishes and fast foods								
Mixed dishes								
Beef and vegetable stew, from home recipe	1 cup	245	220	16	15	11	71	292
Beef potpie, from home recipe, baked, piece, ⅓ of 9-in diam pie	1 piece	210	515	21	39	30	42	596
Chicken a la king, cooked, from home recipe	1 cup	245	470	27	12	34	221	760
Chicken and noodles, cooked from home recipe	1 cup	240	365	22	26	18	103	600
Chicken chow mein								
Canned	1 cup	250	95	7	18	Tr	8	725
From home recipe	1 cup	250	255	31	10	10	75	718
Chicken potpie, from home recipe, baked, piece, ⅓ of 9-in diam pie	1 piece	232	545	23	42	31	56	594
Chile con carne with beans, canned	1 cup	255	340	19	31	16	28	1354
Chop suey with beef and pork, from home recipe	1 cup	250	300	26	13	17	68	1053
Macaroni (enriched) and cheese								
Canned	1 cup	240	230	9	26	10	24	730
From home recipe[u]	1 cup	200	430	17	40	22	44	1086
Spaghetti (enriched) in tomato sauce with cheese								
Canned	1 cup	250	190	6	39	2	3	955
From home recipe[u]	1 cup	250	260	9	37	9	8	955
Spaghetti (enriched) with meatballs and tomato sauce								
From home recipe	1 cup	248	330	19	39	12	89	1009

Tr, Trace amount.
[u]Made with margarine.

Food Item	Serving size	Grams	Calories	Protein (g)	Carbohydrate (g)	Fat (g)	Cholesterol (mg)	Sodium (mg)
Poultry and poultry products								
Chicken								
Fried, flesh, with skin[v]								
Batter dipped								
Breast, ½ breast (5.6 oz with bones)	4.9 oz	140	365	35	13	18	119	385
Drumstick (3.4 oz with bones)	2.5 oz	72	195	16	6	11	62	194
Flour coated								
Breast, ½ breast (4.2 oz with bones)	3.5 oz	98	220	31	2	9	87	74
Drumstick (2.6 oz with bones)	1.7 oz	49	120	13	1	7	44	44
Roasted, flesh only								
Breast, ½ breast (4.2 oz with bones and skin)	3.0 oz	86	140	27	0	3	73	64
Drumstick (2.9 oz with bones and skin)	1.6 oz	44	75	12	0	2	41	42
Turkey, roasted, flesh only								
Dark meat, piece, 2½ by 1⅝ by ¼ in	4 pieces	85	160	24	0	6	72	67
Light meat, piece, 4 by 2 by ¼ in	2 pieces	85	135	25	0	3	59	54
Light and dark meat								
Chopped or diced	1 cup	140	240	41	0	7	106	98
Pieces (1 slice white meat, 4 by 2 by ¼ in and 2 slices dark meat, 2½ by 1⅝ by ¼ in)	3 pieces	85	145	25	0	4	65	60
Soups, sauces, and gravies								
Soups								
Canned, condensed								
Prepared with equal volume of milk								
Clam chowder, New England	1 cup	248	165	9	17	7	22	992
Cream of chicken	1 cup	248	190	7	15	11	27	1047
Cream of mushroom	1 cup	248	205	6	15	14	20	1076
Tomato	1 cup	248	160	6	22	6	17	932
Prepared with equal volume of water								

Tr, Trace amount.
[v]Fried in vegetable shortening.

Food Item	Serving size	Grams	Calories	Protein (g)	Carbohydrate (g)	Fat (g)	Cholesterol (mg)	Sodium (mg)
Soups, sauces, and gravies—cont'd								
Bean with bacon	1 cup	253	170	8	23	6	3	951
Beef noodle	1 cup	244	85	5	9	3	5	952
Chicken noodle	1 cup	241	75	4	9	2	7	1106
Chicken rice	1 cup	241	60	4	7	2	7	815
Clam chowder, Manhattan	1 cup	244	80	4	12	2	2	1808
Cream of chicken	1 cup	244	115	3	9	7	10	986
Cream of mush-room	1 cup	244	130	2	9	9	2	1032
Minestrone	1 cup	241	80	4	11	3	2	911
Pea, green	1 cup	250	165	9	27	3	0	988
Tomato	1 cup	244	85	2	17	2	0	871
Vegetable beef	1 cup	244	80	6	10	2	5	956
Sauces								
From dry mix								
Cheese, prepared with milk	1 cup	279	305	16	23	17	53	1565
Hollandaise, pre-pared with water	1 cup	259	240	5	14	20	52	1564
Gravies								
Canned								
Beef	1 cup	233	125	9	11	5	7	1305
Chicken	1 cup	238	190	5	13	14	5	1373
Mushroom	1 cup	238	120	3	13	6	0	1357
Sugars and sweets								
Candy								
Caramels, plain or chocolate	1 oz	28	115	1	22	3	1	64
Chocolate								
Milk, plain	1 oz	28	145	2	16	9	6	23
Milk, with almonds	1 oz	28	150	3	15	10	5	23
Milk, with peanuts	1 oz	28	155	4	13	11	5	19
Milk, with rice cereal	1 oz	28	140	2	18	7	6	46
Fudge, chocolate, plain	1 oz	28	115	1	21	3	1	54
Gumdrops	1 oz	28	100	Tr	25	Tr	0	10
Hard candy	1 oz	28	110	0	28	0	0	7
Jelly beans	1 oz	28	105	Tr	26	Tr	0	7
Marshmallows	1 oz	28	90	1	23	0	0	25
Custard, baked	1 cup	265	305	14	29	15	278	209
Honey, strained or extracted	1 cup	339	1030	1	279	0	0	17
	1 tbsp	21	65	Tr	17	0	0	1
Jams and preserves	1 tbsp	20	55	Tr	14	Tr	0	2
	1 packet	14	40	Tr	10	Tr	0	2
Jellies	1 tbsp	18	50	Tr	13	Tr	0	5
	1 packet	14	40	Tr	10	Tr	0	4
Popsicle, 3-fl-oz size	1 popsicle	95	70	0	18	0	0	11
Puddings								
Canned								
Chocolate	5-oz can	142	205	3	30	11	1	285
Tapioca	5-oz can	142	160	3	28	5	Tr	252
Vanilla	5-oz can	142	220	2	33	10	1	305

Tr, Trace amount.

Food Item	Serving size	Grams	Calories	Protein (g)	Carbohydrate (g)	Fat (g)	Cholesterol (mg)	Sodium (mg)
Sugars and sweets—cont'd								
Puddings—cont'd								
Dry mix, prepared								
with whole milk								
Chocolate								
Instant	½ cup	130	155	4	27	4	14	440
Regular								
(cooked)	½ cup	130	150	4	25	4	15	167
Rice	½ cup	132	155	4	27	4	15	140
Tapioca	½ cup	130	145	4	25	4	15	152
Vanilla								
Instant	½ cup	130	150	4	27	4	15	375
Regular								
(cooked)	½ cup	130	145	4	25	4	15	178
Sugars,								
Brown, pressed								
down	1 cup	220	820	0	212	0	0	97
White								
Granulated	1 cup	200	770	0	199	0	0	5
	1 tbsp	12	45	0	12	0	0	Tr
	1 packet	6	25	0	6	0	0	Tr
Syrups								
Chocolate-flavored								
syrup or topping								
Thin type	2 tbsp	38	85	1	22	Tr	0	36
Fudge type	2 tbsp	38	125	2	21	5	0	42
Vegetables and vegetables products								
Asparagus, green								
Cooked, drained								
From raw								
Cuts and tips	1 cup	180	45	5	8	1	0	7
From frozen								
Cuts and tips	1 cup	180	50	5	9	1	0	7
Beans								
Lima, immature								
seeds, frozen,								
cooked, drained								
Thick-seeded								
types (Ford								
hooks)	1 cup	170	170	10	32	1	0	90
Beets								
Cooked, drained								
Diced or sliced	1 cup	170	55	2	11	Tr	0	83
Black-eyed peas,								
immature seeds,								
cooked and drained								
From raw	1 cup	165	180	13	30	1	0	7
Broccoli								
Raw	1 spear	151	40	4	8	1	0	41
Spears, cut into								
½-in pieces	1 cup	155	45	5	9	Tr	0	17
Brussels sprouts,								
cooked, drained								
From raw, 7-8								
sprouts, 1¼ to								
1½-in diam	1 cup	155	60	4	13	1	0	33

Tr, Trace amount.

Food Item	Serving size	Grams	Calories	Protein (g)	Carbohydrate (g)	Fat (g)	Cholesterol (mg)	Sodium (mg)
Vegetables and vegetables products—cont'd								
Cabbage, common varieties								
Raw, coarsely shredded or sliced	1 cup	70	15	1	4	Tr	0	13
Carrots								
Raw, without crowns and tips, scraped								
Whole, 7½ by 1⅛ in, or strips, 2½ to 3 in long	1 carrot or 18 strips	72	30	1	7	Tr	0	25
Cooked, sliced, drained								
From raw	1 cup	156	70	2	16	Tr	0	103
Cauliflower								
Raw (flowerets)	1 cup	100	25	2	5	Tr	0	15
Cooked, drained								
From raw (flowerets)	1 cup	125	30	2	6	Tr	0	8
Celery, pascal type, raw								
Stalk, large outer, 8 by 1½ in (at root end)	1 stalk	40	5	Tr	1	Tr	0	35
Corn, sweet								
Cooked, drained								
From raw, ear 5 by 1¾ in	1 ear	77	85	3	19	1	0	13
From frozen	1 ear	63	60	2	14	Tr	0	3
Cucumber, with peel, slices, ⅛ in thick (large, 2⅛-in diam; small, 1¾-in diam)	6 large or 8 small slices	28	5	Tr	1	Tr	0	1
Eggplant, cooked, steamed	1 cup	96	25	1	6	Tr	0	3
Lettuce, raw								
Butterhead, as Boston types:								
Head, 5-in diam	1 head	163	20	2	4	Tr	0	8
Leaves	1 outer or 2 inner leaves	15	Tr	Tr	Tr	Tr	0	1
Crisphead, as iceberg								
Pieces, chopped or shredded	1 cup	55	5	1	1	Tr	0	5

Tr, Trace amount.

Food Item	Serving size	Grams	Calories	Protein (g)	Carbohydrate (g)	Fat (g)	Cholesterol (mg)	Sodium (mg)
Vegetables and vegetable products—cont'd								
Looseleaf (bunching varieties including romaine or cos), chopped or shredded pieces	1 cup	56	10	1	2	Tr	0	5
Mushrooms								
Raw, sliced or chopped	1 cup	70	20	1	3	Tr	0	
Cooked, drained	1 cup	156	40	3	8	1	0	3
Onions								
Raw								
Chopped	1 cup	160	55	2	12	Tr	0	3
Cooked (whole or sliced), drained	1 cup	210	60	2	13	Tr	0	17
Peas, edible pod, cooked, drained	1 cup	160	65	5	11	Tr	0	6
Peas, green								
Canned, drained solids	1 cup	170	115	8	21	1	0	372[w]
Frozen, cooked, drained	1 cup	160	125	8	23	Tr	0	139
Potatoes, cooked								
Baked (about 2 per lb, raw)								
With skin	1 potato	202	220	5	51	Tr	0	16
Flesh only	1 potato	156	145	3	34	Tr	0	8
Boiled (about 3 per lb, raw)								
Peeled after boiling	1 potato	136	120	3	27	Tr	0	5
Peeled before boiling	1 potato	135	115	2	27	Tr	0	7
French fried, strip, 2 to 3½ in long, frozen								
Oven heated	10 strips	50	110	2	17	4	0	16
Fried in vegetable oil	10 strips	50	160	2	20	8	0	108
Potato products, prepared								
Au gratin								
From dry mix	1 cup	245	230	6	31	10	12	1076
From home recipe	1 cup	245	325	12	28	19	56	1061
Hashed brown, from frozen	1 cup	156	340	5	44	18	0	53
Mashed								
From home recipe								
Milk added	1 cup	210	160	4	37	1	4	606
Milk and margarine added	1 cup	210	225	4	35	9	4	620
Potato salad, made with mayonnaise	1 cup	250	360	7	28	21	170	1323

Tr, Trace amount.
[w]For regular pack; special dietary pack contains 3 mg sodium.

Food Item	Serving size	Grams	Calories	Protein (g)	Carbohydrate (g)	Fat (g)	Cholesterol (mg)	Sodium (mg)
Vegetables and vegetable products—cont'd								
Scalloped								
From dry mix	1 cup	245	230	5	31	11	27	835
From home recipe	1 cup	245	210	7	26	9	29	821
Potato chips	10 chips	20	105	1	10	7	0	94
Pumpkin								
Cooked from raw, mashed	1 cup	245	50	2	12	Tr	0	2
Radishes, raw, stem ends, rootlets cut off	4 radishes	18	5	Tr	1	Tr	0	4
Sauerkraut, canned solids and liquid	1 cup	236	45	2	10	Tr	0	1560
Spinach								
Raw, chopped	1 cup	55	10	2	2	Tr	0	43
Cooked, drained								
From raw	1 cup	180	40	5	7	Tr	0	126
From frozen (leaf)	1 cup	190	55	6	10	Tr	0	163
Sweet potatoes								
Cooked (raw, 5 by 2 in; about 2½ per lb)								
Baked in skin, peeled	1 potato	114	115	2	28	Tr	0	11
Boiled, without skin	1 potato	151	160	2	37	Tr	0	20
Tomatoes								
Raw, 2⅗-in diam (3 per 12 oz pkg)	1 tomato	123	25	1	5	Tr	0	10
Tomato juice, canned	1 cup	244	40	2	10	Tr	0	881[x]
Tomato products, canned								
Paste	1 cup	262	220	10	49	2	0	170[y]
Sauce	1 cup	245	75	3	18	Tr	0	1482[z]
Vegetable juice cocktail, canned	1 cup	242	45	2	11	Tr	0	883
Miscellaneous items								
Catsup	1 cup	273	290	5	69	1	0	2845
	1 tbsp	15	15	Tr	4	Tr	0	156
Chili powder	1 tsp	2.6	10	Tr	1	Tr	0	26
Mustard, prepared, yellow	1 tsp or individual packet	5	5	Tr	Tr	Tr	0	63
Olives, canned								
Green	4 medium or 3 extra large	13	15	Tr	Tr	2	0	312
Ripe, Mission, pitted	3 small or 2 large	9	15	Tr	Tr	2	0	68

Tr, Trace amount.
[x]For added salt; if none is added, sodium content is 24 mg.
[y]With no added salt; if salt is added, sodium content is 2070 mg.
[z]With salt added.

Food Item	Serving size	Grams	Calories	Protein (g)	Carbohydrate (g)	Fat (g)	Cholesterol (mg)	Sodium (mg)
Miscellaneous items—cont'd								
Pickles, cucumber								
Dill	1 pickle	65	5	Tr	1	Tr	0	928
Sweet	1 pickle	15	20	Tr	5	Tr	0	107
Salt	1 tsp	5.5	0	0	0	0	0	2132

Tr, Trace amount.

Appendix C Nutritional Information for Selected Fast-Food Restaurants

Item	Serving (oz)	(g)	Calories	Protein (g)	Carbohydrate (g)	Total fat (g)	Dietary fiber (g)	Cholesterol (mg)	Sodium (mg)
Restaurant: Arby's									
Regular Roast Beef	5	147	353	22.2	31.6	14.8	1	39	588
Beef 'N Cheddar	7	197	455	25.7	27.7	26.8	1	63	955
Chicken Breast Sandwich	7	184	493	23.0	47.9	25.0	1	91	1019
Roast Chicken Club	8	234	610	31.0	40.0	33.0	1	80	1500
Turkey Deluxe	7	197	375	23.8	32.5	16.6	2	39	1047
Ham 'N Cheese	6	156	292	22.9	19.2	13.7	1	45	1350
Super Roast Beef	8	234	501	25.1	50.4	22.1	1	40	798
French Fries	3	71	246	2.1	29.8	13.2	2	0	114
Restaurant: Burger King									
Whopper/Everything	10	270	628	27.0	46.0	36.0	2	90	880
Whopper/Cheese	10	294	706	32.0	47.0	43.0	2	113	1164
Hamburger	4	108	272	15.0	29.0	12.0	1	37	509
Cheeseburger	4	121	318	17.0	30.0	15.0	1	48	651
Bacon Double Cheese-burger	6	160	515	33.0	27.0	31.0	1	104	728
Hamburger Deluxe	5	138	344	15.0	30.0	17.0	1	41	486
Cheeseburger Deluxe	5	151	390	17.0	31.0	20.0	2	52	628
Ocean Catch Filet	7	194	488	19.0	45.0	25.0	2	77	592
Chicken Specialty Sand-wich	8	229	685	26.0	56.0	40.0	2	82	1423
Chicken Tenders™	3	90	236	20.0	10.0	10.0	1	47	636
French Fries	4	111	341	3.0	24.0	13.0	3	14	160
Onion Rings	3	86	302	4.02	28.0	16.0	2	0	665
Breakfast Croissan'wich/ Bacon	4	118	355	14.0	20.0	24.0	1	249	762
Breakfast Croissan'wich/ Sausage	6	159	538	20.0	20.0	40.0	1	293	1042
Breakfast Croissan'wich/ Ham/Egg/Cheese	5	144	346	19.0	19.0	21.0	1	241	962
Breakfast Bagel Sandwich/ Bacon	6	169	438	20.0	46.0	20.0	2	274	905
Breakfast Bagel Sandwich/ Sausage/Egg/Cheese	7	210	626	27.0	49.0	36.0	2	318	1137
Breakfast Bagel Sandwich/ Ham/Egg/Cheese	7	196	418	23.0	46.0	15.0	2	287	1130
Scrambled Egg Platter	7	211	549	17.0	44.0	30.0	3	370	808
Scrambled Egg Platter/ Sausage	9	260	768	26.0	47.0	53.0	3	412	1271

Information for all restaurants, except Jack In The Box, from Ross Laboratories, Columbus, Ohio, 43216, from *Dietetic Currents*, 18:4, 1991. Information for Jack in the Box from Boyle MA, Zyla G: *Personal nutrition*, ed 2, St Paul, Minn, 1992, West Publishing,

Item	Serving (oz)	(g)	Calories	Protein (g)	Carbohydrate (g)	Total fat (g)	Dietary fiber (g)	Cholesterol (mg)	Sodium (mg)
Restaurant: Burger King—cont'd									
Scrambled Egg Platter/ Bacon	8	221	610	21.0	44.0	39.0	3	373	1043
French Toast Sticks	5	141	538	10.0	53.0	32.0	2	80	537
Great Danish	3	71	500	5.0	40.0	36.0	3	6	288
Vanilla Shake	10	284	334	9.0	51.0	10.0	0	39	205
Chocolate Shake	10	284	326	9.0	49.0	10.0	1	33	202
Apple Pie	4	125	311	3.0	44.0	14.0	2	4	412
Chicken Salad	9	258	142	20.0	8.0	4.0	2	50	440
Chef Salad	10	273	178	17.0	7.0	9.0	2	120	570
Garden Salad	8	223	95	6.0	8.0	5.0	2	15	125
Side Salad	5	135	25	1.0	5.0	0.0	2	0	20
Thousand Island Dressing	2	63	290	1.0	15.0	26.0	0	36	470
Bleu Cheese Dressing	2	59	300	3.0	2.0	32.0	0	40	600
Reduced Calorie Italian	2	59	170	0.0	3.0	18.0	0	3	762
French Dressing	2	64	290	0.0	23.0	22.0	1	2	400
Bacon Bits	0.1	3	16	1.0	0.0	1.0	0	5	1
Croutons	0.3	7	31	1.0	5.0	1.0	0	0	90
Restaurant: Dairy Queen									
Cone, Small	3	85	140	3.0	22.0	4.0	0	10	45
Cone, Regular	5	142	240	6.0	38.0	7.0	0	15	80
Cone, Large	8	213	340	9.0	57.0	10.0	0	25	115
Cone, Small, Chocolate-Dipped	3	92	190	3.0	25.0	9.0	2	10	55
Cone, Regular, Chocolate-Dipped	6	156	340	6.0	42.0	16.0	3	20	100
Cone, Large, Chocolate-Dipped	8	234	510	9.0	64.0	24.0	4	30	145
Chocolate Sundae, Small	4	106	190	3.0	33.0	4.0	1	10	75
Chocolate Sundae, Regular	6	177	310	5.0	56.0	8.0	1	20	120
Chocolate Sundae, Large	9	248	440	8.0	78.0	10.0	2	30	165
Chocolate Shake, Small	9	241	409	8.0	69.0	11.0	1	30	150
Chocolate Shake, Regular	15	418	710	14.0	120.0	19.0	2	50	260
Chocolate Shake, Large	17	489	831	16.0	140.0	22.0	2	60	304
Chocolate Malt, Small	9	241	438	8.0	77.0	10.0	2	30	150
Chocolate Malt, Regular	15	418	760	14.0	134.0	18.0	3	50	260
Chocolate Malt, Large	17	489	889	16.0	157.0	21.0	3	60	304
Float	14	397	410	5.0	82.0	7.0	0	20	85
Peanut Buster Parfait	11	305	740	16.0	94.0	34.0	6	30	250
Parfait	10	283	430	8.0	76.0	8.0	1	30	140
Freeze	14	397	500	9.0	89.0	12.0	0	30	180
Mr Misty, Small	9	248	190	0.0	48.0	0.0	0	0	10
Mr Misty, Regular	12	330	250	0.0	63.0	0.0	0	0	10
Mr Misty, Large	16	439	340	0.0	84.0	0.0	0	0	10
Mr Misty Kiss	3	89	70	0.0	17.0	0.0	0	0	10
Mr Misty Freeze	15	411	500	9.0	91.0	12.0	0	30	140
Mr Misty Float	15	411	390	5.0	74.0	7.0	0	20	95
Buster Bar	5	149	448	10.0	41.0	29.0	6	10	175
Fudge Nut Bar	5	142	406	8.0	40.0	25.0	2	10	167
Dilly Bar	3	85	210	3.0	21.0	13.0	1	10	50
DQ Sandwich	2	60	140	3.0	24.0	4.0	0	5	40
Chipper Sandwich	4	113	318	5.0	56.0	7.0	0	13	170
Heath Blizzard, Regular	14	404	800	15.0	125.0	24.0	3	65	325
Single Hamburger	5	148	360	21.0	33.0	16.0	1	45	630
Double Hamburger	7	210	530	36.0	33.0	28.0	1	85	660
Triple Hamburger	10	272	710	51.0	33.0	45.0	1	135	690
Single Hamburger/Cheese	6	162	410	24.0	33.0	20.0	1	50	790

Item	Serving (oz)	(g)	Calories	Protein (g)	Carbohydrate (g)	Total fat (g)	Dietary fiber (g)	Cholesterol (mg)	Sodium (mg)
Restaurant: Dairy Queen—cont'd									
Double Hamburger/Cheese	8	239	650	43.0	34.0	37.0	1	95	980
Triple Hamburger/Cheese	11	301	820	58.0	34.0	50.0	1	145	1010
Hot Dog	4	100	280	11.0	21.0	16.0	1	45	830
Hot Dog/Chili	5	128	320	13.0	23.0	20.0	1	55	985
Hot Dog/Cheese	4	114	330	15.0	21.0	21.0	1	55	990
Super Hot Dog	6	175	520	17.0	44.0	27.0	1	80	1365
Super Hot Dog/Chili	8	218	570	21.0	47.0	32.0	2	100	1595
Super Hot Dog/Cheese	7	196	580	22.0	45.0	34.0	1	100	1605
Fish Filet	6	177	430	20.0	45.0	18.0	1	40	674
Fish Filet/Cheese	7	191	483	23.0	46.0	22.0	1	49	870
Chicken Breast Filet	7	202	608	27.0	46.0	34.0	2	78	725
Chicken Breast Filet/ Cheese	8	216	661	30.0	47.0	38.0	2	87	921
All White Chicken Nuggets	4	99	276	16.0	13.0	18.0	1	39	505
BBQ Nugget Sauce	1	28	41	0.0	9.0	0.7	0	0	130
French Fries, Small	3	71	200	2.0	25.0	10.0	2	10	115
French Fries, Large	4	113	320	3.0	40.0	16.0	3	15	185
Onion Rings	3	85	280	4.0	31.0	16.0	3	15	140
Restaurant: Domino's Pizza (2 slices of each pizza)									
Cheese Pizza	6	168	376	21.6	56.3	10.0	6	19	483
Pepperoni Pizza	7	187	460	24.1	55.6	17.5	5	28	825
Sausage/Mushroom Pizza	7	200	430	24.2	55.3	15.8	8	28	552
Veggie Pizza	9	261	498	31.0	60.0	18.5	8	36	1035
Deluxe Pizza	8	234	498	26.7	59.2	20.4	7	40	954
Double Cheese/Pepperoni Pizza	8	227	545	32.1	55.2	25.3	8	48	1042
Ham Pizza	7	186	417	23.2	58.0	11.0	2	26	805
Restaurant: Jack in the Box									
Breakfast Jack Sandwich	4	126	307	18	30	13	<1	203	871
Canadian Crescent	5	134	472	19	25	31	<1	226	851
Sausage Crescent	6	156	584	22	28	43	<1	187	1012
Supreme Crescent	5	146	547	20	27	40	<1	178	1053
Pancakes Breakfast Platter	8	231	612	15	87	22	<1	99	888
Scrambled Egg Breakfast Platter	9	249	662	24	52	40	<1	354	1188
Hamburger	3	98	276	13	30	12	<1	29	521
Cheeseburger	4	113	323	16	32	15	<1	42	749
Jumbo Jack	7	205	485	26	38	26	<1	64	905
Jumbo Jack w/Cheese	9	246	630	32	45	35	<1	110	1665
Bacon Cheeseburger Supreme	8	231	724	34	44	46	<1	70	1307
Swiss and Baconburger	8	231	643	33	31	43	<1	99	1354
Ham and Swiss Burger	7	203	638	36	37	39	<1	117	1330
Chicken Supreme	8	228	601	31	39	36	<1	60	1582
Double Cheeseburger	5	149	467	21	33	27	—	72	842
Tacos									
Regular	3	81	191	8	16	11	<1	21	460
Super	5	135	288	12	21	17	<1	—	—
French Fries	2	68	221	2	27	12	<1	8	164
Hash Brown Potatoes	2	62	116	2	11	7	<1	3	211
Onion Rings	4	108	382	5	39	23	<1	27	407
Milkshakes									
Chocolate	11	322	330	11	55	7	0	25	270
Strawberry	12	328	320	10	55	7	0	25	240
Vanilla	11	317	320	10	57	6	0	25	230
Apple Turnover	4	119	410	4	45	24	<1	15	350

Item	Serving (oz)	(g)	Calories	Protein (g)	Carbohydrate (g)	Total fat (g)	Dietary fiber (g)	Cholesterol (mg)	Sodium (mg)
Restaurant: Kentucky Fried Chicken									
Nuggets	1	16	46	2.8	2.2	2.9	0	12	140
Barbeque Sauce	1	28	35	0.3	7.1	0.6	0	0	450
Sweet and Sour Sauce	1	28	58	0.1	13.0	0.6	0	0	148
Chicken Littles Sandwich	2	47	169	5.7	13.8	10.1	0	18	331
Buttermilk Biscuit	2	65	235	4.5	28.0	11.9	1	1	655
Mashed Potatoes/Gravy	4	98	71	2.4	11.9	1.6	1	0	339
French Fries, Regular	3	77	244	3.2	31.1	11.9	2	2	139
Corn-on-the-cob	5	143	176	5.1	31.9	3.1	7	0	21
Coleslaw	3	91	119	1.5	13.3	6.6	1	5	197
Original Recipe Chicken									
Wing	2	55	178	12.2	6.0	11.7	0	64	372
Breast	4	115	283	27.5	8.8	15.3	0	93	672
Drumstick	2	57	146	13.1	4.2	8.5	0	67	275
Thigh	4	104	294	17.9	11.1	19.7	1	123	619
Extra Crispy Chicken									
Wing	2	65	254	12.4	9.3	18.6	0	67	422
Breast	5	135	342	33.0	11.7	19.7	1	114	790
Drumstick	2	69	204	13.6	6.1	13.9	0	71	324
Thigh	4	119	406	20.0	14.4	29.8	1	129	688
Restaurant: Long John Silver's Seafood Shoppe									
Three-piece Fish Light/ Paprika (Baked)	5	134	120	28.0	1.0	1.0	0	110	120
Three-piece Fish/Lemon Crumb (Baked)	5	141	150	29.0	4.0	1.0	0	110	370
Three-piece Fish/ Scampi Sauce (Baked)	5	148	170	28.0	2.0	5.0	0	110	270
Shrimp/Scampi Sauce (Baked)	5	148	120	15.0	2.0	5.0	0	205	610
Chicken Light/Herbs (Baked)	4	117	140	25.0	1.0	4.0	0	70	670
Rice Pilaf	5	142	210	5.0	43.0	2.0	1	0	570
Green Beans	4	113	30	1.0	6.0	1.0	3	5	540
Garden Vegetables	4	113	120	4.0	16.0	6.0	5	5	95
Coleslaw	3	98	140	1.0	20.0	6.0	1	15	260
Breadstick	1	34	110	3.0	18.0	3.0	1	0	120
Small Salad	2	54	8	1.0	2.0	0.0	1	0	0
Restaurant: McDonald's									
Egg McMuffin	5	138	290	18.2	28.1	11.2	1	226	740
Hotcakes/Butter/Syrup	6	176	410	8.2	74.4	9.2	2	21	640
Scrambled Eggs	4	100	140	12.4	1.2	9.8	0	399	290
Pork Sausage	2	48	180	8.4	0.0	16.3	0	48	350
English Muffin/Butter	2	59	170	5.4	26.7	4.6	1	9	270
Hashbrown Potatoes	2	53	130	1.4	14.9	7.3	2	9	330
Biscuit/Biscuit Spread	3	75	260	4.6	31.9	12.7	1	1	730
Biscuit/Sausage	4	123	440	13.0	31.9	29.0	1	49	1080
Biscuit/Sausage/Egg	6	180	520	19.9	32.6	34.5	1	275	1250
Biscuit/Bacon/Egg/Cheese	6	156	440	17.5	33.3	26.4	1	253	1230
Sausage McMuffin	4	117	370	16.5	27.3	21.9	1	64	830
Sausage McMuffin/Cheese	6	167	440	22.6	27.9	26.8	1	263	980
Apple Danish	4	115	390	5.8	51.2	17.9	2	25	370
Iced Cheese Danish	4	110	390	7.4	42.3	21.8	1	47	420
Cinnamon Raisin Danish	4	110	440	6.4	57.5	21.0	2	34	430
Raspberry Danish	4	117	410	6.1	61.5	15.9	2	26	310
Apple Bran Muffin	3	85	190	5.0	46.0	0.0	2	0	230
Blueberry Muffin	3	85	170	3.0	40.0	0.0	1	0	220

Item	Serving (oz)	(g)	Calories	Protein (g)	Carbohydrate (g)	Total fat (g)	Dietary fiber (g)	Cholesterol (mg)	Sodium (mg)
Restaurant: McDonald's—cont'd									
Chicken McNuggets	4	113	290	19.0	16.5	16.3	1	65	520
Hot Mustard Sauce	1	30	70	0.5	8.2	3.6	0	5	250
Barbeque Sauce	1	32	50	0.3	12.1	0.5	0	0	340
Sweet and Sour Sauce	1	32	60	0.2	13.8	0.2	0	0	190
Hamburger	4	102	260	12.3	30.6	9.5	1	37	500
Cheeseburger	4	116	310	15.0	31.2	13.8	1	53	750
McLean Deluxe	7	203	310	20.0	34.0	10.0	2	37	650
Quarter Pounder	6	166	410	23.1	34.0	20.7	1	86	660
Quarter Pounder/Cheese	7	194	520	28.5	35.1	29.2	1	118	1150
Big Mac	8	215	560	25.2	42.5	32.4	1	103	950
Filet-O-Fish	5	142	440	13.8	37.9	26.1	1	50	1030
McDLT	8	234	580	26.3	36.0	36.8	2	109	990
McChicken	7	190	490	19.2	39.8	28.6	1	43	780
Chef Salad	10	283	230	20.5	7.5	13.3	2	128	490
Garden Salad	8	213	110	7.1	6.2	6.6	2	83	160
Chicken Salad Oriental	9	244	140	23.1	5.0	3.4	2	78	230
Side Salad	4	115	60	3.7	3.3	3.3	1	41	85
Bleu Cheese Dressing	1	14	70	0.5	1.2	6.9	0	6	150
French Dressing	1	14	58	0.1	2.7	5.2	0	0	180
Ranch Dressing	1	14	83	0.2	1.3	8.6	0	5	130
1000 Island Dressing	1	14	78	0.2	2.4	7.5	0	8	100
Lite Vinaigrette Dressing	1	14	15	0.2	2.0	0.5	0	0	75
Oriental Dressing	1	14	24	0.2	5.8	0.1	0	0	180
Red French Reduced Calorie Dressing	1	14	40	0.1	5.2	1.9	0	0	110
Caesar Dressing	1	14	60	0.4	0.6	6.1	0	7	170
Peppercorn Dressing	1	14	80	0.2	0.5	8.7	0	7	85
French Fries, Small	2	68	220	3.1	25.6	12.0	2	9	110
French Fries, Medium	3	97	320	4.4	36.3	17.1	3	12	150
French Fries, Large	4	122	400	5.6	45.9	21.6	3	16	200
Apple Pie	3	83	260	2.2	30.0	14.8	2	6	240
Vanilla Low-fat Milk Shake	11	293	290	10.8	60.0	1.3	0	10	170
Chocolate Low-fat Milk Shake	11	293	320	11.0	66.0	1.7	1	10	240
Strawberry Low-fat Milk Shake	11	293	320	10.7	67.0	1.3	0	10	170
Soft Serve Cone	3	86	140	3.9	21.9	4.5	0	16	70
Strawberry Sundae	6	171	210	5.7	49.2	1.1	1	5	95
Hot Fudge Sundae	6	169	240	7.3	50.5	3.2	1	6	170
Hot Caramel Sundae	6	174	270	6.6	59.3	2.8	0	13	180
McDonaldland Cookies	2	56	290	4.2	47.1	9.2	1	0	300
Chocolaty Chip Cookies	2	56	330	4.2	41.9	15.6	0	4	280
Restaurant: Pizza Hut									
Pan Pizza, 2 slices									
Cheese	7	205	492	30.0	57.0	18.0	5	34	940
Pepperoni	8	211	540	29.0	62.0	22.0	5	42	1127
Supreme	9	255	589	32.0	53.0	30.0	7	48	1363
Super Supreme	9	257	563	33.0	53.0	26.0	6	55	1447
Thin 'n Crispy Pizza, 2 slices									
Cheese	5	148	398	28.0	37.0	17.0	4	33	867
Pepperoni	5	146	413	26.0	20.0	20.0	4	46	986
Supreme	7	200	459	28.0	41.0	22.0	5	42	1328
Super Supreme	7	203	463	29.0	44.0	21.0	5	56	1336

Item	Serving (oz)	(g)	Calories	Protein (g)	Carbohydrate (g)	Total fat (g)	Dietary fiber (g)	Cholesterol (mg)	Sodium (mg)
Restaurant: Pizza Hut—cont'd									
Hand-Tossed Pizza, 2 slices									
Cheese	8	220	518	34.0	55.0	20.0	7	55	1276
Pepperoni	7	197	500	28.0	50.0	23.0	6	50	1267
Supreme	8	239	540	32.0	50.0	26.0	7	55	1470
Super Supreme	9	243	556	33.0	54.0	25.0	7	54	1648
Personal Pan Pizza, 1 pizza									
Pepperoni	9	256	675	37.0	76.0	29.0	8	53	1335
Supreme	9	264	647	33.0	76.0	28.0	9	49	1313
Restaurant: Taco Bell									
Bean Burrito/Red Sauce	7	191	356	13.1	54.4	10.2	5	9	888
Beef Burrito/Red Sauce	7	191	403	22.5	39.1	17.3	3	57	1051
Burrito Supreme/Red Sauce	9	241	413	18.0	46.6	17.6	4	33	921
Double Beef Burrito Supreme/Red Sauce	9	255	457	23.7	41.7	21.8		57	1053
Tostada/Red Sauce	6	156	243	9.5	26.6	11.1	6	16	596
Enchirito/Red Sauce	8	213	382	19.8	30.9	19.7	4	54	1243
Pintos and Cheese/Red Sauce	5	128	191	9.0	19.0	8.7	4	16	642
Nachos	4	106	346	7.5	37.5	18.5	4	9	399
Nachos Bellgrande	10	287	649	21.6	60.6	35.3	7	36	997
Taco	28	778	183	10.3	11.0	10.8	1	32	276
Taco Bellgrande	6	163	355	18.3	17.7	23.1	2	56	472
Taco Light	6	170	410	19.0	18.1	28.8	2	56	594
Soft Taco	3	92	228	11.8	17.9	11.9	1	32	516
Soft Taco Supreme	4	124	275	12.6	19.1	16.3	1	32	516
Taco Salad/Salsa	21	595	941	36.0	63.1	61.3	10	80	1662
Taco Salad/Salsa without Shell	19	530	520	30.6	30.0	31.4	6	80	1431
Taco Salad without Shell	19	530	520	29.5	26.3	31.3	6	80	1056
Mexican Pizza	8	223	575	21.3	39.7	36.8	6	52	1031
Taco Sauce	<1	<1	2	0.1	0.4	0.0	0	0	126
Hot Taco Sauce	<1	<1	3	0.1	0.3	0.1	0	0	82
Jalapeno Peppers	5	100	20	1.0	4.0	0.2	1	0	1370
Steak Fajita	5	135	234	14.6	19.5	10.9	1	14	485
Chicken Fajita	5	135	226	13.6	19.8	10.2	1	44	619
Sour Cream	1	21	46	0.6	0.9	4.4	0	16	10
Pico De Gallo	1	28	8	0.3	1.1	0.2	0	1	88
Guacamole	1	21	34	0.4	3.0	2.3	1	0	113
Meximelt	4	106	266	12.9	18.7	15.4	1	38	689
Restaurant: Wendy's									
Junior Hamburger	3	104	260	15.0	32.0	9.0	1	35	570
Junior Cheeseburger	3	116	300	18.0	33.0	13.0	1	35	770
Small Hamburger	4	111	260	15.0	33.0	9.0	1	34	570
Small Cheeseburger	4	125	310	18.0	33.0	13.0	1	34	770
Chicken Sandwich	8	219	430	26.0	41.0	19.0	2	60	725
Big Classic/Cheese	10	295	640	30.0	46.0	38.0	4	100	1370
Plain Single	4	126	340	24.0	30.0	15.0	1	65	500
Single/Everything	8	210	420	26.0	36.0	21.0	1	70	890
Plain Single/Cheese	5	137	410	25.0	29.0	22.0	1	80	710
Garden Salad (Take-Out)	10	227	102	7.0	9.0	5.0	4	0	110
Chef Salad (Take-Out)	12	331	180	15.0	10.0	9.0	4	120	140
New Chili	9	256	220	21.0	23.0	7.0	7	45	750
Taco Salad	28	791	660	40.0	46.0	37.0	9	35	1110
French Fries, Small	3	91	240	3.0	33.0	12.0	2	15	145

Item	Serving (oz)	(g)	Calories	Protein (g)	Carbohydrate (g)	Total fat (g)	Dietary fiber (g)	Cholesterol (mg)	Sodium (mg)
Restaurant: Wendy's—cont'd									
Baked Potatoes									
Plain	9	250	250	6	52	<1	5	0	60
W/bacon and cheese	12	350	570	19	57	30	5	22	1180
W/broccoli and cheese	13	365	500	13	54	25	5	22	430
W/cheese	12	350	590	17	55	34	5	22	450
W/chili and cheese	14	400	510	22	63	20	8	22	610
W/sour cream and chives	11	310	460	7	53	24	5	15	230

Index